Dunmore and Fleischer's

MEDICAL TERMINOLOGY

Exercises in Etymology

Edition III

Dunmore and Fleischer's

MEDICAL TERMINOLOGY

Exercises in Etymology

Edition III

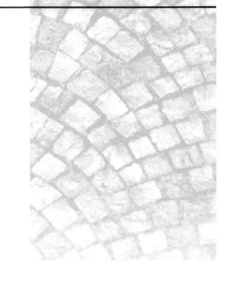

CHERYL WALKER-ESBAUGH, MA
Instructor
Classics and Letters Department
University of Oklahoma

LAINE H. MCCARTHY, MLIS
Clinical Associate Professor
Department of Family and Preventive Medicine
University of Oklahoma Health Sciences Center

RHONDA A. SPARKS, MD
Clinical Assistant Professor
Department of Family and Preventive Medicine
University of Oklahoma Health Sciences Center

F. A. DAVIS COMPANY • Philadelphia

F. A. Davis Company
1915 Arch Street
Philadelphia, PA 19103

Copyright © 2004 by F. A. Davis Company

Printed in the United States of America

Last digit indicates print number: 20 19 18 17 16 15 14

Acquisitions Editor: Andy McPhee
Developmental Editor: Jennifer Pine, David Carroll
Production Editor: Jessica Howie Martin
Cover Designer: Marie Clifton
Art & Design Manager: Louis J. Forgione

As new scientific information becomes available through basic and clinical research, recommended treatments and drug therapies undergo changes. The authors and publisher have done everything possible to make this book accurate, up to date, and in accord with accepted standards at the time of publication. The authors, editors, and publisher are not responsible for errors or omissions or for consequences from application of the book, and make no warranty, expressed or implied, in regard to the contents of the book. Any practice described in this book should be applied by the reader in accordance with professional standards of care used in regard to the unique circumstances that may apply in each situation. The reader is advised always to check product information (package inserts) for changes and new information regarding dose and contraindications before administering any drug. Caution is especially urged when using new or infrequently ordered drugs.

We dedicate this book to Jean-François Vilain, editor emeritus, who got us into this. Thanks, Jean-François. You are an inspiration.

PREFACE

In 1977, Charles W. Dunmore, an associate professor of classics at New York University, and Rita M. Fleischer, from the Latin/Greek Institute at City University of New York, published a novel approach to teaching the challenging language of medicine. Indeed, medicine does have a language all its own, based largely on a vocabulary drawn from ancient Greek and, to a lesser degree, Latin. This approach involved teaching students to recognize the roots of *medical terminology*, the etymology of the words health-care professionals use to communicate with each other and with patients. By teaching students the root elements of medical terminology—the prefixes, suffixes, and combining forms from Greek and Latin—Dunmore and Fleischer sought not only to teach students modern medical terminology but to give them the ability to decipher the evolving language of medicine throughout their careers.

In the third edition of this book, we have continued what Dunmore and Fleischer began. This new edition is organized essentially as Dunmore and Fleischer created it, with some important modifications to make it even more user friendly. The text is organized into interrelated units. Unit 1 (Lessons 1 through 7) includes 7 lessons based on Greek. Unit 2 (Lessons 8 and 9) is composed of 2 lessons based on Latin. Unit 3 (Lessons 10 through 15) takes a body systems approach that combines Greek and Latin elements used to describe the digestive system, respiratory system, and so forth. These first 15 lessons comprise the main body of the text. Each lesson builds and expands on the grammar and vocabulary introduced in the previous lessons.

For students who want additional exposure to medical terminology from a body systems perspective, the 4 lessons in Unit 4 provide just such an opportunity. These lessons include the hematopoietic and lymphatic, musculoskeletal, nervous, and endocrine systems.

Unit 5 stands on its own and provides an overview of *biological nomenclature*, the language used by scientists and physicians to identify the living organisms that exist in our world.

The pronunciation of medical terms follows the same rules that govern the pronunciation of all English words. The consonants *c* and *g* are "soft" before the vowels *e*, *i*, and *y*. That is, they are pronounced like the *c* and *g* of the words *cement* and *ginger*. Before *a*, *o*, and *u*, the consonants are "hard," and are pronounced like the *c* and *g* of *cardiac* and *gas*. The consonant *k* is always "hard," as in *leukocyte*. The long vowels *eta* and *omega* of Greek words are marked with the macrons $\bar{e}$ and $\bar{o}$; this indicates that they are pronounced like the *e* and *o* of *hematoma*. Long *i* is pro-

nounced "eye," as in the *-itis* of *appendicitis*. Words are pronounced with a stronger accent (emphasis) on one syllable. The accent falls on the second to last syllable if that syllable is long. To be considered long, a syllable must contain a short vowel followed by two consonants, a diphthong, or a long vowel (*neph-rī'-tis*). If the second to last syllable is short, the accent falls upon the third syllable from the end of the word (*gen'-ĕ-sis*).

The appendices have been expanded in this edition and include indexes of Latin and Greek suffixes, prefixes, and combining forms, as well as an abbreviated English-to-Greek/Latin glossary and a complete list of terms found in the exercises in Lessons 1 through 15. These appendices provide additional support for students and instructors alike.

The structure of the exercises at the end of each lesson has also changed from previous editions. All 15 of the major lessons contain 3 exercises. The first exercise asks students to analyze 50 terms based on the vocabulary found in that lesson. The second exercise requires students to identify a term based on its definition. The third exercise is a drill-and-review exercise and includes elements from the current and previous lessons.

This approach allows for smooth continuity and ensures that the major body of the text (Lessons 1 through 15) can be covered during a 1-semester course. The exercises in lessons 16 through 19 (Unit 4) are abbreviated and, for the most part, reflect only the material from that specific lesson. This approach allows these lessons to stand alone as additional study material. Lesson 20 (Unit 5), Biological Nomenclature, has also been written as a stand-alone lesson.

Terms in the lessons and exercises have been checked for currency and accuracy and verified in *Taber's Cyclopedic Medical Dictionary*, 19th edition (F.A. Davis Company, Philadelphia, 2001).

All 20 lessons include etymological notes to give students a historical perspective for medical terminology. These notes include tales from ancient Greek and Latin writers, mythical stories of gods and goddesses, excerpts from the writings of famous ancient physicians, such as Hippocrates and Celsus, and more modern stories of scientists and physicians who struggled to identify and accurately label the phenomena they observed.

This text is a workbook. We encourage you to write in this workbook and to make notes and comments that will help you as you work through the lessons and exercises.

Please note that this is not a medical textbook and should not be used for the diagnosis, treatment, prognosis, or etiology of disease. The medical content of this text, although accurate, is incomplete and is included solely to provide students with a context within which to learn medical terminology.

We hope you enjoy using this text to learn the complex and elegant language of medicine and that the knowledge you gain will benefit you throughout your career.

Cheryl Walker-Esbaugh
Laine H. McCarthy
Rhonda A. Sparks

ACKNOWLEDGMENTS

We greatly appreciate the comments and suggestions from a number of people who gave their time and expertise. Special thanks to Drs. John Catlin and Ralph Doty, who, having taught with the second edition of the book, provided valuable insight into its revision and were always available to answer questions; and to Dr. Samuel Huskey, who read several of the revised chapters. Thanks to Dr. Dave McCarthy for reading and commenting on the biological nomenclature lesson and to Danny McMurphy, who patiently read chapter after chapter. Thanks, too, to Tracy Alford for her support and consideration.

We would like to thank F.A. Davis for their generosity in allowing us to use material in *Taber's Cyclopedic Medical Dictionary*, 19th edition. We also thank the editors at Davis for their advice and support. All of the people involved helped to make this a much better work than we could have ourselves. Any errors, of course, are our own.

CONTENTS

DEVELOPMENT OF THE ENGLISH LANGUAGE

In 55 and 54 BC, Julius Caesar invaded Britain. The romanization of Britain, however, did not occur until almost 100 years later, when expeditionary forces were sent out by the Roman emperor Claudius. Although Latin was the official language during the Roman occupation of Britain, Celtic, the native language of the people of Britain, was little affected by it.

The English language began its development as an independent tongue with the migration of Germanic people (Angles, Saxons, and Jutes) from western Europe (modern-day Denmark and northern Germany) across the English Channel to Britain during the 5th and 6th centuries AD. These Germanic invaders, in contact with the Romans from the 1st century BC on, brought with them not only their native tongue but also the Latin words they had borrowed from the Romans. Their language, known as Old English or Anglo-Saxon, was a member of the Germanic family of Indo-European languages and gradually superseded the Celtic dialects in most of southern Britain. Many Old English words have survived, with some linguistic change, to form the basic vocabulary of the English language. Words borrowed from other languages—mostly Latin, French, and Greek—have been added to the English language.

During the 7th century AD, after the establishment of the first monastery in 597 AD, the inhabitants of Britain gradually converted to Christianity. Latin, the language of the Western Church, was spoken, written, and read in the churches, schools, and monasteries. This brought many Latin words into the evolving English language, most having to do with religious matters and many derived from Greek.

Beginning in the 8th century AD, as a result of the Viking invasions, additional words of North Germanic origin entered the English language. Living alongside the Anglo-Saxons and eventually assimilated by them, the Norse and Danish invaders and their language had a marked impact on both England and the English language. It is not surprising that, in 1697 AD, writer Daniel Defoe described English as "your Roman-Saxon-Danish-Norman-English."

The Norman invasion in 1066 AD brought a French-speaking aristocracy to England, and for the next 150 years French was the official spoken and written language of the governing class. In this period, French, with its roots in Latin, existed alongside English but had little effect on it. However, in the 300 years following the expulsion of the Normans from England—from about 1200 to 1500 AD—although English was once again the dominant language, many words were borrowed from French because its vocabulary was far richer. Writers and educated people in England began to look to French as a source of words and concepts lacking in their own language. During these years, the changing English language reached the stage we now know as Middle English.

With the Renaissance (1400–1600 AD) came a revival of classic scholarship. English words began to be formed directly from Latin and Greek and were no longer borrowed through the intermediary of French. Beginning around 1500 AD, for the first time the writings of the ancient Greeks were read in England in their original language. This renewal of interest in Greek and Roman literature and the ideas and concepts expressed in these works created an awareness of the impoverished state of the English language and the difficulty of expressing in English ideas that were easily expressed in Latin or Greek. Words were borrowed extensively from Greek and Latin, both with and without change, and new words were created that combined both Latin and Greek elements. Although most words were borrowed from Latin and Greek, others were borrowed from French and Italian. The English of this period is now known as Modern English.

The extensive borrowing of words from Latin and Greek that began about 1500 AD continued for hundreds of years, and continues to this day. As new advances were made in the fields of medicine and science during and after the Renaissance (and continuing up to the present day), words were needed to describe these new discoveries and inventions. Medical scientists turned to the early Greek and Roman physicians, especially Hippocrates, Galen, and Celsus, whom they greatly admired, and borrowed words from their medical treatises. These ancient scientists had an extensive medical vocabulary, which they used to describe their observations and theories. Hippocrates, for example, used the terms *apoplexy, hypochondria, dysentery, ophthalmia*, *epilepsy*, and *asthma* to describe certain physical features and conditions that he observed. Modern physicians and scientists, who could not find an appropriate word to describe diseases that were unknown to early physicians, turned to the vocabulary of the ancient languages and created suitable terms.

The language used by Linnaeus, as well as by other scientists and scholars of the Renaissance and the period following, that is, the period after 1500 AD, is called New Latin. Scientists and writers, schooled in Classical Latin, tried to emulate the classical writers and to revive the style of Cicero and others. The term New Latin refers to words that have been created in the form of, and on the analogy of, Latin words (e.g., *natrium*, the chemical name for sodium, borrowed from Arabic) or to the use of new meanings applied to extant Latin words (e.g., the word cancer, from *cancer*, crab, or the word bacillus, from *bacillus*, a small rod or staff). New Latin is a rich source of biological terms. *Trichinella spiralis*, the species of *Trichinella* that causes trichinosis, and *Salmonella*, the genus of microorganisms named after the American pathologist Daniel E. Salmon, are two of the many examples of New Latin found in this text.

HIPPOCRATES

Hippocrates, born in 460 BC, was a Greek physician who lived on the Aegean island of Cos. Although he is the most famous of the ancient physicians and is recognized as the "father of medicine," very little is actually known about him or his life. The *Hippocratic Corpus*, a work of about 60 medical treatises attributed to Hippocrates, most likely reflects the work of many physicians rather than that of Hippocrates alone. Hippocrates is recognized for separating superstition from medicine. Unlike other physicians of his time, he believed that illness had a rational explanation, rather than being the result of divine anger or possession by evil spirits, and could therefore be treated. Hippocrates based his medical writings on his observation and study of the human body. He was the first to attempt to record his experiences as a physician for future reference. The Hippocratic Oath, although it cannot be directly attributed to him, is said to reflect his philosophy and principles.

THE HIPPOCRATIC OATH

"I swear by Apollo the physician, and Aesculapius, and Hygeia, and Panacea, and all the gods and goddesses, that according to my ability and judgment, I will keep this oath and its stipulation—to reckon him who taught me this art equally dear to me as my parents, to share my substance with him, and to relieve his necessities if required; to look upon his offspring in the same footing as my own brothers, and to teach them this art if they shall wish to learn it, without fee or stipulation, and that by precept, lecture, and every other mode of instruction, I will impart

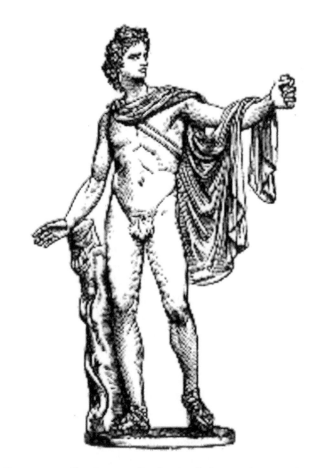

Figure 1. Apollo. (From Bulfinch's *Mythology—The Age of Fable,* with permission. Available at *http://www.bulfinch.org*).

a knowledge of the art to my own sons, and those of my teachers, and to disciples bound by a stipulation and oath according to the law of medicine, but to none other.

"I will follow that system of regimen which, according to my ability and judgment, I consider for the benefit of my patients, and abstain from whatever is deleterious and mischievous. I will give no deadly medicine to anyone if asked, nor suggest any such counsel; and in like manner I will not give to a woman a pessary to produce abortion. With purity and with holiness I will pass my life and practice my art. I will not cut persons laboring under the stone, but will leave this to be done by men who are practitioners of this work. Into whatever houses I enter, I will go into them for the benefit of the sick and I will abstain from every voluntary act of mischief and corruption; and, further, from the seduction of females or males, of freemen and slaves. Whatever, in connection with my professional practice, or not in connection with it, I see or hear, in the life of men, which ought not to be spoken of abroad, I will not divulge, as reckoning that all such should be kept secret.

While I continue to keep this Oath unviolated, may it be granted to me to enjoy life and the practice of this art, respected by all men, in all times. But, should I trespass and violate this Oath, may the reverse be my lot." (From *Taber's Cyclopedic Medical Dictionary*, ed 19. FA Davis, Philadelphia, 2001, pp 949–950, with permission.)

GALEN

Galen (129–199 AD) was born in Pergamum in Asia Minor. After studying medicine at the Asclepium, the famed medical school in his native town, and in Smyrna and Alexandria, he came to Rome in 162 AD, where, except for brief interruptions, he remained until his death, writing philosophical treatises and medical books. His fame and reputation brought him to the attention of the emperor Marcus Aurelius, who appointed him court physician. Galen wrote extensively on anatomy, physiology, and general medicine, relying on his training, the best that was available, and on his dissection of human corpses and experiments on living animals. It was the work of Galen, more than any other medical writer, that profoundly influenced the physicians of the early Renaissance. His theories on the flow of blood in the human body remained unchallenged until the discovery of the circulation of the blood by William Harvey in the 17th century.

CELSUS

Aulus Cornelius Celsus was a Roman encyclopedist who, under the reign of the emperor Tiberius (14–37 AD), wrote a lengthy work dealing with agriculture, military tactics, medicine, rhetoric, and possibly philosophy and law. Apart from a few fragments, only his eight books on medicine still exist. It is suggested that Celsus was not a professional physician but rather a layman writing for other laymen. It appears, especially in his treatises on surgery, that he had little first-hand experience in the field of medicine and relied on material selected from other sources. Celsus was highly esteemed during the Renaissance, possibly as a result of his style of writing.

GREEK-DERIVED MEDICAL TERMINOLOGY

GREEK ALPHABET

Name of Letter	Capital	Lower-case	Trans-literation	Name of Letter	Capital	Lower-case	Trans-literation
alpha	A	α	a	xi	Ξ	ξ	x
beta	B	б or β	b	omicron	O	o	o short
gamma	Γ	γ	g	pi	Π	π	p
delta	Δ	δ	d	rho	P	ρ	r
epsilon	E	ϵ	e short	sigma	Σ	σ or s	s
zeta	Z	ζ	z	tau	T	τ	t
eta	H	η	e long	upsilon	Y	υ	y
theta	Θ	θ	th	phi	Φ	ϕ or φ	f, ph
iota	I	ι	i	chi	X	x	ch as in German "echt"
kappa	K	κ	k, c				
lambda	Λ	λ	l				
mu	M	μ	m	psi	Ψ	ψ	ps
nu	N	ν	n	omega	Ω	ω	o long

Source: Taber's Cyclopedic Medical Dictionary, ed 19, F. A. Davis, Philadelphia, 2001, p 2368, with permission.

GREEK NOUNS AND ADJECTIVES

A man who is wise should consider health the most valuable of all things to mankind and learn how, by his own intelligence, to help himself in sickness.

[Hippocrates, *Regimen in Health* 9]

In the mid-8th century BC, the Greeks borrowed the art of writing from the Phoenicians, a Semitic-speaking people of the Levant who inhabited the region in the area of modern Lebanon. The Phoenician system of writing had to be adapted to the Greek language because there were characters representing sounds in the Semitic language that did not exist in Greek, and sounds in Greek for which there were no characters in the Semitic system. In their adaptation of these Phoenician characters, the Greeks began to distinguish between long and short vowels, representing long e by *eta* [H] and short e by *epsilon* [E], and long and short o by *omega* [W] and *omicron* [O], respectively. However, the distinction was carried no further, and no differentiation in writing was made between the long and short vowels a, i, and u. In transliterating Greek words, a macron (‾) will be used to mark the long vowels $\bar{e}$ and $\bar{o}$ in this text:

Greek	Meaning	Example
xēros	dry	**xeroderma**
splēn	spleen	**splenomegaly**
phōnē	voice	**phonology**
thōrax	chest cavity	**thoracentesis**

During and after the 1st century BC, many Greek words were borrowed by the Romans and, in the process of being borrowed, assumed the spelling of Latin words. It has been the practice since then, in the coining of English words from Greek, to use the form and spelling of Latin, even if the word never actually appeared in the Latin language.

The letter *k* was little used in Latin, and Greek *kappa* was transliterated in that language as *c*, which always had the hard sound of *k*. Most English words derived from Greek words containing a *kappa* are spelled with *c*:

Greek	Meaning	Example
kyanos	blue	**cyanotic**
mikros	small	**microscope**
kolon	colon	**colitis**
skleros	hard	**arteriosclerosis**

There are exceptions, and the *kappa* is retained as *k* in some words:

Greek	Meaning	Example
leukos	white	**leukemia**
kinēsis	motion	**dyskinesia**
karyon	kernel	**karyogenesis**
kēlē	swelling	**keloid**

Some words are spelled with either *k* or *c*: **keratocele, ceratocele** (*kerat-*, horn); **synkinesis, syncinesis** (*kin-*, move); cinematics, kinematics (*kinēma*, motion).

In Latin the letter *k* is rarely used and is found only in the following:

- *Kalendae*, the Calends, the first day of the month, and its derivatives *Kalendalis*, *Kalendaris*, *Kalendarium*, and *Kalendarius*
- *Karthago*, Carthage, the Phoenician city in North Africa
- *kalo* (archaic), call
- *koppa* (archaic), Greek symbol for 90

Greek words beginning with *rho* [*r*] were always accompanied by a strong expulsion of breath called **rough breathing** (also called aspiration). In transliterating Greek words and in the formation of English derivatives, this rough breathing is indicated by an *h* after the *r*:

Greek	Meaning	Example
rhombos	rhombus	**rhombencephalon**
rhodon	rose	**rhodopsin**
rhiza	root	**rhizoid**
rhythmos	rhythm	**rhythmic**

There are exceptions: **rhachis, rachis; rhachischisis, rachischisis** (*rhachis*, spine). Words beginning with *rho* [*r*] usually double the *r* when following a prefix or another word element, and the **rough breathing** [*h*] follows the second *r* (note: the following words are from Greek verbs):

Greek	Meaning	Example
rhe-	flow	**diarrhea**
rhag-	burst forth	**hemorrhage**
rhaph-	sew	**cystorrhaphy**

When Greek words containing diphthongs were borrowed and used in Latin, the diphthongs *ai, ei, oi,* and *ou* were changed to the Latin spelling of these sounds, but these Latin diphthongs usually undergo a further change in English:

Greek	Latin	English	Greek Example	Meaning	English Example
ai	*ae*	*e*	*haima*	blood	**hematology***
			aitia	cause	**etiology***
ei	*ei*	***ei* or *i***	*cheir*	hand	**cheirospasm, dyschiria**
			leios	smooth	**leiomyofibroma**
			meion	less	**miotic**
oi	*oe*	*e*	*oidema*	swelling	**edema***
			oistros	desire	**estrogen**
ou	*u*	*u*	*gloutos*	buttock	**gluteal**

*British spelling usually retains the Latin diphthongs *ae* and *oe*: haematology, aetiology, oedema, oestrogen, and so forth.

In the Greek language, words beginning with the sound of the rough breathing [*h*] often lost their aspiration when another word element preceded the aspirated word (except after the prefixes *anti-, apo-, epi-, hypo-, kata-,* and *meta-*). However, the spelling of English derivatives of such words varies, and the aspiration is often retained:

Greek	Meaning	Example
hidros	sweat	**chromidrosis, hyperhidrosis**

Greek is an **inflected** language. This means that words have different endings to indicate their grammatical function in a sentence. The inflection of nouns, pronouns, and adjectives is called **declension**. Greek nouns are declined in five grammatical cases in both singular and plural: nominative, genitive, dative, accusative, and vocative. There are three declensions of Greek nouns, each having its own set of endings for the cases. Nouns are cited in dictionaries and vocabularies in the form of the nominative singular, often called the **dictionary form**.

Nouns of the first declension, mostly feminine, end in *-ē* or *-ā*, and sometimes in short *-a*. Second-declension nouns, mostly masculine or neuter, end in *-os* if masculine, and in *-on* if neuter. Third-declension nouns will be discussed in Lesson 2.

The base of nouns of the first and second declensions is found by dropping the ending of the nominative case, resulting in the **combining form**, to which suffixes and other combining forms are added to form words.

Greek	Meaning	Example
nephros	kidney	**nephr**-itis
neuron	nerve	**neur**-otic
psōra	sore	**psor**-iasis
psychē	mind	**psych**-osis

Rarely, the entire word is used as the combining form: **colonoscopy** (*kolon*, colon), **neuronitis** (*neuron*, nerve).

If a suffix or a combining form that begins with a consonant is attached to a combining form that ends in a consonant, then a vowel, called the **connecting vowel**, usually **o** and sometimes **i** or **u** (especially with words derived from Latin), is inserted between the two forms.*

leuk-**o**-cyte

neur-**o**-blast

psych-**o**-neurosis

calc-**i**-penia

vir-**u**-lent

Exceptions occur when suffixes beginning with *s* or *t* follow an element ending with *p* or *c*:

eclamp-sia

apoplec-tic

epilep-tic

nephremphraxis (for **nephremphrac-sis**)

Adjectives agree in gender, number, and case with the noun they modify. They are cited in dictionaries and

*Medical dictionaries and English dictionaries usually give the connecting vowel as part of the combining form, as in leuko-, neuro-, psycho-, and so forth.

vocabularies in the form of the nominative singular masculine. The dictionary form of most Greek adjectives ends in -*os*, and the combining form is found by dropping this ending. There are some adjectives that end in -*ys*, and the combining form of these is found by dropping the -*s* or, rarely, the -*ys*:

Greek	Meaning	Example
leukos	white	**leuk**-emia
kyanos	blue	**cyan**-osis
tachys	swift	**tachy**-pnea
glykys	sweet	**glyc**-emia

When Greek nouns are used in English, they usually appear in one of four ways:

1. In the original vocabulary form:

kolon	**colon**
mania	**mania**
omphalos	**omphalos**
psychē	**psyche**

2. With the ending changed to the Latin form:

aortē	**aorta**
bronchos	**bronchus**
kranion	**cranium**
tetanos	**tetanus**

3. With the ending changed to silent -e:

gangraina	**gangrene**
kyklos	**cycle**
tonos	**tone**
zōnē	**zone**

4. With the ending dropped:

organon	**organ**
orgasmos	**orgasm**
spasmos	**spasm**
stomachos	**stomach**

PREFIXES

Prefixes modify or qualify in some way the meaning of the word to which they are affixed. It is often difficult to assign a single specific meaning to each prefix, and often it is necessary to adapt a meaning that fits the particular use of a word. A complete list of prefixes is found in Appendix B.

a- (**an-** before a vowel or *h*): not, without, lacking, deficient:

a-biogenesis	**an**-algesia
a-sthenia	**an**-hydrous
cardi-**a**-sthenia	**an**-hidrosis

anti- (**ant-** often before a vowel or *h*; hyphenated before *i*): against, opposed to, preventing, relieving:

anti-biotic	**anti**-retroviral
anti-histamine	**anti**-septic
anti-toxin	**ant**-acid

di- (rarely **dis-**): two, twice, double:

di-phonia	**di**-ataxia
di-plegia	**dis**-diaclast

dys-: difficult, painful, defective, abnormal:

dys-menorrhea	**dys**-pepsia
dys-pnea	**dys**-genesis
dys-ostosis	**dys**-trophy

ec- (**ex-** before a vowel): out of, away from:

ec-tasis	**ex**-encephalia
ec-topic	**ex**-ophthalmos

The prefix **ex-** in most words is derived from Latin: **excrete, exhale, extensor, exudate,** and so forth.

ecto- (**ect-** often before a vowel): outside of:

ecto-derm	**ecto**-plasm
ecto-cornea	**ect**-ostosis

en- (**em-** before *b, m,* and *p*): in, into, within:

en-cephalitis	**em**-metropia
em-bolism	**em**-physema

endo-, ento- (**end-, ent-** before a vowel): within:

endo-genous	**ento**-cele
endo-metritis	**end**-odontics
endo-cardium	**ent**-optic

epi- (**ep-** before a vowel or *h*): upon, over, above:

epi-cardium	**epi**-demic
epi-dermis	**ep**-encephalon

exo-: outside, from the outside, toward the outside:

exo-cardia	**exo**-genous
exo-crine	**exo**-thermal

hemi-: half, partial; (often) one side of the body:

hemi-cardia	**hemi**-paralysis
hemi-plegia	**hemi**-gastrectomy

hyper-: over, above, excessive, beyond normal:

hyper-hidrosis	**hyper**-lipemia
hyper-glycemia	**hyper**-parathyroidism

hypo- (**hyp-** before a vowel or *h*): under, deficient, below normal:

hypo-chondria	**hyp**-algesia
hypo-dermic	**hyp**-acousia

mono- (**mon-** before a vowel or *h*): one, single:

mono-blast	**mono**-chromatic
mon-ocular	**mono**-neuritis

peri-: around, surrounding:

peri-angiitis	**peri**-laryngitis
peri-cardiac	**peri**-odontology

syn- (**sym-** before *b*, *p*, and *m*; the *n* assimilates or is dropped before *s*): together, with, joined:

syn-apse	**sym**-pathy
syn-thetic	**sym**-melia
sym-biosis	**sy**-stolic

Note that words can have more than one prefix and that a prefix can follow a combining form:

hyper-exo-phoria	cardi-**ec**-tomy
cardi-**a**-sthenia	**dys-anti**-graphia

SUFFIXES

Suffixes are elements that are added to combining forms. Suffixes form nouns, adjectives, and verbs or adverbs. Most of these nouns are abstract; that is, they indicate a state, quality, condition, procedure, or process. In medical terminology, most conditions indicated by these suffixes are pathological or abnormal: **psoriasis, hepatitis, pneumonia, myopia, astigmatism,** and so forth. Some nouns indicating procedures or processes are **thoracocentesis, appendectomy, gastroscopy,** and **gastropexy.** A complete list of suffixes is found in Appendix C.

-a: forms abstract nouns: state, condition:

dyspne-**a**	anasarc-**a**
erythroderm-**a**	rhinorrhe-**a**

-ac (rare): forms adjectives: pertaining to, located in:

cardi-**ac**	ile-**ac**
celi-**ac**	ischi-**ac**

-ia: forms abstract nouns; often the suffix **-ia** appears as **-y**: state, condition:

anem-**ia**	hypertroph-**y**
pneumon-**ia**	microcephal-**y**

-iac (rare): forms nouns: person afflicted with:

hemophil-**iac**	insomn-**iac**
hypochondr-**iac**	man-**iac**

-iasis: forms abstract nouns: disease, abnormal condition, abnormal presence of: often used with the name of a parasitic organism to indicate infestation of the body by that organism. When used with **lith-** [Gr. *lithos*, stone]: formation and/or presence of calculi in the body:

elephant-**iasis**	ancylostom-**iasis**
nephrolith-**iasis**	schistosom-**iasis**

-ic: forms adjectives: pertaining to, located in; words ending in **-ic** can be used as both adjectives and nouns and, as nouns, often indicate a drug or agent:

analges-**ic**	hypoderm-**ic**
gastr-**ic**	tox-**ic**

Words ending in **-ic** can refer to a person suffering from a certain disability or condition:

parapleg-**ic**	anorex-**ic**

-in, -ine: form names of substances:

adrenal-**in**	chlor-**ine**
antitox-**in**	epinephr-**ine**

-ist: forms nouns: a person interested in:

cardiolog-**ist**	hematolog-**ist**
dermatolog-**ist**	orthodont-**ist**

-itic: forms adjectives: pertaining to; pertaining to inflammation; words ending in **-itic** can be used as both adjectives and nouns and, as nouns, often indicate a drug or agent:

antineur-**itic**	arthr-**itic** (Fig. 1–1)
laryng-**itic**	nephr-**itic**

-itis: forms nouns indicating an inflamed condition: inflammation:

gastr-**itis**	laryng-**itis**
hepat-**itis**	periton-**itis**

-itides is the plural form for words ending in **-itis**:

arthr-**itides**	dermat-**itides**

-ium (rarely **-eum**): forms nouns: membrane, connective tissue:

endometr-**ium**	pericard-**ium**
epicran-**ium**	periton-**eum**

In a few words **-ium** names a region of the body:

epigastr-**ium**	hypogastr-**ium**
hypochondr-**ium**	hyponych-**ium**

-ma: forms nouns: (often) abnormal or diseased condition. The combining form for nouns ending in **-ma** is **-mat-**. Sometimes the final **-a** drops off the noun:

ede-**ma**	ede-**mat**-ogenic
trau-**ma**	trau-**mat**-ic
phleg-**m**	phleg-**mat**-ic
sper-**m**	sper-**mat**-ic

-osis: forms nouns: abnormal or diseased condition:*

nephr-**osis**	scler-**osis**
neur-**osis**	sten-**osis**

*See the Etymological Notes in this lesson for other uses of -osis.

-otic: forms adjectives from nouns ending in **-osis**: pertaining to:

nephr-**otic**	scler-**otic**
neur-**otic**	sten-**otic**

-sia: forms abstract nouns: state, condition:

amne-**sia**	dyspha-**sia**
ecta-**sia**	hypacu-**sia**

-sis: forms abstract nouns: state, condition:

antisep-**sis**	paraly-**sis**
eme-**sis**	prophylaxis (prophylac-**sis**)

-tic: forms adjectives from nouns ending in **-sis**: pertaining to; words ending in **-tic** can be used as both adjectives and nouns and, as nouns, often indicate a drug or agent:

antisep-**tic**	paraly-**tic**
eme-**tic**	prophylac-**tic**

Words ending in **-itic** or **-tic** can refer to a person suffering from a certain disability or condition:

neuro-**tic**	arthr-**itic**

-y: forms abstract nouns. See **-ia**.

Words can have more than one suffix. Sometimes the suffix **-iac** or **-ic** is affixed to the noun-forming suffix **-sia**

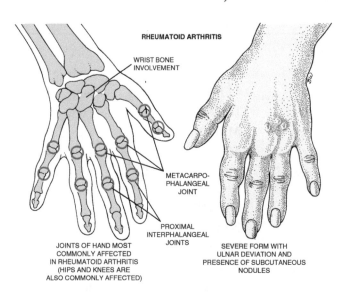

Figure 1–1. Rheumatoid arthritis. (From Taber's Cyclopedic Medical Dictionary, ed 19. F. A. Davis, Philadelphia, 2001, p 167, with permission.)

or **-sis**. When this occurs, the only vestige left of the noun-forming suffix is the **-s**:

amne-**sia**	amne-**s-ic**, amne-**s-iac**

A suffix can appear in the middle of a word affixed to a combining form:

hemat-**in**-emia	hepat-**ic**-o-enterostomy

VOCABULARY

The following is a list of combining forms derived from Greek. (When the meaning of the original Greek word differs from its modern meaning, the original meaning of the word is placed in brackets.) For a complete list of combining forms used in this text, see Appendix A.

Greek	Combining Form	Meaning	Example
akantha	**ACANTH-**	thorn, spine	**acanth**-ocytosis
algos	**ALG-**	pain	my-**alg**-ia
algēsis	**ALGES-**	sensitivity to pain	**alges**-ia
allos	**ALL-**	other, divergence, difference from	**all**-oplasia
angeion	**ANGI-**	(blood) vessel, duct	**angi**-ocarditis
arteria	**ARTERI-**	[air passage] artery (Fig.1–2)	**arteri**-ogram
arthron	**ARTHR-**	joint	**arthr**-itis
bios	**BI-**	life	**bi**-ology
bradys	**BRADY-**	slow	**brady**-rhythmia
kardia	**CARDI-**	heart	**cardi**-ogram
kephalē	**CEPHAL-**	head	**cephal**-algia
kranion	**CRANI-**	skull (Fig. 1–3)	epi-**crani**-um
kytos	**CYT-**	[hollow container] cell	leuko-**cyt**-e
enkephalon	**ENCEPHAL-**	brain (a combination of *en*, in, and *kephalē*, head)	**encephal**-itis
erythros	**ERYTHR-**	red, red blood cell	**erythr**-ocyte

Greek	Combining Form	Meaning	Example
leptos	**LEPT-**	thin, fine, slight	**lept**-omeninges
leukos	**LEUK-**	white, white blood cell	**leuk**-emia
lithos	**LITH-**	stone, calculus	angio-**lith**
logos	**LOG-**	word, study	bio-**log**-y
malakos	**MALAC-**	soft	**malac**-osteon
mesos	**MES-**	middle, secondary, partial, mesentery	**mes**-oderm
metron	**-METER, METR-**	measure, measuring device (Words ending in -**meter** indicate instruments for measuring.)	bio-**metr**-y / cyto-**meter**
nephros	**NEPHR-**	kidney	**nephr**-ectomy
neuron	**NEUR-**	[tendon] nerve, nervous system	**neur**-ology
osteon	**OSTE-**	bone	**oste**-oporosis
prosōpon	**PROSOP-**	face	**prosop**-ospasm
prōtos	**PROT-**	first, primitive, early	**prot**-oneuron
skleros	**SCLER-**	hard	**scler**-oderma
stenos	**STEN-**	narrow	**sten**-ocephaly
stereos	**STERE-**	solid, having three dimensions	**stere**-otropism
tachys	**TACHY-**	rapid	**tachy**-cardia
toxon	**TOX(I)-**	poison	**tox**-in

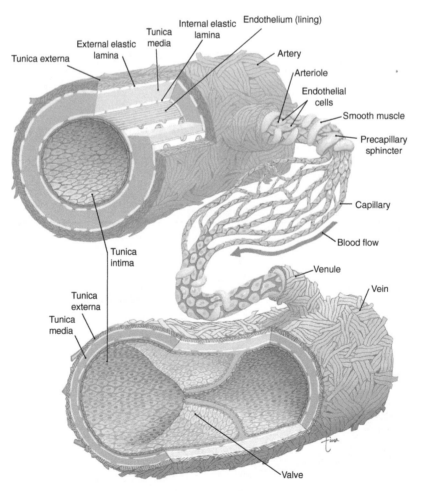

Figure 1–2. Structure of an artery. (From Scanlon, VC, and Sanders, T: Essentials of Anatomy and Physiology, ed 4. F. A. Davis, Philadelphia, 2003, p 279, with permission.)

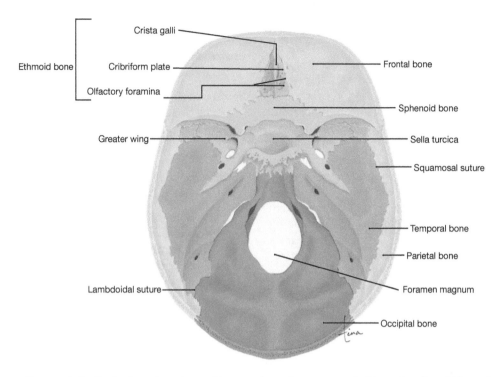

Figure 1–3. Skull. Superior view with top of cranium removed. (From Scanlon, VC, and Sanders, T: Essentials of Anatomy and Physiology, ed 4. F. A. Davis, Philadelphia, 2003, p 111, with permission.)

SUFFIX FORMS

Many combining forms are used with certain suffixes so commonly that this combination can be called a **suffix form**. Some common suffix forms include the following:

Combining Form	Suffix Form	Meaning	Example
LOG-	-logy	study, science, the study or science of	cardio-**logy**
	-logist	one who specializes in a certain study or science	neuro-**logist**
MALAC-	-malacia	the softening (of tissues) of	nephro-**malacia**
SCLER-	-sclerosis	the hardening (of tissues) of	arterio-**sclerosis**
STEN-	-stenosis	the narrowing (of a part of the body)	angio-**stenosis**
TOX-	-toxic	poisonous (to an organ)	cardio-**toxic**
	-toxin	a substance poisonous to (a part of the body)	neuro-**toxin**

ETYMOLOGICAL NOTES

Throughout its history, the English language has been enriched by borrowing words from other languages, particularly Latin, Greek, and French. Borrowing from French began as early as the period of the Norman conquest of England and reached its high point during and immediately after the Renaissance. Because French is based largely on Latin and because many Latin words are derived from Greek, various French words have Greek origins. One such word is **migraine**, a severe form of headache, usually unilateral. The French word *migraine*, the British word *megrim*, and the Italian word *emicránia* are derived from the Latin word *hemicrania*, which was borrowed from the Greek word *hemikrania*, meaning "pain on one side of the head," from the prefix *hēmi* (half) and *kranion* (skull).

The ancient Greeks used to smear poison on their arrowheads for use in hunting, and this poison was called *toxicon pharmakon* (*toxon*, bow, archery; *pharmakon*, drug), thus providing the modern word **toxic**. A **toxicologist** is one who is skilled in the study of poisons, whereas a **toxophilite** is a lover (*philos*) of archery. **Toxicity** means the extent, quality, or degree of being poisonous; toxicity is also used to describe poisonous effects (**neurotoxicity**).

The suffix **-osis** indicates an abnormal condition: **neurosis**, **psychosis** (*psychē*, mind). When affixed to a combining form indicating an organ or a part of the body, it usually indicates a noninflammatory diseased condition: **nephrosis**, **endometriosis** (*endo*, within, *mētra*, uterus). Following the combining form **cyt-** (cell) it means an abnormal increase in number of the type of cell indicated: **leukocytosis**, **erythrocytosis**. Following the combining form for an adjective, it indicates the abnormality characterized by the meaning of the adjective: **stenosis**: narrowing of a passage; **sclerosis**: hardening of tissues; **cyanosis** (*kyanos*, blue): bluish discoloration of a part.

There are a few words ending in **-osis** that have special meanings:

anastomosis: a surgical or pathological connection between two passages

exostosis: a bony growth arising from the surface of a bone

aponeurosis: a sheet of tissue connecting muscles to bones

symbiosis: the living together in close association of two organisms of different species

antibiosis: the association between two organisms in which one is harmful to the other

The adjectival form for words ending in **-osis** is **-otic**: **neurosis**, **neurotic**; **psychosis**, **psychotic**; **nephrosis**, **nephrotic**; **symbiosis**, **symbiotic**.

The word **etiology** is from the Greek noun *aitia* (cause, origin) with the suffix form **-logy**. The etiology of a disease or an abnormal condition is its cause or origin. In medical dictionaries it is usually abbreviated **etiol**.

Exercise 1: Analyze and Define

Analyze and define each of the following words. In this and in succeeding exercises, analysis should consist of separating the words into prefixes (if any), combining forms, and suffixes or suffix forms (if any) and giving the meaning of each. Be certain to differentiate between nouns and adjectives in your definitions. Consult a medical dictionary for the current meanings of these words. Use a separate paper if you need more room for an answer.

1. abiosis _____

2. acanthocyte _____

3. allostery _____

4. analgesic _____

5. analgia _____

6. angiostenosis _____

7. antibiotic _____

8. antitoxin _____

9. arteriostosis _____

10. arthritides _____

11. arthritis _____

12. arthrosclerosis _____

13. arthrosteitis _____

14. biotoxin _____

15. bradycardia _____

16. diencephalon _____

17. dysarthrosis _____

18. encephalalgia _____

19. encephalomalacia _____

20. endoneurium _____

21. endosteum _____

22. endotoxin _____

23. epicardium _____

24. epicranium _____

25. erythrocytosis _____

26. erythroprosopalgia _____

27. exocardia _____

28. exotoxin _____

29. hemialgia _____

30. hypalgesia _____

31. hyperalgesia _____

32. leptocephalia _____

33. leukotoxin _____

34. lithiasis _____

35. mesocardia _____

36. nephrolithiasis _____

37. nephrosclerosis _____

38. neuritis _____

39. ostalgia _____

40. osteometry _____

41. osteomalacia _____

42. pericarditis _____

43. periosteum _____

44. prosoponeuralgia _____

45. protobiology _____

46. scleriasis _____

47. stenocephaly _____

48. stereology _____

49. synalgic _____

50. toxicosis _____

Exercise 2: Word Derivation

Give the word derived from Greek elements that matches each of the following. It is not necessary to give combining terms for words in parentheses. Verify your answer in a medical dictionary. **Note that the wording of the dictionary definition may vary from the wording below.**

1. Inflammation (of the tissues) around a blood vessel _____

2. Softening of the heart (muscle) _____

3. Hardening of the arteries _____

4. Pertaining to the heart _____

5. Living together of two organisms _____

6. Membrane around the heart _____

7. Pertaining to poison _____

8. (Abnormal) narrowing (of a passage) _____

9. (Abnormal) rapidity of the heart _____

10. (Severe) pain along the course of a nerve _____

11. Study of the skull _____

12. Instrument for estimating the size of calculi _____

13. Congenital absence of one-half of the brain _____

14. Specialist in the study of bones _____

15. Headache   _____

16. Substance that is poisonous to kidney (tissue)   _____

17. Measurement of a solid body   _____

18. Instrument for counting and measuring cells   _____

19. Increased heart rate alternating with slow rate   _____

20. White blood cell   _____

Exercise 3: Drill and Review

The meaning of each of the following words can be determined from its etymology. Determine the meaning of each word. Verify your answer in a medical dictionary.

1. acanthocytosis   _____

2. acardia   _____

3. angiitis   _____

4. angiocarditis   _____

5. angiolith   _____

6. angiosclerosis   _____

7. angiosis   _____

8. antiarthritic   _____

9. anticytotoxin   _____

10. antilithic   _____

11. arteriolith   _____

12. arteritis _____

13. arthroneuralgia _____

14. atoxic _____

15. cardioangiology _____

16. craniomalacia _____

17. craniosclerosis _____

18. cytobiology _____

19. cytotoxin _____

20. dysostosis _____

21. ectocardia _____

22. encephalic _____

23. encephalolith _____

24. endangiitis _____

25. endangium _____

26. endarteritis _____

27. endocranium _____

28. erythroleukemia _____

29. erythrotoxin _____

30. exencephalia _____

31. hemianalgesia   _____

32. hyperalgia   _____

33. hypologia   _____

34. lithonephritis   _____

35. malacosteon   _____

36. mesocephalic   _____

37. monocyte   _____

38. nephralgia   _____

39. neurosclerosis   _____

40. neurotoxin   _____

41. osteosclerosis   _____

42. periarteritis   _____

43. periarthritis   _____

44. perinephrium   _____

45. periosteitis   _____

46. sclerencephalia   _____

47. stenosis   _____

48. synarthrosis   _____

49. toxicology   _____

50. toxin   _____

NOUNS OF THE THIRD DECLENSION

The learning of medicine can be compared to the growth of plants in the earth. Our inherent ability is the soil. The precepts of our teachers are the seeds. Learning from childhood is like the seeds falling into the plowed land at the proper season. The place of learning is like the nourishment that arises from the surrounding air to the seeds that are planted. Love of work is the labor. Time strengthens all of these things so that their nurture is completed.

[Hippocrates, *Law* 3]

Nouns of the third declension are somewhat different from those of the first and second declensions in that this class of nouns usually has two combining forms: one formed from the nominative singular, the dictionary form, and the other from a case other than the nominative. For this reason, Greek dictionaries and vocabularies cite the genitive singular, which usually ends in *-os*, along with the nominative case of these nouns. The combining form is found by dropping the ending *-os*. Sometimes the base of the genitive case is the same as the nominative case: *cheir, cheiros* (hand), and there is only one combining form. But usually they differ:

derma, dermatos	skin	**derm**-algia hypo-**derm**-ic **dermat**-ology **dermat**-itis
gastēr, gastros	stomach	**gastr**-ic **gastr**-itis epi-**gaster**

Sometimes the nominative singular, the dictionary form of a noun, is itself a word without a prefix or suffix:

derma:	the skin
hepar:	the liver
meninx:	one of the coverings of the brain and spinal cord
soma:	the body

PREFIXES

amphi-, ampho-: on both sides, around, both:
    amphi-bious   **ampho**-cyte

ana-: up, back, against:
    ana-tomy   **ana**-gen

apo-: away from:
    apo-crine   **apo**-ptosis

cata- (**cat-** before a vowel or *h*): downward, disordered:

cata-bolism   **cat**-hode

dia- (**di-** before a vowel): through, across, apart:

dia-clasis   **di**-optometer

eso-: within, inner, inward:

eso-gastritis   **eso**-tropia
eso-phoria   **eso**-sphenoiditis

eu-: good, normal, healthy:

eu-thyroid   **eu**-phoria
eu-pepsia   **eu**-thanasia

heter-, **hetero-**: different, other, relationship to another:

hetero-chromia   **heter**-esthesia
hetero-sexual   **heter**-metropia

homo-, **homeo-**: same, likeness:

homo-topic   **homo**-genize
homeo-stasis   **homeo**-pathic

meta- (**met-** before a vowel or *h*): change, transformation, after, behind:

meta-bolism   **met**-encephalon
meta-morphosis   **met**-hemoglobin

para- (often **par-** before a vowel): alongside, around, abnormal, beyond:

para-thyroid   **par**-acusia
para-metrium   **par**-onychia

pro-: before:

pro-dromal   **pro**-gnosis
pro-gnathous   **pro**-phylaxis

pros-, **prosth-**: in place of:

pros-thesis   **prosth**-odontics

SUFFIXES

-al: a Latin-derived adjectival suffix: pertaining to, located in:

bronchi-**al**   parenter-**al**
hypogloss-**al**   psychologic-**al**

-ase: forms names of enzymes:

amyl-**ase**   lip-**ase**
lact-**ase**   malt-**ase**

-asia, **-asis** (rare): form abstract nouns: state, condition:

metachrom-**asia**   xer-**asia**
phlegm-**asia**   blepharochal-**asis**

-ema: forms abstract nouns: state, condition. The combining form of nouns ending in **-ema** is **-emat-**:

emphys-**ema**   emphys-**emat**-ous
eryth-**ema**   eryth-**emat**-ous

-esis: forms abstract nouns: state, condition, procedure:

amniocent-**esis**   diur-**esis**
vasopar-**esis**   sudor-**esis**

-etic: forms adjectives, often from nouns ending in **-esis**: pertaining to:

diaphor-**etic**   gen-**etic**
diur-**etic**   sympath-**etic**

-ics, **-tics**: form nouns indicating a particular science or study: science or study of:

geriatr-**ics**   ortho-**tics**
pediatr-**ics**   therapeu-**tics**

-ism: forms abstract nouns: state, condition, quality:

astigmat-**ism**   phototrop-**ism**
thyroid-**ism**   synerg-**ism**

-ismus: forms abstract nouns: state, condition; muscular spasm:

esophag-**ismus**   strab-**ismus**
laryng-**ismus**   pharyng-**ismus**

-oid, (rarely) **-ode**, **-id**: form both nouns and adjectives indicating a particular shape, form, or resemblance: like, resembling:

aden-**oid**   nemat-**ode**
arachn-**oid**   lip-**id**

oma: forms abstract nouns: usually tumor; occasionally disease. The combining form of nouns ending in **–oma** is **–omat-**; the plural often is **–omata**:

carcin-**oma**   carcin-**omat**-osis
xanth-**oma**   xanth-**omata**

-ose: a Latin-derived adjectival suffix; also used to form names of chemical substances: full of, resembling:

ventr-**ose**   fruct-**ose**
varic-**ose**   gluc-**ose**

-ous: a Latin-derived adjectival suffix: pertaining to, characterized by, full of:

bili-**ous**   atrich-**ous**
ven-**ous**   venom-**ous**

tics: See **-ics**.

-us: a Latin noun-forming ending: condition, person (sometimes a malformed fetus):

hypothalam-**us**   microphthalm-**us**
hydrocephal-**us**   tetan-**us**

Verb-Forming Suffix

-ize: a commonly used Greek-derived suffix that means
"to make, become, cause to be, subject to, engage in."

hypnot-**ize**　　　　　　internal-**ize**

PRECEDING HYPHENS

Combining forms preceded by a hyphen (e.g., -em-) are found only following a prefix or another combining form: anemia, leukemia, and so forth.

CHEMICAL SUBSTANCES

There are many suffixes used to form names of chemical substances. Some of these are:

-ate	(chlor-**ate**)
-ide	(brom-**ide**)
-ite	(nitr-**ite**)
-one	(testoster-**one**)

COLI-, CYSTI-, CHOLECYST-

Words beginning with or containing **coli-** usually refer to the colon bacillus, *Escherichia coli.*

Words containing **cyst(i)-** usually refer to the urinary bladder.

Words containing **cholecyst-** refer to the gallbladder.

VOCABULARY

Greek	Combining Form	Meaning	Example
akron	ACR-	[highest point] extremities (particularly the hands and feet)	**acr**-odermatitis
amblys	AMBLY-	dull, faint	**ambly**-acousia
karkinos	CARCIN-	[crab] (Fig 2–1) carcinoma, cancer	**carcin**-oma
kēlē	-CEL-*	hernia, tumor, swelling	hydro-**cel**-e
cheir	CHEIR-, CHIR-	hand	**cheir**-ospasm
cholē	CHOL(E)-	bile, gall	**chol**-olith
kolon	COL(I)-, COLON-	colon	**colon**-oscope
kyanos	CYAN-	blue	**cyan**-otic
kystis	CYST(I)-, -CYSTIS	bladder, cyst	**cyst**-itis
diploos	DIPLO-	double, twin	**diplo**-bacillus
enteron	ENTER-	(small) intestine	**enter**-algia
ergon	ERG-	action, work	**erg**-ometer
gastēr, gastros	GASTR-	stomach	**gastr**-ectomy
haima, haimatos	HEM-, HEMAT-, -EM-	blood	**hem**-orrhage
hēpar, hēpatos	HEPAR-, HEPAT-	liver	**hepat**-itis
lipos	LIP-	fat	**lip**-osuction
makros	MACR-	(abnormally) large or long	**macr**-opodia
megas, megalou†	MEGA-, MEGAL-	(abnormally) large or long	**mega**-colon
melas, melanos	MELAN-	dark, black	**melan**-in
mikros	MICR-	(abnormally) small	**micr**-obe
nyx, nyctos	NYCT-	night	**nyct**-algia
odynē	ODYN-	pain	**odyn**-ophagia
onkos	ONC-	tumor	**onc**-ologist
pachys	PACHY-	thick	**pachy**-derma
pseudēs	PSEUD-	false	**pseud**-arthritis
pyon	PY-	pus	**py**-emia
sarx, sarcos	SARC-	flesh, soft tissue	**sarc**-olysis
spasmos	SPASM-	spasm, involuntary muscular contraction	neuro-**spasm**
splēn	SPLEN-	spleen	**splen**-omegalia
stoma, stomatos	STOM-, STOMAT-	mouth, opening	**stomat**-odynia

*See the Etymological Notes in this lesson for uses of -CEL-.
†The forms of this adjective are irregular.

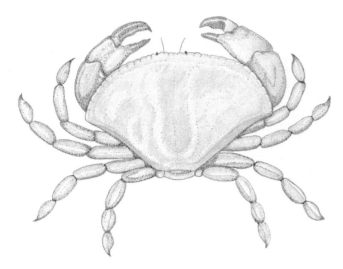

Figure 2–1. Coral crab. The Greek word *karkinos,* as well as the Latin word *cancer,* meant crab. The Greek and Roman medical writers used these words to name any spreading, ulcerous growth on the body. Hippocrates also used the word *karkinoma* (carcinoma) to refer to a growth of this sort. (Drawing by Laine McCarthy.)

ETYMOLOGICAL NOTES

The word **surgeon** has come into English indirectly from two Greek words: *cheir* (hand) and *ergon* (action, work) (Fig. 2–2). The Greek verb *cheirourgoun,* meaning to work with the hands, and the noun *cheirourgos,* one who works with his hands, were applied to the surgeon. The words came into Latin as *chīrurgus.* Celsus, the Roman writer of the 1st century AD, had this to say about the surgeon:

> A surgeon (chirurgus) should be a young man, or certainly one not long out of youth. He should have a strong and steady hand, one which never trembles, and he should be able to use both the right and left hand equally well. He must have a sharp and keen eye and be of a firm spirit, feeling a sense of pity deep enough that he wishes to cure his patient, but not so sensitive as to be so influenced by his cries of pain that he acts in haste or cuts less than necessary; on the contrary, he should go about everything just as if he were not at all affected by the moans that he hears. [*De Medicina,* Preface 4]

The Latin word *chirurgus* came into Old French as *cirurgien* and was used in English as early as the 13th century in the form *sorgien.* Among the subsequent forms of the word in English were *surgeyn, surgyen, surgien,* and ultimately *surgeon.* However, a collateral form of the word also developed, giving rise to the spelling *chirurgeon.* In 1760, Samuel Johnson wrote to Boswell concerning a friend, "I am glad that the chirurgeon at Coventry gives him so much hope." The modern French word for surgeon is *chirurgien,* and the Italian word is *chirúrgo.*

The Greek noun *ergon* has given rise to the words **syn-**

ergy and **synergism**. *Taber's Cyclopedic Medical Dictionary* (2001) defines synergy, synergism as "An action of two or more agents or organs working with each other, cooperating. Their action is combined and coordinated." From the same root come the words **synergia**, **synergic**, **synergetic**, and **synergist**.

The Greek word *stoma* (mouth, opening) has a specialized use in medical terminology. In surgical procedures, an **anastomosis** (*ana-,* up, back) is the formation of a passage between any two normally distinct spaces or organs. An **arteriovenous anastomosis** is an opening between an artery and a vein. Words ending in **-stomy** indicate such surgical procedures. An **enteroenterostomy** is the creation of a communication between two noncontiguous segments of the intestine. A **colostomy** is the formation of a more or less permanent passage between the colon and the surface of the abdomen. This opening is known as a **stoma**. The plural of **stoma** is **stomata** or, less preferably, **stomas**.

The suffix **-oma** often indicates an abnormal or diseased condition, such as **trachoma**, a chronic contagious form of conjunctivitis, or **glaucoma**, a destructive disease of the eye caused by increased intraocular pressure. However, it usually denotes an abnormal growth of tissue (neoplasm) or a tumor (Latin *tumor,* swelling). *Taber's Cyclopedic Medical Dictionary* (2001) defines tumor as "1. A swelling or enlargement; one of the four classic signs of inflammation. 2. An abnormal mass." Tumors are generally benign, but there are exceptions. **Sarcoma** is a malig-

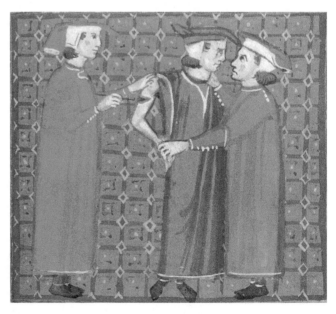

Figure 2–2. Operating on the upper arm. Manuscript illustration for *Chirurgia* by Theodoric of Cervia, 13th century AD. (From Special Collections, University of Leiden, Netherlands: Leiden, University Library, ms. Voss. Lat. F. 3, fol. 43r. with permission.)

nant tumor originating in connective tissue such as muscle (**myosarcoma**; Greek *mys*, muscle) or bone (**osteosarcoma**). If the tumor arises in the muscular tissue of a blood vessel, it is called **angiosarcoma** or **hemangiosarcoma**. A sarcoma containing nerve cells is called **neurosarcoma**.

The word element to which the suffix **-oma** is affixed indicates either the location of the growth or its nature: **hepatoma**, tumor of the liver; **nephroma**, tumor of a kidney; **cholangioma**, a tumor of the bile ducts; **hemangioma**, a tumor of the blood vessels—that is, the swelling consists of dilated blood vessels; **hematoma**, a swelling that contains blood; this occurs when ruptured blood vessels flood the nearby tissues. **Melanoma** is a malignant tumor composed of cells of **melanin**, the substance that gives pigmentation to the hair, skin, and other tissues. **Melanomatosis** is the formation of numerous melanomas on or beneath the skin.

The Greek noun *onkos* meant bulk, mass. This word has given rise to the combining form indicating a swelling or tumor: **mastoncus**, tumor of the breast (*mastos*, breast). **Oncology** is the branch of medicine dealing with tumors.

Another combining form indicating an abnormal swelling comes from the noun *kēlē*. The form **-cele**, which is generally used as a suffixed element of a word, usually means hernia, the protrusion of an organ or part of an organ through the wall of the cavity that normally contains it: **gastrocele**, hernia of the stomach; **cystocele**, hernia of the bladder; **rectocele**, hernia of the rectum into the vagina. Sometimes a word ending in **-cele** indicates a swelling caused by an abnormal accumulation of fluid, as in **uro-cele**, an accumulation of urine in the scrotal sac; **hydrocele**, an accumulation of serous fluid in a saclike structure such as the scrotum in a newborn male child; or **galactocele**, a milk-filled tumor caused by obstruction of a milk duct. A **keloid** is a scarlike growth of tissue on the skin (**kel-** is an alternate form of **cel-**, from Greek *kēlē*).

The term **cyst** refers to either a cyst or the bladder (Fig. 2–3). *Taber's Cyclopedic Medical Dictionary* (2001) defines cyst as "A closed sac or pouch, with a definite wall, that contains fluid, semifluid, or solid material. It is usually an abnormal structure resulting from developmental anomalies, obstruction of ducts, or parasitic infection." There are many types of cysts, including the following: **dermoid cyst**, a cyst containing elements of hair, teeth, or skin; **ovarian cyst**, a sac that develops in the ovary; **sebaceous cyst**, a cyst of the sebaceous, or oil-secreting, glands of the skin. **Cystalgia** is pain in the bladder and **cholecystitis** is inflammation of the gallbladder. Words containing **cholecyst-** refer to the gallbladder. In ophthalmology, the **dacryocyst** is the lacrimal sac and the **phacocyst** is the capsule of the crystalline lens of the eye. Some words containing **cyst-** refer to the growth called a cyst: **cystoid**.

Words beginning with, ending in, or containing **coli-** refer to the colon bacillus *Escherichia coli*, named after the German physician Theodor Escherich (1857–1911). **Colinephritis** is inflammation of the kidney caused by the presence of *Escherichia coli* (usually abbreviated *E. coli*).

Some words beginning with, ending in or containing **-gaster** refer to embryonic structures: **archigaster**, **epigaster**.

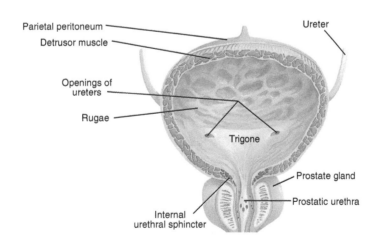

Figure 2–3. Urinary bladder. (From Scanlon, VC, and Sanders, T: Essentials of Anatomy and Physiology, ed 3. F. A. Davis, Philadelphia, 1999, p 414, with permission.)

Exercise 1: Analyze and Define

Analyze and define each of the following words. In this and in succeeding exercises, analysis should consist of separating the words into prefixes (if any), combining forms, and suffixes or suffix forms (if any) and giving the meaning of each. Be certain to differentiate between nouns and adjectives in your definitions. Consult a medical dictionary for the current meanings of these words. Use a separate paper if you need more room for an answer.

1. acromegaly _____

2. allodynia _____

3. amphocyte _____

4. anastomosis _____

5. anemic _____

6. anergia _____

7. anodyne _____

8. arthropyosis _____

9. asynergy _____

10. cheirology _____

11. cholelithiasis _____

12. colicystitis _____

13. coloenteritis _____

14. colonalgia _____

15. colostomy _____

16. cyanosis _____

17. cystoma _____

18. dysentery _____

19. endogastritis _____

20. enterocholecystostomy _____

21. enterodynia _____

22. epigastrium _____

23. eucholia _____

24. gastrocele _____

25. gastrolithiasis _____

26. hematoma _____

27. heparin _____

28. hepatosplenitis _____

29. heteroprosopus _____

30. hyperemia _____

31. lipemia _____

32. melanoma _____

33. metabiosis _____

34. microbe* _____

35. microcephalia _____

36. nephrocystanastomosis _____

* The *b* in microbe is the only surviving part of the Greek noun *bios*. The final *-e* is an English noun-forming suffix.

37. nephropyosis _____

38. nyctalgia _____

39. pachycephalic _____

40. paracanthoma _____

41. parenteral _____

42. proencephalus _____

43. protogaster _____

44. pseudoanemia _____

45. pyonephrosis _____

46. sarcocarcinoma _____

47. spasm _____

48. splenomegaly _____

49. stomatitis _____

50. synergy _____

Exercise 2: Word Derivation

Give the word derived from Greek elements that matches each of the following. It is not necessary to give combining forms for words in parentheses. Verify your answer in a medical dictionary. **Note that the wording of the dictionary definition may vary from the wording below**.

1. Hernia of the bladder _____

2. Inflammation of the kidneys and bladder _____

3. Enlargement of the liver _____

4. Resembling pus _____

5. Blue, gray, slate, or purple discoloration of the skin _____

6. Excessively large mouth _____

7. Inflammation (of tissues) around the gallbladder _____

8. Pain in the stomach and intestine _____

9. Fat cell _____

10. Blue or purple discoloration of the extremities _____

11. Apparatus for measuring work _____

12. Condition of having two heads _____

13. Able to live both on land and in water _____

14. Spasm of the hand muscles (writer's cramp) _____

15. Inflammation of the colon _____

16. Around the liver _____

17. Science of health and hygienic living _____

18. (Pathological) softening of any structures of the mouth _____

19. Device for measuring (the degree of sensitivity to) pain _____

20. Fleshy tumor (of the testicle) _____

Exercise 3: Drill and Review

The meaning of each of the following words can be determined from its etymology. Determine the meaning of each word. Verify your answer in a medical dictionary.

1. acromicria _____

2. allochiria _____

3. antianemic _____

4. arthrodynia _____

5. cephalodynia _____

6. cholangioma _____

7. cholecystenterostomy _____

8. colicolitis _____

9. colinephritis _____

10. colonitis _____

11. cystoid _____

12. cystolith _____

13. dyscephaly _____

14. endocystitis _____

15. endostoma _____

16. enterocystocele _____

17. enteromegaly _____

18. enterostenosis _____

19. erythrism _____

20. gastrology _____

21. hemangioma _____

22. hemangiomatosis _____

23. hemarthrosis _____

24. hemocytology _____

25. hepatomalacia _____

26. hepatomelanosis _____

27. heterotoxin _____

28. hypoliposis _____

29. leukocytoid _____

30. lipocele _____

31. macrocardius _____

32. macrocheiria _____

33. megalocystis _____

34. melanomatosis _____

35. mesogastrium _____

36. microlithiasis _____

37. microstomia _____

38. oncology   _____

39. ostempyesis   _____

40. pachyostosis   _____

41. paracolitis   _____

42. periangiocholitis _____

43. periosteoma   _____

44. protoleukocyte   _____

45. pseudocyst   _____

46. pyemic   _____

47. pyocephalus   _____

48. splenocele   _____

49. stenostomia   _____

50. toxemia   _____

BUILDING GREEK VOCABULARY I: NOUNS AND ADJECTIVES

For those who have a fever, if jaundice occurs on the seventh, the ninth, the eleventh, or the fourteenth day, it is a good sign, provided the right hypochondrium does not become rigid. Otherwise it is a bad sign.

[Hippocrates, *Aphorisms* 4.64]

VOCABULARY

Greek	Combining Form	Meaning	Example
arachnē	**ARACHN-**	spider, web; arachnoid membrane	**arachn**-ophobia
chlōros	**CHLOR-**	green	**chlor**-ine
chondros	**CHONDR-**	cartilage	costo-**chondr**-al
daktylos	**DACTYL-**	finger, toe	**dactyl**-ospasm
derma, dermatos	**DERM(AT)-, -DERMA**	skin (Fig. 3–1)	**dermat**-oplasty
helkos	**(H)ELC-**	ulcer	**helc**-osis
hidrōs, hidrōtos	**HIDR(OT)-, -IDR-**	sweat	**hidr**-opoiesis
histos	**HIST(I)-***	[web] tissue	**hist**-oblast
hydōr, hydatos	**HYDR-†**	water, fluid	**hydr**-olysis
hypnos	**HYPN-**	sleep	**hypn**-osis
ikteros	**ICTER-**	jaundice	**icter**-ohepatitis
is, inos	**IN-, INOS-**	fiber, muscle	**in**-otropic

* The combining form HISTI- is from the diminutive noun *histion*.
† This combining form is slightly irregular.

Greek	Combining Form	Meaning	Example
isos	IS-	equal, same, similar, alike	**is**-ocytosis
mēninx, mēningos (plural, *mēninges*)	MENING-, -MENINX	meningeal membrane, meninges	**mening**-itis
mys, myos	MY(S)-	[mouse] muscle	**my**-okinesis
mykēs, mykētos	MYC(ET)-	[mushroom] fungus	**mycet**-hemia
myelos	MYEL-	bone marrow, spinal cord	**myel**-ocyte
narkē	NARC-	stupor, numbness	**narc**-olepsy
nekros	NECR-	corpse; dead	**necr**-olysis
oligos	OLIG-	few, deficient	**olig**-ospermia
onyx, onychos	ONYCH-	fingernail, toenail	**onych**-omycosis
pous, podos	POD-	foot	**pod**-iatrist
polios	POLI-	[gray] gray matter of the brain and spinal cord	**poli**-ovirus
polys	POLY-	many, excessive	**poly**-morphic
poros	POR-	passage, opening, duct, pore, cavity	osteo-**por**-osis
psychē	PSYCH-	[soul] mind	**psych**-iatric
sōma, sōmatos	SOM(AT)-, -SOMA	body	**somat**-ization
sthenos	STHEN-	strength	**sthen**-ia
trachēlos	TRACHEL-	neck, cervix	**trachel**-omyitis
xanthos	XANTH-	yellow	**xanth**-ochromia

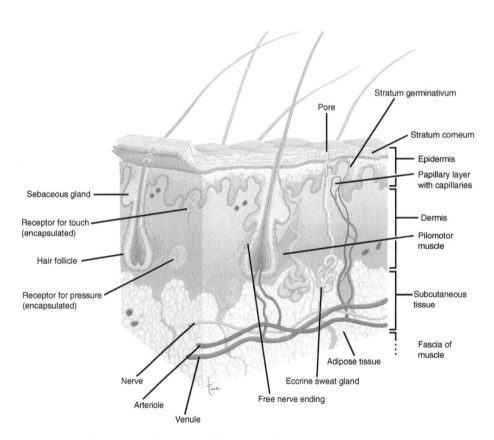

Figure 3–1. Skin section. (From Scanlon, VC, and Sanders, T: Essentials of Anatomy and Physiology, ed 4. F. A. Davis, Philadelphia, 2003, p 85, with permission.)

ETYMOLOGICAL NOTES

Arachne, in Greek mythology, was a young girl of Maeonia, a land of Asia Minor, who became so skilled in the art of weaving that she challenged Athena, a goddess unequaled at the loom, to a contest (Fig. 3–2). Ovid, the 1st century BC Roman poet, tells us the story in the *Metamorphoses*, a poem that deals with mythological metamorphoses.

Athena took up the challenge, and the two, goddess and girl of humble origins, began to weave their tapestries. The goddess began by depicting the Acropolis in Athens with the 12 Olympian gods seated on their lofty thrones in serene majesty, with Jove [Zeus] in their midst. Then, so that Arachne might know what reward she could expect for her mad presumption, she wove in the four corners scenes showing punishments meted out to mortals who had dared to challenge the gods.

Arachne, in her tapestry, wove pictures of the gods in various disguises seducing mortal women. Athena could find no flaw in Arachne's work but, indignant at her success, tore the tapestry showing the celestial crimes, and with her shuttle struck Arachne again and again. The wretched girl could bear the punishment no longer and bound a noose around her neck and hanged herself. Ovid tells us that as Arachne hung there, Athena felt pity and lifted her, saying:

> Live, wicked girl, but hang forever; and so that you may never feel secure in time to come, let this same punishment fall upon all your generations, even to remote posterity.

And as the goddess turned to leave, she sprinkled Arachne with the juices from Hecate's herb, and the girl's hair, touched by the poison, fell off, and her nose and ears fell off, and her head became shrunken, and her whole body was tiny. There was nothing left but belly and slender fingers clinging to her side as legs. And as a spider she still spins and practices her ancient art. [Ovid, *Metamorphoses* 6.136–145]

The arachnoid membrane, or **arachnoidea**, is a thin, delicate membrane, the intermediate of the three that enclose the brain and spinal cord. The outer, tough, fibrous membrane is the dura mater (Latin, hard mother), sometimes called the **pachymeninx**, or simply the dura. The innermost of the three meninges is the pia mater (devout mother). The arachnoidea is separated from the dura by the subdural (Latin *sub*, under) space, and from the pia by the subarachnoid space. **Subdural hematoma** is caused by venous blood oozing into the subdural space of the brain. It is usually the result of trauma, and even a comparatively trivial injury can result in severe and steady headaches and sometimes coma. Symptoms of subdural hematoma may not be apparent for a period of several days or even several weeks after the initial injury.

Meningitis is inflammation of the meninges of the brain or spinal cord, and there are several types, the most common of which is acute bacterial meningitis. This may be caused by one of several bacteria; however, regardless of the causative organism, the resulting disorders are similar. Classic symptoms are headache, fever, stiff neck, and lethargy. Unfortunately, typical manifestations of the disease are not seen in infants aged 3 months to 2 years, and, although antibiotics have reduced the fatality rate to less than 10 percent for cases recognized early, undiagnosed meningitis remains a lethal disease, with the prognosis for life progressively more bleak the younger the patient.

The combining form MYEL- refers to either bone marrow or the spinal cord. A **myeloma** is a tumor originating in the bone marrow. **Multiple myeloma** is a neoplastic disease characterized by the infiltration of bone and bone marrow by myeloma cells forming multiple tumor masses that lead to pathological fractures. **Poliomyelitis**, inflammation of the gray matter of the spinal cord, is also known as infantile paralysis, or simply polio. Until recently this was a dread paralytic infection of childhood, but in recent years it has become rare as a result of the development of first, the Salk vaccine by Dr. Jonas E. Salk (1914–1995) and later, the Sabin vaccine by Dr. Albert B. Sabin (1906–1993), an American physician born in Russia.

Jaundice is a condition that manifests itself externally by a yellow staining of the skin caused by the deposition of bile pigments. The word jaundice is from the French *jaunisse*, which is from the Latin *galbinus* meaning yellowish-green in color. Another term for jaundice is **icterus**, from the Greek *ikteros* (jaundice). Pliny the Elder, the 1st-century AD Roman writer whose 37-volume *Natural*

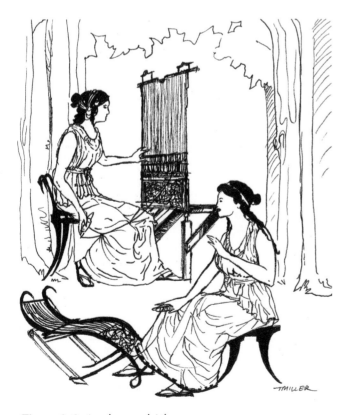

Figure 3–2. Arachne and Athena.

History provides us with an encyclopedia of geography, botany, zoology, and other information, writes on jaundice, which was called the royal disease (*rēgius morbus*):

There are certain remedies for jaundice: a dram of dirt from the ears and teats of sheep mixed with a pinch of myrrh and two cups of wine; the ashes of the head of a dog mixed with honey wine; a millipede in a half-cup of wine; earthworms in vinegar mixed with myrrh; wine in which a hen's feet have been rinsed—but the feet must be yellow and be washed in water first; a partridge's or an eagle's brain in three cups of wine; the ashes of a pigeon in honey wine; the intestines of a pigeon in wine; the ashes of sparrows in honey wine and water.

There is a bird that is called icterus because of its color. People say that if one with jaundice looks at this bird the disease leaves him. But the bird dies. I think that this bird is the one that in Latin is called galgulus (the golden oriole). [Pliny, *Natural History* 30.28]

Interestingly, the phrase "scleral icterus" is used to describe the yellow staining of the sclera (the white part of the eye) often associated with jaundice.

The **hypochondrium** is the soft part of the abdomen beneath the cartilage of the lower ribs, the upper central region of the abdomen over the pit of the stomach and located on either side of the **epigastrium**. This area, in which are situated the gallbladder, liver, and spleen, was thought of as the seat of melancholy. The form **hypochondria**, properly the plural of hypochondrium, entered the English language in the 17th century as an abstract noun meaning a melancholy state for which there is no apparent cause.

Exercise 1: Analyze and Define

Analyze and define each of the following words. In this and in succeeding exercises, analysis should consist of separating the words into prefixes (if any), combining forms, and suffixes or suffix forms (if any) and giving the meaning of each. Be certain to differentiate between nouns and adjectives in your definitions. Consult a medical dictionary for the current meanings of these words. Use a separate paper if you need more room for an answer.

1. achlorhydria _____

2. angiosclerotic myasthenia _____

3. anisocytosis _____

4. antihypnotic _____

5. arachnodactyly _____

6. arteriomyomatosis _____

7. asthenia _____

8. chloroleukemia _____

9. chondralgia _____

10. dermatosclerosis _____

11. dermatomycosis _____

12. helcoma _____

13. hidrosis _____

14. histiocyte _____

15. histiocytosis _____

16. hydronephrosis _____

17. hyperchlorhydria _____

18. hypnotic _____

19. hypnotize _____

20. inosemia _____

21. isodactylism _____

22. macrodactylia _____

23. melanoleukoderma _____

24. meningitis _____

25. mesoderm _____

26. mycethemia _____

27. myoendocarditis _____

28. narcosis _____

29. narcotize _____

30. necrocytotoxin _____

31. necrosis _____

32. neurasthenia _____

33. onychomycosis _____

34. osteochondroma _____

35. pachyderma _____

36. pachyonychia _____

37. perionychium _____

38. poliomyelitis _____

39. polymyositis _____

40. polyp _____

41. pseudoicterus _____

42. psychosis _____

43. psychosomatic _____

44. somatic _____

45. sympodia _____

46. syndactylous _____

47. toxicoderma _____

48. trachelocele _____

49. xanthoma _____

50. xanthosis _____

Exercise 2: Word Derivation

Give the word derived from Greek elements that matches each of the following. It is not necessary to give combining terms for words in parentheses. Verify your answer in a medical dictionary. **Note that the wording of the dictionary definition may vary from the wording below.**

1. Fewer than the normal number of fingers or toes _____

2. Tumor composed of tissue _____

3. Skin cyst _____

4. Study of the (human) body _____

5. Yellowness of the skin _____

6. Lacking water _____

7. Inflammation of fibrous tissue _____

8. Tumor originating in the cells of bone marrow _____

9. Resembling an ulcer _____

10. Muscular weakness _____

11. Having an excessive number of nails _____

12. Numbness following sleep _____

13. Pain in the feet _____

14. Excessive sweating _____

15. Cells of equal size _____

16. Inflammation of the skin accompanied by (thickening and) hardening _____

17. Inflammation of cartilage _____

18. Disease of the intestine resulting from (bacteria or) fungi _____

19. Under the (finger)nail; nail bed _____

20. Pain in the neck _____

Exercise 3: Drill and Review

The meaning of each of the following words can be determined from its etymology. Determine the meaning of each word. Verify your answer in a medical dictionary.

1. acanthosis _____

2. acrohyperhidrosis _____

3. amyosthenia _____

4. anonychia _____

5. antasthenic _____

6. anti-icteric _____

7. antinarcotic _____

8. chondroangioma _____

9. chondrocyte _____

10. chlorosis _____

11. cyanoderma _____

12. dermalgia _____

13. dermatomyoma _____

14. dyshidrosis _____

15. epidermitis _____

16. helcosis _____

17. hematomyelia _____

18. histocyte _____

19. hypnoidal _____

20. icterohepatitis _____

21. icteroid _____

22. isocytotoxin _____

23. lipochondroma _____

24. megalonychosis _____

25. melanonychia _____

26. meningoarteritis _____

27. meningomyelocele _____

28. metamyelocyte _____

29. myeloid _____

30. myodynia _____

31. myolipoma _____

32. myoneural _____

33. myosclerosis _____

34. neurohistology _____

35. neuromyelitis _____

36. osteoporosis _____

37. paronychomycosis _____

38. podencephalus _____

39. podocyte _____

40. polyarthritis _____

41. polyneuritis _____

42. psychometry _____

43. scleronychia _____

44. splenicterus _____

45. symbiotic _____

46. syndactylism _____

47. toxicodermatitis _____

48. trachelismus _____

49. xanthemia _____

50. xanthocyte _____

GREEK VERBS

In the winter eat as much as possible and drink as little as possible. The drink should be undiluted wine, and the food should be bread and roasted meat. Eat as few vegetables as possible during this season. In this way the body will be most dry and hot.

[Hippocrates, *Regimen in Health* 1]

For those who have a fever (pyretos), if deafness occurs, if blood flows from the nose, or if the bowels become disordered, the disease will be cured.

[Hippocrates, *Aphorisms* 4.40]

Greek verbs are **conjugated**. This means that there are different endings for person and number, and sometimes for tense, mood, and voice. A Greek verb normally has six different forms, called principal parts, on which the various tenses are built. Many verbs lack one or more of the principal parts, and verbs are often irregular. Thus, knowing the dictionary form of a verb does not always allow one to predict the other forms.

Greek dictionaries and grammar texts cite verbs in the first person singular. English and medical dictionaries, however, usually cite verbs in the form of the present infinitive, and they are given in this form in this manual. The present infinitive of most verbs ends in *-ein*, but there are other infinitival endings such as *-ai*, *-an*, *-oun*, and *-sthai*. Not all of the principal parts of a verb are used in forming English derivatives, and in this manual only the combining forms of principal parts that have produced English derivatives are given.

Often the entry form of a verb has not yielded any English derivatives. For example, the principal parts of the verb *gignesthai* (come into being) are:

gignomai, genēsomai, egenomēn, gegenēmai, gegona, egenēthēn

The third principal part, which supplies one of the past tenses (the aorist), furnishes the combining form GEN-, as in the words **pathogenic**, **genesis**, **carcinogen**, and so forth. Greek grammar texts often cite the verb *lyein* (loosen, destroy) as an example of a model verb:

lyō, lysō, elysa, lelyka, lelymai, elythēn

The combining form of *lyein* is LY(S)-, as in **analysis** or **hemolysin**.

VOCABULARY

Greek	Combining Form	Meaning	Example
autos	**AUT-**	self	**aut**-ism
krinein	**CRIN-**	[separate] secrete, secretion	endo-**crin**-ology
aisthēsis	**ESTHE(S)-**	sensation, sensitivity, sense	**esthe**-tics
gignesthai	**GEN(E)-, -GEN**	come into being; produce	**gene**-tics
gramma	**GRAM-**	[something written] a record	cardio-**gram**
graphein	**GRAPH-**	write, record	**graph**-ology
iatros	**IATR-**	healer, physician; treatment	**iatr**-ogenic
idios	**IDI-**	of one's self	**idi**-opathic
kinein	**KINE-**	move	**kine**-tics
kinēsis	**KINES(I)-**	movement, motion	**kines**-iology
lyein	**LY(S)-**	destroy, break down	hemo-**lys**-is
myxa	**MYX-**	mucus	**myx**-ocyte
orthos	**ORTH-**	straight, erect; normal	**orth**-odontia
ous, ōtos	**OT-**	ear	**ot**-algia
pathos	**PATH-**	[suffering] disease	**path**-ogen
philein	**PHIL-**	love; have an affinity for	hemo-**phil**-iac
piptein	**PT-**	fall, sag, drop, prolapse	hystero-**pt**-osis
pyr, pyros	**PYR-**	[fire] fever, burning	**pyr**-omania
pyretos	**PYRET-**	fever	anti-**pyret**-ic
pyressein	**PYREX-**	be feverish	**pyrex**-in
rhein	**RHE-**	[run] flow, secrete	diar-**rhe**-a
rhēgnynai	**RHAG-**	[burst forth] flow profusely, hemorrhage	menor-**rhag**-ia
rhēxis	**RHEX-**	rupture	**rhex**-is
rhis, rhīnos	**RHIN-**	nose	**rhin**-oplasty
skopein	**SCOP-**	look at, examine	oto-**scop**-y
sēpein	**SEP-**	[be putrid] be infected	**sep**-sis
tasis	**TA-**	stretching	myo-**ta**-tic
telos	**TEL-**	end, completion	**tel**-angion
tenōn, tenontos	**TEN-, TENON(T)-**	tendon	**ten**-odesis
therapeuein	**THERAP(EU)-**	treat medically, heal	**therapeu**-tics
tomē	**TOM-**	a cutting, slice, incision	**tom**-ography
tonos	**TON-**	[a stretching] (muscular) tone, tension	**ton**-icity

COMPOUND SUFFIX FORMS

Some combining forms of verbs, usually with the addition of a suffix and/or prefix, have become so commonly used in a certain form and meaning as to remain fixed as **compound suffix forms**:

Compound Suffix Form	Meaning	Example
-ectasia, -ectasis	dilation, enlargement	cardi-**ectasia**, nephr-**ectasis**
-ectomy	surgical excision; removal of all (total excision) or part (partial excision) of an organ	gastr-**ectomy**, nephr-**ectomy**

Compound Suffix Form	Meaning	Example
-gen*	substance that produces (something)	antitoxino-**gen**, carcino-**gen**
-genesis	formation, origin	lipo-**genesis**, patho-**genesis**
-genic,	causing, producing, caused	carcino-**genic**
-genous	by, produced by or in	hepato-**genous**†
-gram	a record of the activity of an organ (often an x-ray) (Fig. 4–1)	cardio-**gram**, angio-**gram**
-graph	an instrument for recording the activity of an organ	poly-**graph**, cardio-**graph**
-graphy	(1) the recording of the activity of an organ (usually by x-ray examination)	cholangio-**graphy**, cysto-**graphy**
	(2) a descriptive treatise (on a subject)	spleno-**graphy**, osteo-**graphy**
-lysis	dissolution, reduction, decomposition, disintegration	hemo-**lysis**, pyreto-**lysis**
-lytic	pertaining to dissolution or decomposition, disintegration (forms adjectives from words ending in -*lysis*)	hemo-**lytic**, bacterio-**lytic**
-pathy	disease	neuro-**pathy**, cardio-**pathy**
-ptosis	dropping, sagging, prolapse (of an organ or part)	gastro-**ptosis**, colo-**ptosis**
-rrhagia:‡	profuse discharge, hemorrhage	leuko-**rrhagia**, meningo-**rrhagia**
-rrhea	profuse discharge, excessive secretion	rhino-**rrhea**, myxo-**rrhea**
-rrhexis	bursting (of tissues), rupture	angio-**rrhexis**, entero-**rrhexis**
-scope	an instrument for examining	rhino-**scope**, colpo-**scope**
-scopy	examination	endo-**scopy**, cysto-**scopy**
-tome	a surgical instrument for cutting	adenoma-**tome**, gastro-**tome**
-tomy	surgical incision	cholecysto-**tomy**, abdominohystero-**tomy**

* Strictly speaking, -gen, -gram, and -graph are not suffix forms because there is no suffix on the combining form. It seemed desirable, however, that -gen, -genesis, -genic, and -genous as well as -gram, -graph and, -graphy should be listed together in order to show the relationship between words using these forms.

† Because these suffix forms can mean either producing or produced by, the meaning of some words is ambiguous: pyretogenous means either producing fever or produced by fever.

‡ Words beginning with the letter *r*- [Greek *rho*] usually double this letter when following another element. There are some exceptions: perirhinal, craniorhachischisis (sometimes spelled craniorrhachischisis).

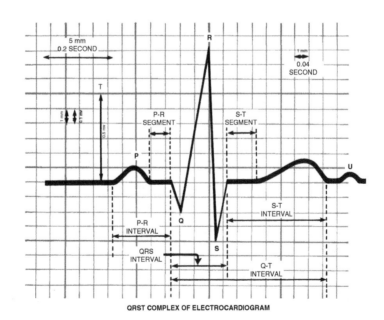

Figure 4–1. QRST complex of electrocardiogram. (From Taber's Cyclopedic Medical Dictionary, ed 19. Philadelphia: F. A. Davis, 2001, p 646, with permission.)

ETYMOLOGICAL NOTES

There is no disease more grievous or severe than that which, by a certain stiffness of the nerves, now draws the head back toward the shoulder blades, now draws the chin down toward the chest, and now holds the neck stretched out immobile. The Greeks call the first *opisthotonos*, the second *emprosthotonos*, and the third *tetanos*. [Celsus, *De Medicina* 4.6]

The name of the disease **tetanus** (Greek *tetanos*) is related linguistically to the nouns *tasis* (stretching), and *tonos* (tension); this acute disease was known to ancient physicians. Hippocrates wrote, "Spasm or tetanus following severe burns is a bad sign." [*Aphorisms* 7.13] Signs of tetanus are stiffness of the muscles of the jaw, esophagus, and neck. For this reason, the disease is often called lockjaw. In the advanced stage, these and other muscles become fixed in a rigid position. If the body is stretched backward in a tetanic spasm, the position is called **opisthotonos** (Greek *opisthen*, in back) (Fig. 4–2); if stretched forward, it is called **emprosthotonos** (*emprosthen*, in front); if stretched to the side, **pleurothotonos** (*pleurothen*, on the side); and if the body is held rigidly stretched in a straight line, the condition is called **orthotonos** (*orthos*, straight, upright).

The causative agent of tetanus is the bacillus *Clostridium tetani*, which takes its name from *klōstēr* (spindle), from the rodlike shape of these bacilli. The suffix *-id* indicates a member of a genus, and *-ium* is a Latin diminutive ending, from the Greek *-ion*. The word *klōstēr* is derived from the verb *klōthein* (spin). Clotho, the Spinner, is the one of the three sisters, the Fates (in Greek *Moirai*, in Latin *Parcae*), who spins the thread of life for each of us. Her sister Lachesis, the Apportioner, determines the length of the thread, and the third sister, Atropos, Irreversible, cuts it (Fig. 4–3).

The adjective *idios* meant of one's self, pertaining to one's own interest. Galen, the 2nd century AD Roman physician, used the term *idiopatheia*, **idiopathy**, to refer to an ailment having a local origin—that is, originating within the body. We speak of an **idiopathic** disease as one without a recognizable cause. There was a noun *idiōma*, meaning a peculiarity or particular feature of something. Our word idiom is ultimately derived from this noun. An *idiōtēs* was a person in private life, as opposed to one holding public office. It came to mean one who was unlearned or unskilled. The word idiot entered the English language early in the 14th century in the sense of a person who was so lacking in mental ability as to be incapable of acting in a rational way: an idiot. In the 16th century, the term "an idiot" mistakenly came to be "a nidiot," and then, through the influence of the pronunciation of the term, the spelling was changed to nidget or nigit. Thomas Heywood, the 17th-century English dramatist, wrote in *The Wise Woman of Hogsdon* (1638), "I think he saith we are a company of fooles and nigits."

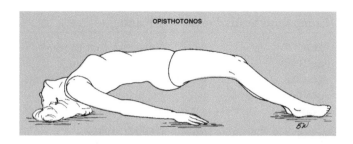

Figure 4–2. Opisthotonos. (From Taber's Cyclopedic Medical Dictionary, ed 19. Philadelphia: F. A. Davis, 2001, p 1449, with permission.)

The **parotid** gland, which runs alongside the ear, is one of the glands that supply saliva to the mouth. Inflammation of this gland, **parotitis**, is the acute, contagious disease commonly known as mumps. The Roman physician Celsus knew of mumps, although there was no Latin name for it.

Parotid swellings (parotides) are likely to occur below the ears, sometimes in periods of health when inflammation occurs here, and sometimes after long fevers when the force of the disease has turned in that direction. [*De Medicina* 6.16]

As a remedy for these swellings he recommended a mixture of pumice, liquid pine resin, frankincense, soda scum, iris, wax, and oil. Pliny, the Roman encyclopedist, recommended a mixture of foxes' testicles and bull's blood, dried

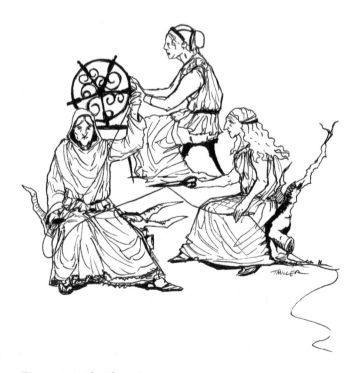

Figure 4–3. The Three Fates.

and pounded together and mixed with the urine of a she-goat, all of this to be poured drop by drop into the ear and followed by an external application of she-goat's dung mixed with axle grease [*Natural History* 28.49].

Rheum, a watery discharge, is from *rheuma, rheumatos,* a word related to the verb *rhein* and meaning "that which flows." The ancient Greek writers used the word to refer to the current of a river, the eruption of lava from a volcano, or to anything that flowed. Hippocrates used it in the sense of a discharge of liquid from the body:

> Those of us with a cold in the head and a discharge (rheuma) from the nostrils generally find that this discharge is more acrid than that which formerly accumulated there and daily passed from the nostrils [*Ancient Medicine* 18].

Rheumatism (*rheumatismos*) was thought to be caused by a flowing of the humors in the body, and was thus named.

The word **ptomaine**, the generic name for certain alkaloid bodies found in decaying animal and vegetable matter, some of which are exceedingly toxic, was coined in 1876 by the Italian scientist Franz Salmi from the Greek *ptōma, ptōmatos* (fallen body, corpse), from the verb *piptein* (fall). Not only was the word incorrectly formed, as it should have been *ptomatine* (*ptomat- + ine*), but popular usage has given it an incorrect pronunciation, rhyming it with domain; it should be pronounced in three syllables, pto-ma-ine.

The ancient Greeks were unaware of the existence of capillaries in the human body simply because they did not have the optical devices with which to see these microscopic vessels. It was not until the 17th century that their existence was demonstrated by the Italian anatomist Marcello Malpighi as a result of his discovery of capillary anastomosis in the lungs. The word **capillary** is from Latin *capillāris*, pertaining to hair (*capillus*). But many terms for abnormal conditions of the capillaries have been formed from the Greek elements *tel-* (end), and *angi-* (vessel), as both the arterial and the venous systems terminate in capillaries. **Telangiosis** is any disease of capillaries, and **telangioma** is a tumor made up of dilated capillaries.

Exercise 1: Analyze and Define

Analyze and define each of the following words. In this and in succeeding exercises, analysis should consist of separating the words into prefixes (if any), combining forms, and suffixes or suffix forms (if any) and giving the meaning of each. Be certain to differentiate between nouns and adjectives in your definitions. Consult a medical dictionary for the current meanings of these words. Use a separate paper if you need more room for an answer.

1. amyxia _____

2. anesthesiology _____

3. angiogram _____

4. arachnolysin _____

5. atelocardia _____

6. autism _____

7. autohemolysis _____

8. cardiotomy _____

9. crinogenic   _____

10. dysgraphia   _____

11. dyskinesia   _____

12. endocrinology   _____

13. gastroscope   _____

14. genetics   _____

15. hemidysesthesia   _____

16. hemophiliac   _____

17. hepatogenous   _____

18. hepatorrhexis   _____

19. histokinesis   _____

20. hypertonus   _____

21. iatrogenesis   _____

22. idiopathic   _____

23. leukorrhagia   _____

24. meningorrhea   _____

25. myectomy   _____

26. myelatelia   _____

27. myotatic   _____

28. myxoma _____

29. necrogenous _____

30. onychorrhexis _____

31. orthodiagraph _____

32. orthosis _____

33. otomycosis _____

34. pachyrhinic _____

35. pathogenic _____

36. ptosis _____

37. pyrexia _____

38. pyrogen _____

39. rhinomycosis _____

40. sepsis _____

41. spasmolytic _____

42. splenectasia _____

43. telangioma _____

44. telangiosis _____

45. tenodynia _____

46. tenontography _____

47. tenontomyotomy _____

48. tenostosis _____

49. therapeutics _____

50. toxolysin _____

Exercise 2: Word Derivations

Give the word derived from Greek elements that matches each of the following. It is not necessary to give combining terms for words in parentheses. Verify your answer in a medical dictionary. **Note that the wording of the dictionary definition may vary from the wording below.**

1. Producing cancer _____

2. (Extreme) slowness of movement _____

3. Rupture of the bladder _____

4. Right living _____

5. Branch of medicine dealing with the ear and nose and their diseases _____

6. Surgical removal of a kidney _____

7. Incomplete development of the foot _____

8. Originating outside (an organ or part) _____

9. Prolapse of the heart _____

10. Producing fever _____

11. Study of (the nature and cause of) disease _____

12. (Thin, watery) discharge from the nose _____

13. Any (congenital or acquired) muscle disease _____

14. Disintegration of the tissues _____

15. Resembling mucus _____

16. White (vaginal) discharge _____

17. Lack of sensation in (one or more of) the extremities _____

18. Inflammation of the ear _____

19. Rupture of a blood vessel _____

20. Deficiency or loss of muscular tone _____

Exercise 3: Drill and Review

The meaning of each of the following words can be determined from its etymology. Determine the meaning of each word. Verify your answer in a medical dictionary.

1. akinesia _____

2. anesthesia _____

3. antihemorrhagic _____

4. apyrexia _____

5. apyrogenic _____

6. atelocheiria _____

7. autoantitoxin _____

8. autosepticemia _____

9. chondrectomy _____

10. cystoscopy _____

11. dermatotherapy _____

12. ectogenous _____

13. encephalomyelopathy _____

14. endotoscope _____

15. epiotic _____

16. erythrocytorrhexis _____

17. gastric atony _____

18. hemangiectasis _____

19. hepatolytic _____

20. histopathology _____

21. hypnogenic _____

22. hypomyxia _____

23. iatrology _____

24. idiogram _____

25. isotonia _____

26. kinesiatrics _____

27. macrotia _____

28. meningorrhagia _____

29. metakinesis _____

30. mycetogenetic _____

31. mycosis _____

32. myotasis _____

33. myxangitis _____

34. myxochondroma _____

35. nephrolithotomy _____

36. oncolysis _____

37. orthopsychiatry _____

38. osteoarthropathy _____

39. osteogen _____

40. otoncus _____

41. ototoxic _____

42. parotic _____

43. polyotia _____

44. pyretolysis _____

45. rhinolithiasis _____

46. rhinorrhea _____

47. sarcolysis   _____

48. telangiitis   _____

49. tenalgia   _____

50. therapy   _____

BUILDING GREEK VOCABULARY II

γνῶθι σαυτόν. Know thyself.

[Thales, 6th-century BC philosopher, as quoted by Diogenes Laertius (3rd century AD), *Lives of the Philosophers.*]

VOCABULARY

Greek	Combining Form	Meaning	Example
akouein	ACOU(S)-, ACU(S)-	hear	**acous**-tics
amnion	AMNI-	fetal membrane, amniotic sac, amnion	**amni**-ocentesis (Fig. 5–1)
*askitēs**	ASC-, ASCIT-	[leather bag] bladder, sac, bag	**ascit**-es
barys	BARY-	heavy, dull, hard	**bary**-lalia
kentein	CENTE-	pierce	cardio-**cente**-sis
chrōma, chrōmatos	CHROM-, CHROMA-, CHROMAT-	color, pigment	**chromat**-ography
dipsa	DIPS-	thirst	**dips**-ophobia
ēkhō	ECHO-	reverberating sound, echo	**echo**-cardiogram
oidēma, oidēmatos	EDEMA, EDEMAT-	swelling	**edemat**-ogenic
emein	EME-	vomit	**eme**-sis
gignōskein	GNO(S)-	know	loga-**gnos**-ia
lalein	LAL-	talk	**lal**-iatry
lapara	LAPAR-	abdomen, abdominal wall	**lapar**-omyitis
legein	LEX-	read	dys-**lex**-ia
mimnēskein	MNE-	remember	**mne**-monics
neos	NE-	new	**ne**-onatal

* See the Etymological Notes in this lesson.

Greek	Combining Form	Meaning	Example
nous	NO-	mind, mental activity, comprehension	para-**no**-ia
oregein	OREC-, OREX-	have an appetite	an-**orex**-ia
oxys	OX(Y)-	acute, pointed; rapid; acid; oxygen	**oxy**-cephalous
phēnai	PHA-	speak, communicate	dys-**pha**-sia
phagein	PHAG-	swallow, eat	**phag**-ocyte
pharmakon	PHARMAC(EU)-*	medicine, drug	**pharmaceu**-tics
phēmē	PHEM-	speech	a-**phem**-ia
phobos	PHOB-	(abnormal) fear	hydro-**phob**-ia
phonē	PHON-	voice, sound	**phon**-ograph
phrassein	PHRAC-, PHRAG-	enclose, obstruct	nephrem-**phrax**-is[†]
phrazein	PHRAS-	speak	poly-**phras**-ia
phrēn	PHREN-	mind; diaphragm	**phren**-ospasm
phylattein	PHYLAC-	protection (against disease)	**phylax**-is
physis	PHYS(I)-	nature, appearance	**physi**-ology
phyton	PHYT-	plant (organism), growth	**phyt**-otoxin
poiein	POIE-	produce, make	leuko-**poie**-sis
sapros	SAPR-	rotten, putrid, decaying	**sapr**-ophilous
stear, steatos	STEAR-, STEAT-	fat, sebum, sebaceous glands	**steat**-adenoma

* The combining form PHARMACEU- is from the Greek adjective *pharmakeutikos* (concerning drugs).
[†] Words ending in -emphraxis are from PHRAC- and -sis.

OX-

The combining form **OX**- indicates the presence of oxygen: anoxia, hypoxia, hypoxemia, and so forth. In a few words, **OXY**- means rapid: oxylalia, oxytocic. Oxycephalous denotes a head that is pointed and cone-like. In some words **OXY**- has the meaning of acid: oxyphil. In a few words, **OXY**- has the meaning of sharp: oxyphonia means an abnormally sharp sound to the voice.

ETYMOLOGICAL NOTES

On August 1, 1774, Joseph Priestley, a British clergyman and experimental chemist, focused the rays of the sun through a magnifying glass onto red oxide of mercury and produced a vapor that he named dephlogisticated air. Scientists of that time commonly believed that all matter contained a substance called phlogiston (Greek *phlogistos*, inflammable), which was released during burning. Priestley, after discovering that his lungs felt particularly light and easy for some time after breathing the vapor, asked, "Who can tell but that, in time, this pure air may become a fashionable article in luxury? Hitherto, only two mice and myself have had the privilege of breathing it."*

Priestley journeyed to Paris in the fall of 1774 and described his experiment to the French scientist Antoine Lavoisier, who renamed the newly discovered vapor oxygen, meaning acid producing.

Oedipus, the tragic hero of Sophocles' *Oedipus the King*, owes his name to the verb *oidein*, meaning to become swollen. An oracle had told Laius, king of Thebes, that if his wife bore him a son, this child would eventually kill him. When a son was born to the queen, Laius pierced the infant's feet and tied them together and gave him to a shepherd to expose on the mountainside. But instead, the child was given to the childless king of Corinth, who brought him up as his own son, naming him *Oidipous* (swollen foot). As is well known, Oedipus (to give his name the Latin spelling) did eventually kill his father and, furthermore, marry Jocasta, his own mother; hence the Freudian term Oedipus complex.

The Greek noun *oidēma* (swelling), from the verb *oidein* (become swollen), has given us the word **edema**, meaning a swelling caused by an accumulation of fluid in tissue. If the condition is generalized over large areas of the body, it is sometimes called **hydrops** (Greek *hydrōps*, from *hydōr*, water) or **dropsy**.

The Greek noun *askos* meant skin or hide, but more commonly referred to a bag or sack made of skin, espe-

*Copyright 1974 by the New York Times Company. Reprinted by permission.

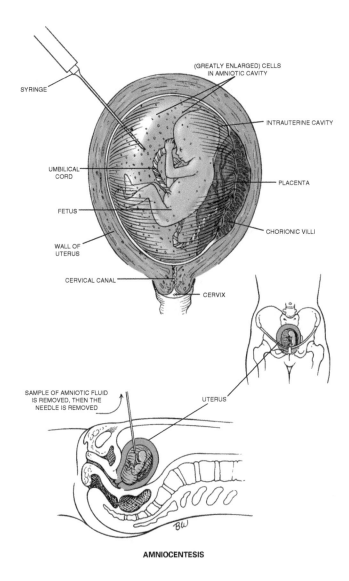

Figure 5–1. Amniocentesis. (From Taber's Cyclopedic Medical Dictionary, Ed 19. Philadelphia: F. A. Davis, 2001, p 89.)

cially a wineskin. Homer tells us that when Odysseus and his men departed from the island of Aeolia, where Aeolus, the Keeper of the Winds, had entertained them for a full month, Aeolus gave Odysseus a bag (*askos*) made of the hide of a 9-year-old ox in which he bound the blustering winds, allowing only the breath of the west wind to blow, thus affording Odysseus and his men a sure passage across the sea. [*Odyssey* 10.19ff]

The ancient Greeks knew of the condition that we call **ascites,** and named it *ascitēs*, the baggy disease, from the baggy aspect of the human body resulting from the accumulation of serous fluid in the peritoneal cavity.

In Greek mythology, Mnemosyne (Memory) was a Titaness, one of the children of Sky and Earth. The 8th-century BC poet Hesiod tells us of the union of Mnemosyne and Zeus:

> For nine nights did all-wise Zeus lie with her, entering her holy bed far away from the immortals. And when a year

had passed and the seasons turned as the months waned, and many days were fulfilled, she bore nine daughters, all of like mind, whose hearts are turned to song and whose spirits are free from care, a little way from the highest peak of snow-clad Olympus. [*Theogony* 56 ff]

These daughters were the nine Muses: Clio, Euterpe, Thalia, Melpomene, Erato, Terpsichore, Polyhymnia, Urania, and Calliope, patron goddesses of the arts.

There was a Greek verb *mimnēskein* (remember), related to the name of the goddess of memory, Mnemosyne, and from it we get such words as **amnesia, amnesty, mnemonic,** and so forth. The Latin nouns *memotia* and *mēns, mentis* (mind) are related to this Greek verb and have given us the words **memory** and **mental**.

The Greek word *amnos* (lamb) had a diminutive form, *amnion*, meaning the innermost of the membranes surrounding the human fetus, and this is the modern meaning of the word. The **amnion** is a thin, transparent sac in which the fetus is suspended, surrounded by the amniotic fluid, or **liquor amnii**, which protects the fetus from injury. The Greek diminutive form *amnion* (little lamb) was probably so named because this membrane resembles the extremely thin and delicate skin of the newborn lamb. **Amniocentesis** is the puncturing of the abdomen with a long, thin, hollow needle, and the removal of a small amount of the amniotic fluid surrounding the fetus. This fluid contains some fetal cells that are grown in a laboratory, then examined microscopically to determine if there is any abnormality in the chromosome number. Each human somatic cell contains 23 pairs of chromosomes, the genetic and hereditary determinants of human beings. Abnormalities in the number of chromosomes in the cells can indicate genetic defects in the unborn fetus.

The often fatal disease **hydrophobia**, which, literally translated, means fear of water, is characterized by excruciating spasms of the throat muscles whenever the victim attempts to drink, even though the victim is at the point of death from dehydration. The incubation period of this disease varies from 10 days to 3 months. If the carrier of the virus, often a dog, squirrel, or bat, is identified, treatment may begin immediately and recovery is normal. The Latin word *rabīes*, which is commonly used for this disease, means simply madness. Celsus wrote about hydrophobia and its cure:

> Certain physicians, after the bite of a rabid dog, send the victims directly to the bath, and there allow them to sweat as long as their strength permits, with the wound kept exposed so that the poison may readily drip from it. Then much undiluted wine is drunk, as this is an antidote to all poisons. After three days of this treatment, the patient is thought to be out of danger. But if the wound is not sufficiently treated there arises a fear of water which the Greeks call *hydrophobia*, an exceedingly distressing disease in which the sufferer is tormented simultaneously by thirst and dread of water. There is little hope for those who are in this state. However, there remains one last remedy: throw the patient unexpectedly into a pool of water when

he is not looking. If he cannot swim, allow him to sink and drink the water and then raise him up; but if he can swim, keep pushing him under so that he becomes filled with water, although unwillingly. In this way both his thirst and his fear of water are removed at the same time. [*De Medicina* 5.27.2]

The ancients believed that the midriff was the seat of the emotions, and thus the word *phrēn* was applied to this area as a physical part of the body and also as the center of the emotions, the heart, or the mind. Homer tells us in the *Odyssey* that Odysseus, after the Cyclops Polyphemus (Fig. 5–2) had made a meal of two of his companions, pondered how to deal with this monster:

And I formed a plan to steal near to him and, drawing my sharp sword from beside my thigh, to strike him in the breast, at the point where the midriff (*phrēn*) holds the liver (*hēpar*). [*Odyssey* 9.299–301]

Later in the poem, Odysseus becomes enraged when one of his companions speaks slightingly of him.

So he spoke, and I pondered in my mind (*phrēn*) whether or not to draw my long sword from beside my thigh and

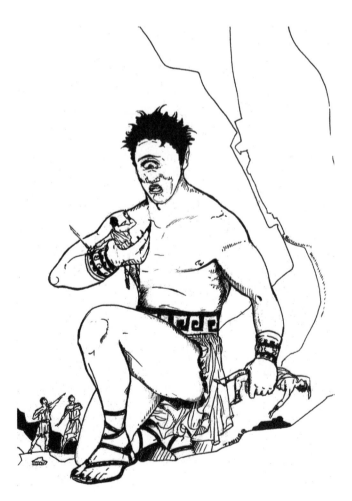

Figure 5–2. The Cyclops Polyphemus.

strike off his head and bring it to the ground, even though he was a kinsman of mine by marriage. [*Odyssey* 10.438–441]

Thus, derivative words of *phrēn* in medical terminology refer to either the diaphragm or the mind or the mental processes. The **phrenic nerve** serves the diaphragm; **tachyphrenia** means abnormally rapid mental activity.

The Greek verb *gignōskein* meant to know or to understand; a secondary meaning was to examine, form an opinion, or determine. From this verb were derived the nouns *gnōsis* (knowledge); *diagnōsis* (means of discerning, opinion, diagnosis); and *gnōmōn* (one who knows, judge).

The verb *phyein* meant to grow according to the laws of nature. From this verb was derived a noun, *physis*, meaning natural growth, the outward form or appearance of anything. The word *physiognōmia* meant the study of one's appearance, a judgment of character from an individual's appearance. Our word is **physiognomy**, the human countenance. From *gnōsis* and *diagnōsis* we get **physiognosis**, diagnosis from one's facial appearance, and **leukodiagnosis**, diagnosis from an examination of leukocytes. Other derivatives of the noun *physis* include **physic**, **physics**, **physical**, and **physician**.

The Greek nouns *phyton* (plant, growth) has given us **phytogenous**, arising or caused by plants; **phytotoxin**, a poison derived from plants; **dermatophyte**, a fungal (that is, plant) organism growing in or on the skin; and **osteophyte**, a bony outgrowth.

In cases where there are swellings (*phymata*) and pains in the joints following fevers, those afflicted are eating too much food. [Hippocrates, *Aphorisms* 7.45]

Horace, the Roman poet of the first century BC, mentions in two of his poems a girl whom he calls Lalage. She is otherwise unknown, and Horace may have made up the name from the Greek verb *lalein* (talk), because his Lalage seems to be fond of chattering.

pone me pigris ubi nulla campis
arbor aestiva recreatur aura,
quod latus mundi nebulae malusque
  Iuppiter urget;

pone sub curru nimium propinqui
solis in terra domibus negata:
dulce ridentem Lalagen amabo,
  dulce loquentem.

[*Odes* 1.22.17–24]

Place me on a barren plain
where no tree grows in the summer breeze,
a land overhung by mists and gloomy skies;

place me in a land too close to the chariot
of the sun, a land barren of homes.
I will love my sweetly laughing,
sweetly chattering Lalage.

Exercise 1: Analyze and Define

Analyze and define each of the following words. In this and in succeeding exercises, analysis should consist of separating the words into prefixes (if any), combining forms, and suffixes or suffix forms (if any) and giving the meaning of each. Be certain to differentiate between nouns and adjectives in your definitions. Consult a medical dictionary for the current meanings of these words. Use a separate paper if you need more room for an answer.

1. achromatosis _____

2. agnosia _____

3. amniography _____

4. anaphylaxis _____

5. anoxia _____

6. aphemia _____

7. ascus _____

8. barylalia _____

9. bradylexia _____

10. cholemesis _____

11. chromophobia _____

12. dermatophyte _____

13. diaphragmitis _____

14. dipsophobia _____

15. dysacousia _____

16. dysmnesia _____

17. echogram _____

18. edema _____

19. emetic _____

20. hypophrenia _____

21. lalopathology _____

22. laparocholecystotomy _____

23. leukopoiesis _____

24. logagnosia _____

25. monophasia _____

26. myelopoiesis _____

27. neostomy _____

28. nephremphraxis _____

29. osteophyte _____

30. oxyacusis _____

31. oxyesthesia _____

32. paracentesis _____

33. paranoid _____

34. paraphemia _____

35. parorexia _____

36. periphrenitis   _____

37. phage   _____

38. phagocytosis   _____

39. phoniatrics   _____

40. phrenicotomy   _____

41. physical   _____

42. physiognosis   _____

43. polyphrasia   _____

44. psychochromesthesia   _____

45. saprobe   _____

46. saprophyte   _____

47. stearodermia   _____

48. steatoma   _____

49. tachyphasia   _____

50. toxophylaxin   _____

Exercise 2: Word Derivation

Give the word derived from Greek elements that matches each of the following. It is not necessary to give combining terms for words in parentheses. Verify your answer in a medical dictionary. **Note that the wording of the dictionary definition may vary from the wording below.**

1. Lack or loss of appetite   _____

2. Excessive vomiting   _____

3. Heavy, thick quality of the voice   _____

4. Loss of memory   _____

5. Difficulty in swallowing   _____

6. Production of blood (cells)   _____

7. Dullness of hearing   _____

8. Surgical opening of the abdomen   _____

9. Abnormal thirst   _____

10. Puncture of a joint (space)   _____

11. Without an amnion   _____

12. Having one color   _____

13. Decreased oxygen (tension) in the blood   _____

14. Causing edema   _____

15. Abnormal flow of speech   _____

16. Poison (produced by or derived) from a plant   _____

17. Denoting a head that is pointed and conelike   _____

18. Vocal weakness   _____

19. Abnormal fear of taking medicines   _____

20. Inability to swallow   _____

Exercise 3: Drill and Review

The meaning of each of the following words can be determined from its etymology. Determine the meaning of each. Verify your answer in a medical dictionary.

 1. acanthoid _____

 2. algophobia _____

 3. amblychromatic _____

 4. amniocentesis _____

 5. amniorrhexis _____

 6. anisochromatic _____

 7. baryophobia _____

 8. centesis _____

 9. chromatogenous _____

10. chromidrosis _____

11. chromotherapy _____

12. dyslalia _____

13. echopathy _____

14. ectophyte _____

15. erythrophage _____

16. erythropoiesis _____

17. euphonia _____

18. gastrophrenic _____

19. hematophyte _____

20. homogenize _____

21. hypacousia _____

22. hyperphrenia _____

23. hypomnesia _____

24. isochromatic _____

25. lalopathy _____

26. laparoenterostomy _____

27. laparomyitis _____

28. leptochromatic _____

29. leukopoietic _____

30. monophagia _____

31. necrophagous _____

32. odynacusis _____

33. oligohydramnios _____

34. onychophagy _____

35. paranoia _____

36. paraphrenitis _____

37. phagocytolysis _____

38. pharmacotherapy _____

39. phonopathy _____

40. phytogenous _____

41. polyphagia _____

42. prophylactic _____

43. pyemia _____

44. saprogenic _____

45. splenemphraxis _____

46. steatolysis _____

47. steatopathy _____

48. steatorrhea _____

49. tachylalia _____

50. tachyphrasia _____

6

BUILDING GREEK VOCABULARY III

NIΨONANOHMHMAMMONANOΨIN: Nίψον ἀνόμημα μὴ μόναν ὄψιν.

Wash your sins, not only your face.

[A palindromic inscription on the sacred font in the courtyard of Hagia Sophia in Istanbul.]

VOCABULARY

Greek	Combining Form(s)	Meaning	Example
anēr, andros	**ANDR-**	man, male	**andr**-ogynous
ankylos	**ANKYL-, ANCYL-**	fused, stiffened; hooked, crooked	**ankyl**-odactylia
Aphrodisios	**APHRODIS(I)-**	[of or pertaining to Aphrodite, Greek goddess of love] sexual desire	**aphrodis**-iac
brachys	**BRACHY-**	short	**brachy**-dactylia
kryptos	**CRYPT-**	hidden, latent	**crypt**-ic
dēmos	**DEM-**	people, population	epi-**dem**-ic
dolichos	**DOLICH-**	long, narrow, slender	**dolich**-omorphic
dromos	**DROM-**	a running	**drom**-omania
Erōs, Erōtos	**ER-, EROT-**	[Eros, son of Aphrodite, Greek goddess of love] sexual desire	**erot**-ic
gynē, gynaikos	**GYN(EC)-**	woman, female	**gynec**-ologic
helmins, helminthos	**HELMINT(H)-**	(intestinal) worm	**helminth**-icide
nēma, nēmatos	**NEMAT-**	thread (worm)	**nemat**-ode
nosos	**NOS-**	disease, illness	**nos**-ophobia
odous, odontos	**ODONT-**	tooth	orth-**odont**-ist
palin	**PALI(N)-**	back, again	**pali**-lalia

63

Greek	Combining Form(s)	Meaning	Example
pas, pantos	**PAN(T)-**	all, entire, every	**pan**-carditis
phoros	**PHOR-**	bearing, carrying	phos-**phor**-us
phōs, phōtos	**PHOS-, PHOT-**	light, daylight	**phot**-osynthesis
plessein	**PLEC-, PLEG-**	strike, paralyze	para-**pleg**-ia
rhachis	**R(H)ACHI-**	spine	**rachi**-tome
schizein	**SCHIZ-, SCHIST-, -SCHISIS**	split, cleft, fissure	**schiz**-ophrenia
spondylos	**SPONDYL-**	vertebra	**spondyl**-arthritis
staxis	**-STAXIS, -STAXIA**	dripping, oozing (of blood)	epi-**staxis**
thanatos	**THAN(AT)-**	death	**thanat**-obiological
tithenai	**THE-**	place, put	syn-**the**-sis
thrix, trichos	**TRICH-**	hair	**trich**-ogen
trophē	**TROPH-**	nourishment	a-**troph**-y

ETYMOLOGICAL NOTES

Trichinosis (Greek *trichinos*, of hair) is a disease caused by ingesting the larvae of the parasitic worm *Trichinella spiralis* as a result of eating raw or insufficiently cooked pork or, rarely, infested bear meat. The larvae penetrate the mucous lining of the intestinal tract and, in a few days, mature and mate, after which the males die. The females begin to discharge their young larvae after about a week, a process that continues for up to 6 weeks. These tiny larvae enter the bloodstream of the host and are carried to the tissues and organs of the body, where they lodge in muscle tissue, causing, among other symptoms, pain, nausea, diarrhea, edema, fever, chills, and general weakness. Most people afflicted with trichinosis recover, although involvement of the respiratory muscles can lead to death.

The name *Trichinella spiralis* is New Latin. This term is applied to words and names that have been coined in modern times in the form of, and on the analogy of, Latin words. In some instances, New Latin has been used for new meanings applied to extant Latin words. In the name *Trichinella spiralis*, -*ella* is a Latin diminutive ending added to the stem of the Greek adjective *trichinos*, and *spiralis* is a modern adjectival formation of the Latin noun *spīra* (coil

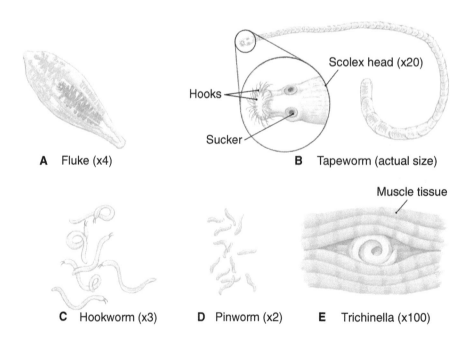

A   Fluke (x4)   **B**   Tapeworm (actual size)

Scolex head (x20)

Hooks

Sucker

Muscle tissue

C   Hookworm (x3)   **D**   Pinworm (x2)   **E**   Trichinella (x100)

Figure 6–1. Representative helminths. (From Scanlon, VC, and Sanders, T: Essentials of Anatomy and Physiology, ed 4. F. A. Davis, Philadelphia, 2003, p 493.)

or spiral), borrowed from the Greek noun *speira*, meaning anything that is coiled or twisted. In the binomial system of biological nomenclature, the generic name is indicated by a capitalized noun; the species is indicated by an adjective agreeing with this noun in gender and number.[*]

The Greek word *trophē* (nourishment) has given us such words as **trophic,** meaning concerned with nourishment. Most of the words in medical terminology that use the form TROPH- have to do with nourishment that is carried to the cells of the body by circulating blood. Any impediment to the flow of blood to a part will result in **hypotrophy** and eventually **atrophy.** Hypotrophy is the gradual degeneration and loss of function of tissue—usually muscle tissue—resulting from a decrease in the flow of blood to that part. Atrophy is a decrease in size of a part resulting from lack of cell nourishment, as in muscle atrophy, which occurs with long periods of non-use of muscles in bedridden individuals. **Hypertrophy** is an increase in the size of an organ or part as a consequence of increased absorption of nutrients. This is usually caused by an increase in functional activity, as in **cardiac hypertrophy,** an increase in the size of the heart resulting from overgrowth of the tissues of the heart muscle. This condition is caused by continued stress beyond normal limits, such as occurs in long-standing hypertension with resultant stress on the heart. One of the four signs of the tetralogy of Fallot (a congenital disorder caused by a defect in the heart that allows blood to pass from the left ventricle to the right) is hypertrophy of the right ventricle. This is caused by the extra stress placed on this part of the heart muscle by the burden of pumping the additional blood that accumulates there.

Hypermyatrophy is unusual wasting of muscle tissue. **Amyotrophy** is muscular atrophy. **Dystrophy** is the name given to any disorder of the body caused by defective nutrition, such as **muscular dystrophy,** a familial disease characterized by progressive atrophy of muscles. **Hemidystrophy** is dystrophy of one side of the body.

The words **euphoria** and **dysphoria** are formed from the Greek compound nouns *euphoria*, a sense of well-being or comfort, and *dysphoria*, a sense of discomfort.

The Greek adjective *ankylos* meant crooked or curved, and the noun *ankylē* meant a joint that was bent and stiffened by disease; both words are derivatives of the noun *ankos* (bend or hollow). **Ankylosis** is abnormal immobility of a joint caused by some pathological changes in the joint or its surrounding tissue. The combining form ANKYL- means a fusion of parts normally separate, as in **ankylochilia** (*cheilos*, lip) and **ankyloproctia** (*prōktos*, anus). **Ankylosing spondylitis** is a progressive condition in which inflammatory changes and new bone formation occur at the site of attachment of tendons and ligaments to bone.

The Greek word *Aphrodisia* meant sexual pleasures, things connected with Aphrodite, the goddess of love (Fig.

*See Unit 5, Biological Nomenclature.

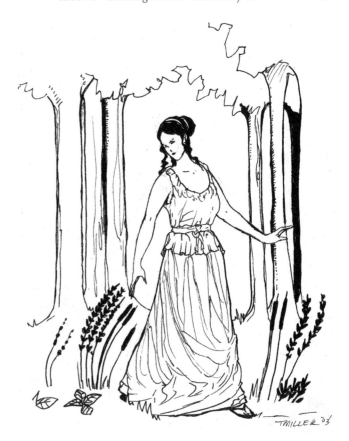

Figure 6–2. Aphrodite.

6–2). There was an adjective *Aphrodisiakos*, from which we get the word **aphrodisiac.** Aphrodite did not confine her amorous attentions to Hephaestus, her husband and god of the forge, but had numerous affairs with immortals and mortals alike. One such relationship, that with Hermes, a Greek god of many functions, resulted in the birth of a son who grew to be a handsome young man resembling both his mother and his father. His name was Hermaphroditus. Ovid, the 1st-century BC Roman poet, tells us an anecdote about this young man.

As the story goes, there was once a naiad, a water nymph, named Salmacis, who dwelled in a pool in Caria, a land of Asia Minor. One day, 15-year-old Hermaphroditus came to the place and Salmacis fell in love with him on sight. A shy young man, he refused her advances. But she waited until he went bathing in the pool and, casting off all her garments, dived in, crying, "I win, he is mine!"

Hermaphroditus resists and denies the nymph the pleasures she has hoped for, but she clings to him, pressing her whole body to him as if they were grown together. *Struggle as hard as you wish, you wicked boy,* she says, *but you will not escape. May the gods grant me this, that no day ever come that will take him from me.* The gods heard her. Their two bodies were joined together, one face and one form for both. Just as one grafts a twig onto a branch and sees them join and grow together, so were these two bodies joined in close embrace, no longer two beings, yet no longer either man or woman, but neither, and yet both. [*Metamorphoses* 4.368ff]

Thus **hermaphrodite** came to mean a person with the genital organs of both sexes.

Hesiod, the Greek poet of the mid-8th century BC, tells us in his *Theogony* (Origin of the Gods) that in the beginning of Creation, Chaos first came into being; then Earth, dark Tartarus in the depths of Earth; and then Eros, "fairest among the deathless gods, who unnerves the limbs and overcomes the counsels of a prudent mind of all gods and men" (*Theogony* 120–123). But in the sense in which he is usually conceived, that of the Latin Cupid, Eros is the creation of later Greek poets. Far from remaining the primeval deity of Hesiod, he grows younger, and from the handsome youth of the 6th to 5th centuries BC, he becomes a wanton, lascivious boy in the Alexandrian period (3rd to 1st centuries), whose arrows kindle passion in the heart. The parentage of the second Eros is in some dispute, but the most commonly held belief makes Aphrodite his mother and either Hermes or Ares, the god of war, his father. Cicero holds to the latter view (*On the Nature of the Gods* 3.23). His Latin name, Cupid (*cupīdō*, desire), gives us the word **cupidity**; his Greek name gives us **erotic, eroticism**, and so forth.

To the ancient Greeks, Thanatos was the god of death. Thanatos appears as a character on the stage in the opening scene of Euripides' tragedy *Alcestis*, when he comes to claim Alcestis, the lovely young wife of King Admetus, for whom she has offered to die. Admetus had offended the goddess Artemis, and she decreed that he must die on a certain date—unless someone would voluntarily die for him. When Admetus could find no one to make this sacrifice, Alcestis agreed to take his place. But this was a tragedy with a happy ending, for the great hero Heracles went to the underworld and succeeded in taking Alcestis away from Thanatos, and the drama ends with Heracles leading Alcestis back to her husband.

Homer, in the *Iliad* (16.666 ff), tells us that when Zeus' son, Sarpedon, was killed in the fighting before the walls of Troy, the god ordered Apollo to remove Sarpedon's body from the field of battle and entrust it to Sleep (Hypnos) and his twin brother Death (Thanatos), who would return it to Sarpedon's home in Lycia. This legend is the subject of the painting on a famous ancient Greek vase, the Euphronios vase, now in the Metropolitan Museum of Art in New York City. Sleep and Death are depicted lifting the body of Sarpedon while Apollo looks on.

Exercise 1: Analyze and Define

Analyze and define each of the following words. In this and in succeeding exercises, analysis should consist of separating the words into prefixes (if any), combining forms, and suffixes or suffix forms (if any) and giving the meaning of each. Be certain to differentiate between nouns and adjectives in your definitions. Consult a medical dictionary for the current meanings of these words. Use a separate paper if you need more room for an answer.

1. amyotrophia _____

2. androgynous _____

3. ankylodactylia _____

4. ankylosis _____

5. antaphrodisiac _____

6. apoplexy _____

7. atrophy _____

8. autoerotism _____

9. brachycephalous _____

10. chromatophore _____

11. cryptanamnesia _____

12. demography _____

13. dermonosology _____

14. diaphoresis _____

15. diplegia _____

16. dolichocephalic _____

17. dysphoria _____

18. dystrophy _____

19. endemic _____

20. endodontitis _____

21. epistaxis _____

22. erogenous _____

23. euphoria _____

24. euthanasia _____

25. gynandroid _____

26. gynecopathy _____

27. helminthiasis _____

28. hemidiaphoresis _____

29. hermaphrodite _____

30. heterodromus _____

31. homoerotic _____

32. hydrorrhachis _____

33. hypertrichosis _____

34. mesodont _____

35. nematology _____

36. nosophyte _____

37. odontonecrosis _____

38. osteosynthesis _____

39. palindromia _____

40. pancarditis _____

41. pandemic _____

42. paraplegia _____

43. photodysphoria _____

44. photosynthesis _____

45. prosopoplegia _____

46. schistocytosis _____

47. schizonychia _____

48. spondylolysis _____

49. thanatophobia _____

50. trichogen _____

Exercise 2: Word Derivation

Give the word derived from Greek elements that matches each of the following. It is not necessary to give combining terms for words in parentheses. Verify your answer in a medical dictionary. **Note that the wording of the dictionary definition may vary from the wording below.**

1. Resembling a male _____

2. Absence of hair _____

3. Abnormal shortness of the fingers and toes _____

4. Congenital deformity in which the head is inapparent _____

5. (Abnormally) long colon _____

6. Producing sexual excitement _____

7. Paralysis of the stomach _____

8. Resembling the female (of the species) _____

9. Study of worms _____

10. Pertaining to nutrients carried in the blood _____

11. Science (of description or classification) of diseases _____

12. Study of death _____

13. Hemorrhage from a tooth (socket) _____

14. Fear of everything _____

15. Around a vertebra _____

16. Dissolution or disintegration under stimulus of light rays _____

17. Inflammation of the spine _____

18. (Congenital) fissure of the face _____

19. Relating to (the processes of) life and death _____

20. Concerned with nourishment _____

Exercise 3: Drill and Review

The meaning of each of the following words can be determined from its etymology. Determine the meaning of each word. Verify your answer in a medical dictionary.

1. amblychromasia _____

2. anaphrodisiac _____

3. androgynoid _____

4. antatrophic _____

5. anthelmintic _____

6. aphrodisiac _____

7. brachycheilia _____

8. chondrodystrophy _____

9. chromophore _____

10. craniorachischisis _____

11. cryptogenic _____

12. endocrinotherapy _____

13. erotophobia _____

14. exodontia _____

15. gastroschisis _____

16. gynandrism _____

17. gynecophonus _____

18. gynoplasty _____

19. helminthemesis _____

20. hypertrophy _____

21. hypotrichosis _____

22. melanophore _____

23. metachromasia _____

24. microdontism _____

25. nematoid _____

26. nephrohypertrophy _____

27. nosomycosis _____

28. odontodynia _____

29. odontogenic _____

30. oligodontia _____

31. onychatrophia _____

32. osteochondrodystrophy _____

33. palilalia _____

34. palingraphia _____

35. panasthenia _____

36. panoptosis _____

37. periodontal _____

38. photogenic _____

39. plegaphonia _____

40. protopathic _____

41. rachitome _____

42. rhachialgia _____

43. sclerotrichia _____

44. spondylarthritis _____

45. spondylopyosis _____

46. symphysodactyly _____

47. synthetic _____

48. toxonosis _____

49. trichophagia _____

50. trophedema _____

BUILDING GREEK VOCABULARY IV

The art of medicine would never have been discovered, nor would there have been any medical research—for there would have been no need for medicine—if sick men had benefited by the same manner of living and by the same food and drink of men in health.

[Hippocrates, *Ancient Medicine* 3]

VOCABULARY

Greek	Combining Form(s)	Meaning	Example
adēn	ADEN-	gland	**aden**-oids
aēr	AER-	air, gas	**aer**-obe
blennos	BLENN-	mucus	**blenn**-orrhea
koilia	CEL(I)-	abdomen	**celi**-ocentesis
cheilos	CH(E)IL-	lip	**cheil**-oschisis
chronos	CHRON-	time, timing	**chron**-ic
klān	CLA(S)-, -CLAST	break (up), destroy	polio-**clast**-ic
desis	-DESIS	binding	syn-**desis**
desmos	DESM-	[binding] ligament, connective tissue	**desm**-ocyte
dynamis	DYNAM-	force, power, energy	**dynam**-ic
gēras	GER-	old age	**ger**-iatrics
gnathos	GNATH-	(lower) jaw	pro-**gnath**-ous
ischein	ISCH-, -SCHE-	suppress, check	**isch**-emia
kleptein	KLEPT-	steal	**klept**-omania
leios	LEI-	smooth	**lei**-otrichous
lēpsis	LEP-	attack, seizure	epi-**lep**-tic
mainesthai	MAN-	be mad	**man**-iac
melos	MEL-	limb	**mel**-algia
morphē	MORPH-	form, shape	meta-**morph**-osis
nomos	NOM-	law	**nom**-ogram
omphalos	OMPHAL-	navel, umbilicus	**omphal**-oncus

Greek	Combining Form(s)	Meaning	Example
pais, paidos	**PED-**	child	**ped**-iatrics (British: paediatrics)
penia	**PEN-**	decrease, deficiency	leuko-**pen**-ia
pexis	**-PEX-**	fixing, (surgical) attachment	gastro-**pex**-y
plassein	**PLAS(T)-**	form, develop	a-**plas**-ia
presbys	**PRESBY-**	old, old age	**presby**-opia
prostatēs	**PROSTAT-**	[one who stands before] prostate gland	**prostat**-itis
ptyein	**PTY-**	spit	**pty**-sis
ptyalon	**PTYAL-**	saliva	**ptyal**-in
rhaptein	**-RRHAPH-**	suture	cardio-**rrhaph**-y
sitos	**SIT-**	food	**sit**-otoxin
histanai	**STA(T)-**	stand, stop	**sta**-sis
taxis	**TAX-**	(muscular) coordination	a-**tax**-ia
thermē	**THERM-**	heat, (body) temperature	**therm**-ometer
tropē	**TROP-**	turning	**trop**-ism

-PLASTY, -TROPISM

Words ending in -**plasty** (molding, surgically forming) refer to plastic or restorative surgery: rhino-**plasty**, angio-**plasty** (Fig. 7–1).

Words ending in -**tropism** refer to the turning of living organisms toward (positive tropism) or away from (negative tropism) an external stimulus: photo-**trop-ism**, aero-**trop-ism**.

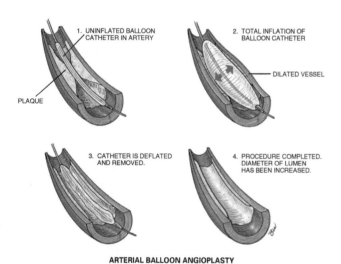

ARTERIAL BALLOON ANGIOPLASTY

1. UNINFLATED BALLOON CATHETER IN ARTERY
PLAQUE
2. TOTAL INFLATION OF BALLOON CATHETER
DILATED VESSEL
3. CATHETER IS DEFLATED AND REMOVED.
4. PROCEDURE COMPLETED. DIAMETER OF LUMEN HAS BEEN INCREASED.

Figure 7–1. Arterial balloon angioplasty. (From Taber's Cyclopedic Medical Dictionary, ed 19. F. A. Davis, Philadelphia, 2001, p 116, with permission.)

Table 7–1. Comparative Thermometric Scale

	Celsius*	Fahrenheit
Boiling point of water	100°	212°
	90	194
	80	176
	70	158
	60	140
	50	122
	40	104
Body temperature	37°	98.6°
	30	86
	20	68
	10	50
Freezing point of water	0°	32°
	–10	14
	–20	–4

*Also called *Centigrade*.
Source: From Taber's Cyclopedic Medical Dictionary, ed. 19. F. A. Davis, Philadelphia, 2001, p 2084, with permission.

INSTRUMENTS

Words ending in -**clast** indicate an instrument or device for breaking or crushing: litho-**clast**

Words ending in -**stat** indicate a device or agent for stopping the flow of something: hemo-**stat**

Words ending in -**meter** (Lesson 1) indicate an instrument for measuring: cephalo-**meter**

Words ending in -**tome** (Lesson 4) indicate a device for cutting or excising: gastro-**tome**

ETYMOLOGICAL NOTES

The verb *mainesthai* (to be mad) is one of several words in both Greek and Latin that have the root MN-, all having to do with mental processes: Greek, *mimnēskein* (remember) (cf. *Mnemosyne* (Memory), *manteia* (prophetic power), *manthanein* (learn), *ma(n)thematikos* (mathematical), *mantis* (prophet or prophetic); and Latin, *mēns, mentis* (mind), *mentiō, mentiōnis* (mention), *mentīrī* (lie, cheat). In the beginning of the *Iliad*, Apollo rains his arrows upon the Greek camp. Agamemnon, the leader of the Greek army, refuses to return the girl whom he has taken captive to her father, a priest of Apollo. Achilles rises in the assembly and speaks:

> Come, let us consult some seer (*mantis*) or priest, or some interpreter of dreams—for dreams are sent by Zeus—who can tell us why Phoebus Apollo has conceived such anger [*Iliad* 1.62–64].

Tiresias, the famous blind prophet of Thebes, had a daughter, Manto, who also became a famous seer. Manto is also the name of an Italian nymph who had the gift of prophecy and who founded the city of Mantua in Lombardy, the birthplace of Virgil.

Theocritus, the 3rd-century BC Greek bucolic poet, called the orthopterous insect *Mantis religiosa* (praying mantis) the prophetic grasshopper (*mantis kalamaia*). Perhaps this insect was given its Latin name because of its posture, holding its forelegs in a position that suggests hands folded in prayer (Fig 7–2). [*Idylls* 10.18]

The narcotic drug morphine takes its name from Morpheus, the Greco-Roman god of dreams (Greek *morphē*, form, shape). Morpheus was one of the thousand sons of Sleep. Morphine takes its name from Morpheus because of the dreams induced by it, especially by opium, from which morphine is derived. The Roman poet Ovid tells us that Morpheus is the cleverest of all of Sleep's sons in imitating the form of humans:

> No other is more skilled than he in simulating the gait, the countenance, and the speech of mortals, or in assuming their clothing and the words that each is accustomed to use [*Metamorphoses* 11.635–638].

The *Metamorphoses*, Ovid's greatest work, was written before his banishment, for unknown reasons, to Tomis on the Black Sea in 8 AD by the emperor Augustus. A long poem (11,990 lines), the *Metamorphoses* tells stories from Greek mythology and Near Eastern legend, all involving a change in shape or form. The poem begins with the creation of the universe and ends with the transformation of Julius Caesar into a star after his death. The poet declares his intentions at the opening of the work:

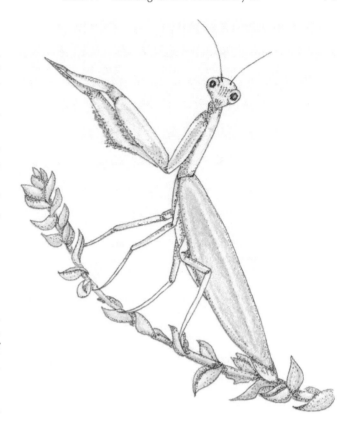

Figure 7–2. Praying mantis. (Drawing by Laine McCarthy, 2000.)

> My purpose is to tell of bodies changed to new forms.
> Gods—for it is you who made the changes—
> give me inspiration for this poem
> that runs from the beginning
> of the world down to our own days.

The verb *ptyein* and its derivative noun *ptyalon*, both meaning spit, are examples of onomatopoeia (*onoma, onomatos*, name, *poiein*, make), the formation of words in imitation of sounds. One of the best-known examples of this from antiquity is found in a fragment of the *Annales* by the 2nd-century BC Roman poet Ennius, whose works are mostly lost:

> *At tuba terribili sonitu taratantara dixit.*

> But the trumpet, with a terrible sound, went *taratantara*.

The prostate gland was called *prostatēs* (*pro-*, in front of, *histanai*, stand) by the early Greek physicians because of its location in front of the bladder and urethra.

The term "stat" used in hospitals is from Latin *statim* meaning immediately.

Exercise 1: Analyze and Define

Analyze and define each of the following words. In this and in succeeding exercises, analysis should consist of separating the words into prefixes (if any), combining forms, and suffixes or suffix forms (if any) and giving the meaning of each. Be certain to differentiate between nouns and adjectives in your definitions. Consult a medical dictionary for the current meanings of these words. Use a separate paper if you need more room for an answer.

1. adenoids _____

2. aerobe _____

3. aerotropism _____

4. alloplasia _____

5. ankylochilia _____

6. aplasia _____

7. arthroclasia _____

8. ataxophobia _____

9. blennadenitis _____

10. celiocentesis _____

11. cheiloschisis _____

12. cholestasia _____

13. chronognosis _____

14. cystopexy _____

15. desmoneoplasm _____

16. dolichomorphic _____

17. dysstasia _____

18. enteropexy _____

19. erythromelalgia _____

20. erythropenia _____

21. exomphalos _____

22. geriatrics _____

23. gnathalgia _____

24. hematomphalocele _____

25. hemiataxia _____

26. hemodynamics _____

27. hyperthermalgesia _____

28. hypoplasia _____

29. idiotropic _____

30. ischesis _____

31. kleptomania _____

32. leiomyoma _____

33. macrocheilia _____

34. myotenontoplasty _____

35. narcolepsy _____

36. nomogram _____

37. omphaloncus _____

38. osteoclast _____

39. pancytopenia _____

40. parasite _____

41. pedatrophy _____

42. pericardiorrhaphy _____

43. polyadenomatosis _____

44. presbyiatrics _____

45. prognathous _____

46. sitophobia _____

47. stasis _____

48. syndesmopexy _____

49. tenodesis _____

50. thermanesthesia _____

Exercise 2: Word Derivation

Give the word derived from Greek elements that matches each of the following. It is not necessary to give combining terms for words in parentheses. Verify your answer in a medical dictionary. **Note that the wording of the dictionary meaning may vary from the wording below.**

1. Device for excising a gland _____

2. Condition in which (paired) limbs are (noticeably) unequal _____

3. Resembling mucus _____

4. Abdominal tumor _____

5. Excision of (part of) the lip _____

6. Connective tissue cell _____

7. Any disease affecting ligaments _____

8. Caused by (an increase of) energy _____

9. Destructive to cells _____

10. Physician who specializes in the care of elderly people _____

11. Condition marked by possession of the same form _____

12. (Morbid) fear of stealing _____

13. Suture of (a wound in) the abdominal wall _____

14. (Abnormal) decrease of white blood cells _____

15. Abnormal smallness of the (lower) jaw _____

16. Defective formation of the spinal cord _____

17. Umbilical hemorrhage _____

18. Plastic surgery of the nose _____

19. Any poison (developed) in food _____

20. Measurement of temperature _____

Exercise 3: Drill and Review

The meaning of each of the following words can be determined from its etymology. Determine the meaning of each word. Verify your answer in a medical dictionary.

1. adenoidectomy _____

2. aerotitis _____

3. aerothermotherapy _____

4. anerythroplasia _____

5. angiorrhaphy _____

6. aptyalia _____

7. atelognathia _____

8. blennemesis _____

9. celiac _____

10. cheilophagia _____

11. chronobiology _____

12. cryptolith _____

13. desmorrhexis _____

14. dynamic _____

15. endoparasite _____

16. enterosepsis _____

17. gastropexy _____

18. geriatric _____

19. gnathoschisis _____

20. hemostasis _____

21. hidradenitis _____

22. hydropenia _____

23. hypoptyalism _____

24. ischemia _____

25. leiotrichous _____

26. leptomeninges _____

27. maniacal _____

28. melalgia _____

29. myodynamometer _____

30. myoischemia _____

31. nephrotropic _____

32. nomography _____

33. odontoclasis _____

34. omphalorrhexis _____

35. oreximania _____

36. pachycheilia _____

37. pediatrician _____

38. pedomorphism _____

39. periomphalic _____

40. phototropism _____

41. phrenohepatic _____

42. prostatodynia _____

43. pseudoedema _____

44. ptyalolithiasis _____

45. schistocelia _____

46. scleradenitis _____

47. sitotoxism _____

48. stereotropism _____

49. synchilia _____

50. tenorrhaphy _____

LATIN-DERIVED MEDICAL TERMINOLOGY

LATIN NOUNS AND ADJECTIVES
LATIN VERBS

ROMAN NUMERALS

A line placed over a letter increases its value one thousand times.

1 I	6 VI	11 XI	40 XL	90 XC	5000 $\overline{V}$
2 II	7 VII	12 XII	50 L	100 C	10,000 $\overline{X}$
3 III	8 VIII	15 XV	60 LX	500 D	100,000 $\overline{C}$
4 IV	9 IX	20 XX	70 LXX	1000 M	1,000,000 $\overline{M}$
5 V	10 X	30 XXX	80 LXXX	2000 MM	

Source: Taber's Cyclopedic Medical Dictionary, ed 19. F. A. Davis, Philadelphia, 2001, p 2368, with permission.

LESSON 8

LATIN NOUNS AND ADJECTIVES

Just as agriculture promises nourishment to healthy bodies, so does the practice of medicine promise health to the sick.

[Celsus, *De Medicina*, Prœmium 1]

Latin, like Greek, is an **inflected** language, and nouns, pronouns, and adjectives have different endings to indicate their grammatical function in a sentence. Latin nouns are divided into five classifications, or groups, called **declensions,** and in each of these declensions the endings of the various grammatical cases are substantially different in both singular and plural. The first three of the declensions produce most English derivatives.

Nouns of the first declension, mostly feminine, have the ending *-a* in the nominative singular, the vocabulary form of the noun. The combining form of these nouns is found by dropping the final *-a*. Latin nouns of the first declension appear in English in either their vocabulary form or with the final *-a* dropped or changed to silent *-e*.

Latin Noun	Meaning	English Derivative
fistula	pipe	**fistula**
vāgīna	sheath	**vagina**
tībia	shin bone	**tibia**
axilla	armpit	**axilla**
larva	ghost	**larva**
lympha	clear water	**lymph**
forma	shape	**form**
palma	palm	**palm**
tunica	garment	**tunic**
membrāna	skin	**membrane**

ūrīna	urine	**urine**
sūtūra	seam	**suture**
tuba	trumpet	**tube**
valva	folding door	**valve**

The nominative plural of first-declension nouns is *-ae*: *antenna, antennae*; *larva, larvae*; *vertēbra, vertēbrae*. The genitive singular of first-declension nouns ends in *-ae*. This form is sometimes found in descriptive terminology and can be translated by the word "of": **os coxae** (*os*, bone; *coxa*, hip), bone of the hip; **cervix vesicae** (*cervix*, neck; *vēsīca*, bladder), neck of the bladder.

Nouns of the second declension are either masculine or neuter. Masculine nouns in the nominative end in *-us* and neuter nouns end in *-um*. The combining form of these nouns is found by dropping this ending. Nouns of the second declension are usually found in the vocabulary form, but sometimes the ending is dropped or changed to silent *-e*.

Latin Noun	Meaning	English Derivative
bacillus	small staff	**bacillus**
cuneus	wedge	**cuneus**
fungus	mushroom	**fungus**
humerus	upper arm	**humerus**
globus	sphere	**globe**

digitus	finger	**digit**
ileum	groin	**ileum**
ōvum	egg	**ovum**
cerebrum	brain	**cerebrum**
palātum	palate	**palate**
intestīnum	intestine	**intestine**

The nominative plural of second-declension masculine nouns is *-ī*: *bacillus, bacillī; fungus, fungī*; and the plural of neuter nouns is *-a*: *cilium, cilia; ovum, ova*. The genitive singular of second-declension nouns ends in *-i*. This form is sometimes found in descriptive terminology: **cervix uteri** (*cervix*, neck; *uterus*, womb), neck of the uterus; **labium cerebri** (*labium*, lip, margin; *cerebrum*, brain), margin of the brain (Figure 8–1). The genitive plural of these nouns ends in *-ōrum*: **icterus neonatorum** (Greek *neos*, new, Latin *nātus*, born), jaundice of newborns.

Latin nouns of the third declension are like Greek third-declension nouns in that it is not always possible to determine the base of these nouns by knowing the nominative singular, the dictionary form. To find the base, it is usually necessary to know the form of some case other than the nominative. For this reason, dictionaries and vocabularies cite, along with the nominative case, the genitive singular, which ends in *-is*. The base is found by dropping this ending. In forming English words, often the nominative case is used alone, and sometimes suffixes are added directly to it. More often, however, the base of these nouns is used to form compound words. Third-declension nouns can be masculine, feminine, or neuter. (In this manual, if the base of a noun is the same as the dictionary form, or if the genitive case is the same as the nominative case, the genitive case is not given in the vocabularies.)

Latin Noun	Combining Form	Meaning	English Derivative
auris (auris)	*AUR-*	ear	**auris, auricle**
latus, lateris	*LATER-*	side	**latus, lateral**
os, ossis	*OSS-*	bone	**os coxae, ossify**
rādix, rādīcis	*RADIC-*	root	**radix, radical**
sopor (sopōris)	*SOPOR-*	sleep	**sopor, soporific**
vās (vāsis)	*VAS-*	vessel	**vas deferens, vascular**

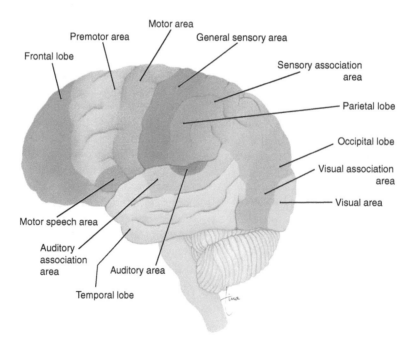

Figure 8–1. Cerebrum (left hemisphere). (From Scanlon, VC, and Sanders, T: Essentials of Anatomy and Physiology, ed 4. F. A. Davis, Philadelphia, 2003, p 170, with permission.)

LATIN GENITIVE ENDINGS

	Genitive Ending	Example	Meaning
First Declension			
Singular	*-ae*	**vesicae**	of the bladder
Second Declension			
Singular	*-ī*	**uteri**	of the uterus
Plural	*-ōrum*	**neonatorum**	of newborns
Third Declension			
Singular	*-is*	**dentis**	of the tooth

GENITIVE SINGULAR

The genitive singular of nouns of the first, second, and third declensions is sometimes found in descriptive terminology and can be translated by the word "of": **corona capitis** (*corōna*, crown, *caput, capitis*, head), crown of the head.

The nominative plural of masculine and feminine nouns of the third declension ends in *-ēs*: *cervix, cervīcis* (neck): **cervix** (plural, **cervices**); *nāris, nāris* (nostril): **naris** (plural, **nares**); *rēn, rēnis* (kidney): **ren** (plural, **renes**) and the plural of neuter nouns ends in *a*: *corpus, corporis* (body): **corpus** (plural, **corpora**); *genus, generis* (kind): **genus** (plural, **genera**); *viscus, visceris* (internal organ): **viscus** (plural, **viscera**).

There are a few nouns of the fourth and fifth declensions in medical terminology. Most fourth-declension nouns are masculine and end in *-us* in the nominative singular, with the plural ending in *-ūs*: *meātus* (passage): **meatus** (plural, **meatus**), **meatoscopy**, **meatotomy**; *plexus* (a braid): **plexus** (plural, **plexus** or **plexuses**). Neuter nouns of the fourth declension end in *ū* in the nominative singular: *genū* (knee): **genupectoral**, pertaining to the knees and chest (*pectus, pectoris*, chest). The nominative plural of fourth-declension neuter nouns ends in *-ua*: *cornū* (horn): **cornu** (plural, **cornua**). The nominative singular of fifth-declension nouns ends in *-ēs*: *cariēs* (decay); *rabiēs* (madness); *scabiēs** (itch). Most fifth-declension nouns are feminine; the plural is identical to the singular in the nominative case.

*Most fifth-declension nouns end in *-iēs* in the nominative singular and plural.

LATIN NOMINATIVE SINGULAR AND PLURAL ENDINGS

	Singular	Example	Plural	Example
First and second declensions				
Masculine	*-us*	**fungus**	*-ī*	**fungi**
Feminine	*-a*	**larva**	*-ae*	**larvae**
Neuter	*-um*	**ovum**	*-a*	**ova**
Third declension				
Masculine/Feminine	*s**	**cervix**	*-ēs*	**cervices**[†]
Neuter	**	**viscus**	*-(i)a*	**viscera**[‡]
Fourth declension				
Masculine	*-us*	**meatus**	*-ūs*	**meatus**
Neuter	*-u*	**genu**	*-ua*	**genua**
Fifth declension				
Feminine	*-ēs*	**rabies**	*-ēs*	**rabies**

* Third-declension nouns have a variety of endings in the nominative singular.
[†]Latin *cervix, cervicis*.
[‡]Latin *viscus, visceris*.

LATIN ADJECTIVES

There are two classes of Latin adjectives: they are either of the first and second declension, with endings like those of masculine, feminine, and neuter nouns of the first and second declensions; or of the third declension. Latin dictionaries and grammar texts cite first- and second-declension adjectives by using the masculine singular, ending in *-us*, as the entry form, and following it with the feminine and neuter endings *-a* and *-um*; *bonus, -a, -um* (good); *magnus, -a, -um* (large); *medius, -a, -um* (middle). In this manual, adjectives of this class are cited only in the form of the masculine nominative singular, ending in *-us*, the dictionary form. There are some adjectives of the first and second declension with masculine forms ending in *-er*, but with the feminine and neuter forms ending in *-a* and *–um*, respectively: *asper, aspera, asperum* (rough); *tener, tenera, tenerum* (tender). Some adjectives ending in *-er* drop the *-e-* in the feminine and neuter: *integer, integra, integrum* (whole); *ruber, rubra, rubrum* (red).

Third-declension adjectives usually have two terminations: *-is* for the masculine and feminine and *-e* for the neuter: *gravis, -e* (severe); *fortis, -e* (strong); *levis, -e* (light). There are some adjectives of the third declension with masculine forms ending in *-er*; these have *-ris* in the feminine and *-re* in the neuter: (*ācer, ācris, ācre* (sharp); *salūber, salūbris, salūbre* (healthful). Some adjectives of the third declension have one form for the masculine, feminine, and neuter genders: *ātrox*, genitive *ātrōcis* (*fierce*), *praegnāns*, genitive *praegnantis* (pregnant); *sapiēns*, genitive *sapientis* (knowing, wise). There are no adjectives of the fourth and fifth declensions.

Latin adjectives usually follow the nouns they modify and agree with them in gender and number:

myasthenia **gravis**

genu **recurvatum**

vena **cava**

LATIN PREFIXES

Latin prefixes, like Greek prefixes, modify or qualify the meaning of the word to which they are affixed. It is difficult to assign a single specific meaning to each prefix, and often it is necessary to adapt a meaning that will fit the particular use of a word. A word may have more than one prefix and, in compound words, a prefix may follow a combining form. Latin prefixes (and suffixes) are frequently used with Greek combining forms.

ab- (**a-** rarely before certain consonants; **abs-** before *c* and *t*): away from:

ab-ductor	**abs**-cess
ab-lation	**abs**-tract
ab-ortion	**a**-vulsion

ad- (**ac-** before *c*; **af-** before *f*; **ag-** before *g*; **al-** before *l*; **an-** before *n*; **ap-** before *p*; **as-**before *s*; **a-** before *sp*; **at-** before *t*): to, toward:

ad-aptation	**an**-nectent
ad-renaline	**ap**-pendix
ac-cessory	**as**-sist
af-ferent	**a**-spirate
ag-glomerate	**at**-traction
al-literation	**af**-fection

ambi-: both:

ambi-dextrous	**ambi**-opia
ambi-lateral	**ambi**-valence

ante-: before, forward:

ante-febrile	**ante**-pyretic
ante-natal	**ante**-version

bi- (**bin-, bis-**): two, twice, double, both:

bi-furcate	**bin**-aural
bi-lateral	**bin**-ocular
bi-para	**bis**-acromial

circum-: around:

circum-articular	**circum**-ocular
circum-duction	**circum**-renal

con- (**co-** before *h*; **col-** before *l*; **com-** before *e, m*, and *p*; **cor-** before *r*): together, with; thoroughly, very:

con-genital	**com**-mensal
co-hesion	**com**-press
col-lapse	**cor**-rosive
com-edo	**co**-habitation

contra-: against, opposite:

contra-ception	**contra**-indication
contra-fissura	**contra**-lateral

de-: down, away from, absent:

de-generation	**de**-sensitize
de-hydration	**de**-saturation

dis- (**di-** before *g, v*, and usually before *l*; **dif-** before *f*): apart, away:

dis-infect	**di**-vert
dif-fusate	**di**-lation
di-gest	**dif**-fuse

ex- (**e-** before certain consonants; **ef-** before *f*): out of, away from:

ex-halation	**ef**-ferent
ex-pectoration	**e**-visceration

extra- (rarely **extro-**): on the outside, beyond:

extra-sensory	**extro**-vert
extra-vasation	**extro**-version

(1) in- (**il-** before *l*; **im-** before *b, m,* and *p*; **ir-** before *r*): in, into:

in-cubation	**im**-bibition
in-farct	**im**-mersion
in-gestion	**im**-pregnate
il-lumination	**ir**-radiate

(2) in- not:

in-continence	**im**-balance
in-firm	**im**-mune
in-nominate	**im**-potent
il-legal	**ir**-reducible

(3) in-: very, thoroughly:

in-duration	**in**-flammation
in-ebriation	**in**-toxication

infra-: beneath, below:

infra-maxillary	**infra**-umbilical
infra-sternal	**infra**-mammary

inter-: between:

inter-costal	**inter**-meningeal
inter-dental	**inter**-renal

intra- (rarely **intro-**): within:

intra-gastric	**intra**-venous
intra-muscular	**intro**-version

non-: not:*

non-conductor	**non**-toxic
non-protein	**non**-viable

mult- (often **multi-**): many, much, affecting many parts:

mult-angular	**multi**-cuspid
multi-gravida	**multi**-parous

ob- (**oc-** before *c*; **op-** before *p*): against, toward; very, thoroughly:

ob-session	**oc**-cult
oc-clusion	**op**-position

per- (**pel-** before *l*): through; very, thoroughly:

per-manent	**per**-spiration
per-meable	**pel**-lucid

post-: after, following, behind:

post-mortem	**post**-partum
post-nasal	**post**-uterine

pre-: before, in front of:

pre-digestion	**pre**-tibial
pre-gnant	**pre**-urethritis

pro-: forward, in front:

pro-cedure	**pro**-jection
pro-cess	**pro**-tection

re-: back, again:

re-cess	**re**-sonance
re-fraction	**re**-suscitation

retro-: backward, in back, behind:

retro-grade	**retro**-peritoneal
retro-nasal	**retro**-pharyngeal

se-: apart, away from:

se-crete	**se**-gregation
se-duce	**se**-paration

semi-: half:

semi-conscious	**semi**-permeable
semi-normal	**semi**-prone

sub- (**suf-** before *f*; **sup-** before *p*): under:

sub-costal	**suf**-fusion
sub-dural	**sup**-purate

super- (often **supra-**): over, above; excess:

super-ficial	**supra**-mastoid
super-virulent	**supra**-renal

trans-: across, through:

trans-parent	**trans**-thoracotomy
trans-plant	**trans**-vaginal

ultra-: beyond, excess:

ultra-sonic	**ultra**-microtome
ultra-violet	**ultra**-sound

*Non is not a prefix in Latin, but an adverb. Because it is used as a prefix in English, it is included here with prefixes.

Numeric Combining Forms and Prefixes

Combining Form/Prefix	Meaning	Example
uni-	one	**uni**-form
bi-, *bin-*, *bis-*	two, twice, double, both	**bi**-modal, **bin**-aural, **bis**-iliac
*tri-**	three	**tri**-cyclic
quadr-	four	**quadr**-iplegia, **quadr**-uped
quint-	five, fifth	**quint**-ipara, **quint**-uplet
sex-, *sext-*	six, sixth	**sex**-digital, **sext**-an, **sext**-igravida
sept-	seven	**sept**-ivalent, **sept**-uplet
oct-, *octa-*	eight	**oct**-ane, **octa**-hedron, **oct**-ogenarian, **oct**-ipara
non-	nine, ninth	**non**-ose, **non**-igravida
*dec-,** *deca-*	ten, one-tenth	**dec**-inormal, **deca**-meter,

*Derived from Greek.

LATIN SUFFIXES

Suffixes are elements that are added to the combining forms of nouns, adjectives, and verbs to form new words. Nouns are either abstract or concrete. Abstract nouns indicate a state, quality, condition, procedure, or process, whereas concrete nouns give names to objects and agents. Adjectives impart qualities or characteristics to nouns. The Latin language was rich in suffixes, but only those that are in common use in modern medical terminology are presented here.

Most of the abstract noun-forming suffixes that were used in Latin were affixed to verbal stems and are presented in Lesson 9. The suffixes given below are attached to the combining forms of adjectives or nouns. In most instances, Latin suffixes have come into English in a form slightly changed from their original as a result of their transition through French. The following list gives their English form. Note that when the base of a noun or adjective ends in a consonant and the suffix begins with a consonant, a **connecting vowel**, usually **i**, but sometimes **o** or **u**, is inserted.

The Latin language was particularly rich in adjectival suffixes. Only those suffixes that are frequently found are listed here; the less common ones will be identified as they occur. As with the noun-forming suffixes, adjectival suffixes usually come into English in a form slightly changed from their original. The following list gives their English form. Many Latin adjectives end in *-eus*, *-ea*, or *-eum*, which explains the presence of -e- in many English words: **esophageal**, **sanguineous**, **cesarean**, and so forth.

-al: forms adjectives: pertaining to:

dors-**al**   ren-**al**

-an: forms adjectives: pertaining to, located in:

medi-**an**   ovari-**an**

-ar: forms adjectives: pertaining to, located in:

ocul-**ar**   vascul-**ar**

-arium: forms nouns: denotes a place for something:

aqu-**arium**   herb-**arium**

-ary: forms nouns: denotes a place for something:

libr-**ary**   mortu-**ary**

-ary: forms adjectives: pertaining to:

saliv-**ary**   axill-**ary**

-ate: forms adjectives: having the form of, possessing:

cord-**ate**   caud-**ate**

-ia: forms abstract nouns:

somnolent-**ia**   macrolab-**ia**

-ian: forms nouns: indicates an expert in a certain field:

librar-**ian**   mortic-**ian**

-ic: forms adjectives: pertaining to:

pregravid-**ic**   rhythm-**ic**

-id*: forms adjectives: pertaining to:

morb-**id**   rab-**id**

*Note that there is a Greek-derived suffix *-id*, an alternative form of *-oid*, meaning "having the form of": hominid (*homo, hominis*, man).

-ile: forms adjectives: pertaining to, capable of:

sen-**ile**	febr-**ile**

-ine: forms adjectives: pertaining to, located in:

uter-**ine**	amygdal-**ine**
sangu-**ine**	femin-**ine**

-ive: forms adjectives: pertaining to:

tuss-**ive**	palliat-**ive**

-lent: forms adjectives: full of:

somno-**lent**	puru-**lent**

-ose: forms adjectives: full of:

adip-**ose**	varic-**ose**

-ous: forms adjectives: full of:

bili-**ous**	sanguine-**ous**

-ty: forms abstract nouns:

gravi-**ty**	morbidi-**ty**

-y: forms abstract nouns:

memor-**y**	remed-**y**

-AD

The English suffix **-ad** forms adverbs from nouns. These adverbs indicate direction toward a part of the body: **dextrad**, toward the right side (*dextra*, the right hand); **sinistrad**, toward the left side (*sinistra*, the left hand); **cephalad**, toward the head (Greek *kephalē*, head). (See the Etymological Notes in this lesson.)

DIMINUTIVE SUFFIXES

There was a group of suffixes in Latin that formed diminutive nouns from other nouns. These diminutives were nouns of the first or second declension, ending in *-us*, *-a*, or *-um*, depending on the gender of the noun to which they were affixed, and were all characterized by the presence of a single or double *l*. These diminutives usually appear in English in their original Latin form, but the final *-us* is sometimes changed to *-e*, *-culus* to *-cle*, and *-illa* to *-il*. A diminutive suffix expresses the idea of smallness, as in **fibril**, meaning a small fiber.

Examples of Diminutive Suffixes

-cle	ventricle	**-culus**	ventriculus
-ella	rubella	**-ellum**	cerebellum
-il	fibril	**-illa**	fibrilla
-ola	roseola	**-olus**	alveolus
-ule	globule	**-ulus**	calculus

DIMINUTIVE SUFFIXES

Diminutive siffixes are characterized by the presence of a single or double *l* and express the idea of smallness.

Words such as **rubella** (*ruber*, red) and **roseola** (*roseus*, rosy, reddish) are New Latin formations from Latin adjectives of the first and second declensions. These particular words are neuter plural in form; thus, rubella, or German measles, is named for the "little red things," the eruptions that accompany this disease, and roseola, a skin condition marked by maculae or red spots, for the "little reddish things" that characterize this condition. **Variola** (varius, spotted), smallpox, and **varicella** (an irregularly formed diminutive from varius), chickenpox, are similar formations. Often a new genus of bacteria is named by adding the neuter plural suffix -ella to the surname of its discoverer: *Salmonella* (Daniel E. Salmon, 1850–1914), *Brucella* (Sir David Bruce, 1855–1931), *Shigella* (Kiyoshi Shiga, 1870–1957).

NOTE: A word may have more than one suffix: **adiposity**, **morbidity**. Greek prefixes and suffixes may be used with Latin words: **adipositis**, **periocular**. Greek and Latin words may be combined in a single term: **cardiopulmonary** (Greek *kardia*, heart, Latin *pulmō*, *pulmōnis*, lung). Such words are known as **hybrids** (Latin *hybrida*, mongrel). A child born of a Roman father and a foreign mother, or one born of a freeman and a slave, was known as a *hybrida*, a word probably borrowed from the Greek *hybris* (insolence).

Many Latin words and expressions are used in medical terminology in their original form: **medulla oblongata** (*medulla*, marrow; *oblongata* [New Latin], elongated), referring to the lowest part of the brainstem; **cerebellum** (*cerebellum*, little brain), the portion of the brain forming the largest part of the rhombencephalon; **labium oris** (*labium*, lip; *ōs*, *ōris*, mouth), the skin and muscular tissue surrounding the mouth, the lips of the mouth; **auris externa** (*auris*, ear; *externa*, external or outer), the outer ear; **auricle** (*auricle*, little ear), the portion of the external ear not contained within the head.

VOCABULARY

NOTE: Beginning with this lesson, combining forms of Latin words will be printed in ***bold italics***.

Latin	Combining Form(s)	Meaning	Example
abdōmen, abdōminis	*ABDOMIN-*	belly, abdomen	**abdomin**-algia
adeps, adipis	*ADIP-*	fat	**adip**-ose
auris	*AUR-*	ear	**aur**-icular
bacillus	*BACILL-*	[rod, staff] bacillus	**bacill**-emia
bursa (Medieval Latin)	*BURS-*	[leather sack] bursa	**burs**-itis
calx, calcis	*CALC-*	stone, calcium, lime (salts)	**calc**-iferous
calor	*CALOR-*	heat, energy	**calor**-ic
caput, capitis	*CAPIT-*	head	de-**capit**-ate
cerebrum	*CEREBR-*	brain	**cerebr**-al
costa	*COST-*	rib	**cost**-algia
dens, dentis (Fig. 8–2)	*DENT-*	tooth	**dent**-ist
dorsum	*DORS-*	back (of the body)	**dors**-al
externus, -a, -um	*EXTERN-*	outer	**extern**-al
fibra	*FIBR-*	fiber, filament	**fibr**-ous
fistula	*FISTUL-*	(tube, pipe) fistula, an abnormal tubelike passage in the body	**fistul**-ectomy
frīgus, frīgoris	*FRIG-, FRIGOR-*	cold	re-**frig**-erate
insula	*INSUL-*	island*	**insul**-in
internus, -a, -um	*INTERN-*	inner	**intern**-al
meātus	*MEAT-*	passage, opening, meatus (pronounced mee-ate'-us)	**meat**-oscope
nāsus	*NAS-*	nose	**nas**-al
pus, puris	*PUR-*	pus	**pur**-ulent
rādix, rādīcis	*RADIC-, RAD-, RADIX*	root	**radic**-es
rēn, rēnis	*REN-*	kidney	**ren**-ogastric
sanguis, sanguinis	*SANGUI(N)-*	blood	**sangui**-colous
sonus	*SON-*	sound	**son**-ogram
synovia (New Latin)	*SYNOV-*	synovial fluid, synovial membrane or sac	**synov**-ium
tuba	*TUB-*	[trumpet] tube	**tub**-oovaritis
tussis	*TUSS-*	cough	anti-**tuss**-ive
vacca	*VACC-*	cow†	**vacc**-ine
vīrus (Fig. 8–3)	*VIR-, VIRUS-*	[poison, venom] virus‡	**vir**-al
viscus, visceris (plural, *viscera*)	*VISCER-*	internal organ(s)	**viscer**-al

*See the Etymological Notes in this lesson.
†Words containing vaccin- have to do with vaccine.
‡Words like virulent are from the Latin adjective *vīrulentus*, strong, powerful (literally, full of poison).

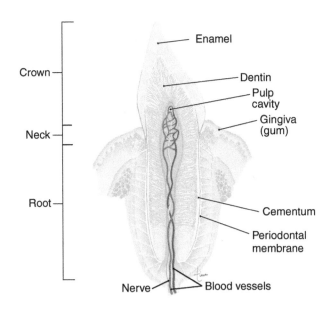

Figure 8–2. Tooth structure (longitudinal section). (From Scanlon, VC, and Sanders, T: Essentials of Anatomy and Physiology, ed 4. F. A. Davis, Philadelphia, 2003, p 352, with permission.)

LATIN PRONUNCIATION

In Latin, all consonants and vowels are pronounced, with no silent letters. The sound of the consonants is the same as in English, except that *c* and *g* are always "hard"; thus, *cancer* is pronounced "kanker," and the *g* of *genus* is pro-nounced like the *g* of gate. The letter *t* is always pro-nounced like the *t* in tin and never has the sound of the *t* in nation. It is customary to pronounce *i* like the *y* in yes and *v* like the *w* in win. Vowels may be long or short and are pronounced as follows:

Short Vowels	Long Vowels	Diphthongs
a as in adrift	$\bar{a}$ as in father	*ae* as ie in tie
e as in bet	$\bar{e}$ as in they	*au* as ou in house
i as in tin	$\bar{i}$ as in machine	*ei* as ei in eight
o as in hot	$\bar{o}$ as in tone	*oe* as oi in boil
u as oo in look	$\bar{u}$ as in rude	

Latin words are accentuated on the penult, the syllable next to last, if that syllable is long. A long syllable is one that contains a long vowel or a diphthong, or one in which the vowel, whether long or short, is followed by two con-sonants. If the second of two consonants is *l* or *r*, the syl-lable need not be considered long; *cerebrum* is accented on the antepenult. If the penult is short, the syllable before that, the antepenult, receives the accent.

NOMINATIVE SINGULAR

The nominative singular, the vocabulary form, of some words (*radix*, *tussis*, *abdomen*, *auris*, and *viscus*, for exam-ple) is used in medical terminology.

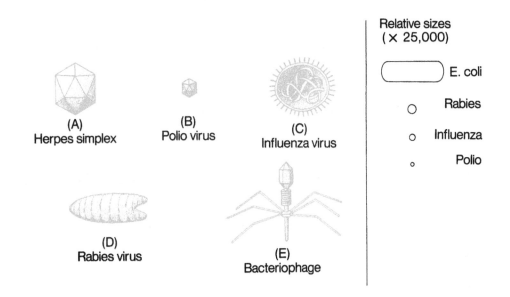

(A) Herpes simplex

(B) Polio virus

(C) Influenza virus

(D) Rabies virus

(E) Bacteriophage

Relative sizes (× 25,000)

E. coli

Rabies

Influenza

Polio

Figure 8–3. Viruses. (From Scanlon, VC, and Sanders, T: Essentials of Anatomy and Physiology, ed 4. F. A. Davis, Philadelphia, 2003, p 489, with permission.)

ETYMOLOGICAL NOTES

As spoken Latin gradually became French, a number of sound changes took place. The sound of an initial Latin *c*, when followed by *a*, usually developed into *ch* in French: Latin *caballus* (horse), French *cheval*; Latin *caldus* (hot), French *chaud*; Latin *castus* (pure), French *chaste*. Latin *cancer* (crab, ulcer) became French *chancre*, which is used with the same spelling in English. A **chancre** is a venereal ulcer, the first outward manifestation of syphilis. This disease takes its name from Syphilus, the hero of a kind of medical poem entitled *Syphilis sive Morbus Gallicus* (Syphilis, or the French Disease) by the Italian physician and poet Girolamo Fracastoro (1484–1553). In this poem, Syphilus suffered from an infectious disease that Fracastoro named syphilis, perhaps from the Greek verb *philein* (love).

Insulin (*insula*, island) takes its name from the islets of Langerhans, cell clusters in the pancreas. These cells are of three types: alpha, beta, and delta, and it is the beta cells that produce the protein hormone insulin, which regulates the metabolism of carbohydrates in the body. Deficient production or utilization of insulin causes **hyperglycemia** (Greek *glykys*, sweet), the characteristic of the disease **diabetes mellitus** (Latin *mel, mellis*, honey), commonly known as sugar diabetes. The islets of Langerhans were named after the German pathologist Paul Langerhans (1847–1888), who first realized their existence and function.

The words **vaccine** and **vaccination** come from the Latin *vacca* (cow). In 1789, Edward Jenner, an English country physician, announced to the world his discovery that injection of the cowpox virus into humans (i.e., vaccination) provided immunity against smallpox. It was known then that people who were employed on dairy farms and who happened to contract the bovine disease cowpox became immune to smallpox. Jenner began his experimentation in 1796 by inoculating a healthy young boy with matter taken from an ulcerating sore on the hand of a milkmaid suffering from cowpox. Later, this boy was inoculated with the smallpox virus and resisted the disease. This was the first vaccination. Smallpox has now virtually disappeared from the United States, Great Britain, and Europe, and in recent years mass vaccinations in Africa and Asia have reduced the incidence of this disease to isolated areas in these continents.

The English words viscous and viscid bear no relationship to the internal organs, the viscera, but are derived from Latin *viscum* (mistletoe) (Fig. 8–4). The ancient Romans prepared a sticky substance from the berries of the mistletoe plant that they spread on branches of trees. Unfortunate birds that perched on those branches were caught and held fast by this glutinous substance, which we call birdlime. The Roman poet Virgil writes of the olden days when men had to toil for their living and hunt for their food:

It was then that men found a way to snare wild beasts in nets, to trap birds with birdlime (*viscum*) and to surround

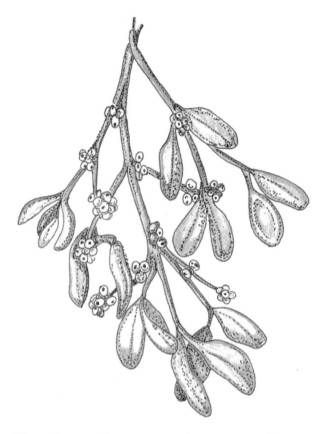

Figure 8–4. Mistletoe. (Drawing by Laine McCarthy, 2001.)

the huge groves of trees with hounds [*Georgics* 1.139–140].

The suffix **-ad**, which indicates direction toward a part of the body, as in the words **dextrad**, toward the right; **sinistrad**, toward the left; or **cephalad**, toward the head, entered the English language early in the 19th century after a proposal by the British scholar James Barclay in his work *New Anatomical Nomenclature* (1803) that it be used as an equivalent of -ward in English: **homeward, forward**, and so forth. The suffix **-ad** did not exist in Latin and seems to have been an adaptation of the prefix *ad-* (toward).

Aureolus Theophrastus Bombastus von Hohenheim (1493–1541), better known as Paracelsus, a name that is supposed to have been bestowed upon him as an indication of his superiority to the Roman physician Celsus, has been called the "precursor of chemical pharmacology and therapeutics, and the most original medical thinker of the 16th century."* The son of a physician, he became professor of medicine at Basle in 1527. He was a pioneer in chemistry who wrote extensively (in Latin) on medicine during a stormy career that ended in a tavern brawl in Salzburg. The word **synovia** is first found in his writing and seems to have been coined by him, perhaps from the Latin *ōvum* (egg) because of the viscous quality of this colorless fluid.

---

*An Introduction to the History of Medicine, Fielding H. Garrison, W. B. Saunders Company, Philadelphia, 1927.

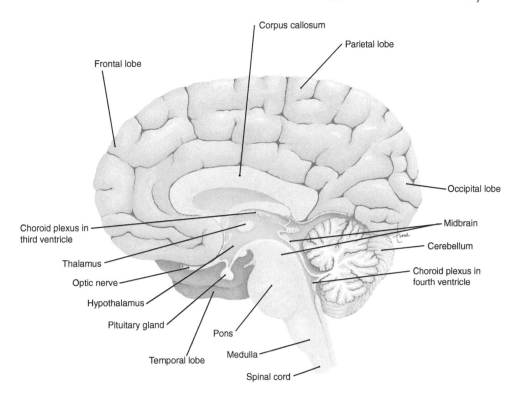

Figure 8–5. Midsagittal section of brain as seen from left. (From Scanlon, VC, and Sanders, T: Essentials of Anatomy and Physiology, ed 4. F. A. Davis, Philadelphia, 2003, p 167, with permission.)

Paracelsus considered synovia the nutritive fluid of the body, but its use by later physicians was restricted to the lubricating fluid secreted within synovial membranes of joints, bursae, and tendon sheaths. The word synovia has no etymology; it seems to have been the invention of Paracelsus.

The word **bursa** is first found in Medieval Latin and is derived from the Greek *byrsa* (skin, hide of an animal). This word meant a leather bag or sack, and later the term *bursa mucosa* was applied to a sac or cavity found in connective tissue and containing synovial fluid. One of the original senses of the word, that of a bag to hold money, is retained in the English words purse (where the letter *p* is unexplained), burse (a scholarship for school or university), bursar, disbursement, and so forth, and in the French *bourse*, meaning purse, and *Bourse*, the stock exchange of Paris. The Burse was the original Royal Exchange in London.

The Latin words *occipitium* and *occiput, occipitis* are compounds of the prefix *ob-* and *caput, capitis* (head), and meant the back part of the head, the **occiput** (Fig. 8–5). Latin *sinciput* was an abbreviated form of *semi-caput* and in Latin meant half of a head, in particular the smoked cheek or jowl of a hog. **Sinciput** now means the fore and upper part of the cranium, or the upper half of the skull. The words *occiput* and *sinciput* show a reduction of the *a* of *caput* to *i* in the nominative case and of the *u* to *i* in the genitive case.

This is believed to be because of a strong stress accent on the first syllable of Latin words that occurred during an early period of the development of the language. Other examples of this vowel reduction can be seen in **biceps**, two-headed, or **triceps**, three-headed, which are also from *caput*. This change can be seen more clearly in Latin verbs and in their derivatives in English.

The word *fistula* (tube, pipe) was used by Ovid in the *Metamorphoses* in a simile to describe how the blood of the unhappy lover Pyramus spurted from his body when he took his own life with a sword. Pyramus and Thisbe were a young couple of Babylon who lived next door to one another. They fell in love, but their parents forbade them to meet. However, they spoke to one another through a chink in the common wall that separated their houses, and at length decided to meet under a mulberry tree that was laden with snow-white berries at the nearby tomb of Ninus, an ancient king of Babylon. The young girl, Thisbe, arrived first at the appointed place that night and, as she waited, a lioness came along, fresh from the kill, to quench her thirst at a nearby pool. Thisbe fled in terror, dropping the thin cloak that she had brought along. When the lioness had drunk her fill, the beast found the cloak and mangled it with her bloodied jaws. Pyramus arrived shortly after and, seeing the bloodstained cloak and thinking that Thisbe had met a cruel death, drew his sword and fell upon it. As he lay there dying,

Cruor emicat alte,
non aliter quam cum vitiato fistula plumbo
scinditur et tenui stridente foramine longas
eiculatur aquas atque ictibus aera rumpit.
[*Metamorphoses* 4.121–124].

The blood gushed forth, just as water bursts through a broken pipe (*fistula*) and, with a strident sound, spurts through the air.

Ovid goes on to say that the fruit of the mulberry tree was stained with the crimson blood. Thisbe came out of her hiding place and found Pyramus with his life's blood ebbing. She fitted the point of the sword to her own breast and fell forward on the blade that was still warm from the blood of her lover. From that day on, the fruit of the mulberry tree reddens as it ripens, a remembrance of the lovers' blood that was shed there.

Exercise 1: Analyze and Define

Analyze and define each of the following words. In this and in succeeding exercises, analysis should consist of separating the words into prefixes (if any), combining forms, and suffixes or suffix forms (if any) and giving the meaning of each. Be certain to differentiate between nouns and adjectives in your definitions. Consult a medical dictionary for the current meanings of these words. Use a separate paper if you need more room for an answer.

1. adipose _____

2. adrenalin _____

3. auricula _____

4. auris externa* _____

5. bacillar _____

6. biceps _____

7. bursae _____

8. calcipenia _____

9. calcium† _____

10. calorimeter _____

*Latin *auris* is a feminine noun.
†This word was coined by Sir Humphry Davy based on the analogy of the names of other metals ending in *-ium*.

11. capitulum _____

12. cerebellum _____

13. costotome _____

14. denticle _____

15. diplobacillus _____

16. dorsad _____

17. externalize _____

18. fibromyoma _____

19. fistula _____

20. frigotherapy _____

21. insulin _____

22. internal _____

23. leiomyofibroma _____

24. meatoscopy _____

25. myelofibrosis _____

26. myofibril _____

27. nasal _____

28. neurotropic virus _____

29. nonose _____

30. occiput _____

31. osteosynovitis _____

32. pertussis _____

33. polyradiculitis* _____

34. postnasal _____

35. quadriplegia _____

36. purulent _____

37. radiculomeningomyelitis _____

38. radix _____

39. renogastric _____

40. retroviruses _____

41. sanguine _____

42. subaural _____

43. synovia _____

44. tubectomy _____

45. tussive _____

46. vaccine _____

47. viremia _____

*Words containing radic- and radicul- usually refer to roots of spinal nerves.

48. viscerotropic _____

49. viscus _____

50. ultrasonogram _____

Exercise 2: Word Derivation

Give the word derived from Greek and/or Latin elements that matches each of the following. Verify your answer in a medical dictionary. **Note that the wording of the dictionary definition may vary from the wording below.**

1. Plastic repair of any tube _____

2. Pertaining to a rib and its cartilage _____

3. Unit of heat _____

4. Pain in the abdomen _____

5. Study of the nose and its diseases _____

6. Agent that prevents or relieves coughing _____

7. Formation of calculi _____

8. Behind the ear _____

9. Cell that stores fat _____

10. (Morbid) fear of bacilli _____

11. Pertaining to the blood supply of the kidneys _____

12. Tumor arising from a synovial membrane _____

13. Calculus formed in a bursa _____

14. Head shaped _____

15. Situated toward the back of the head _____

16. Any disease of the brain _____

17. Device for measuring the size of an opening or a passage _____

18. Excessive amount of insulin (in the blood) _____

19. Development of fibrous tissue _____

20. Generalized enlargement of the internal [abdominal] organs _____

Exercise 3: Drill and Review

The meaning of each of the following words can be determined from its etymology. Determine the meaning of each word. Verify your answer in a medical dictionary.

1. abdominoplasty _____

2. abenteric _____

3. adipectomy _____

4. antepyretic _____

5. auris interna _____

6. avirulent _____

7. binotic _____

8. bursopathy _____

9. cerebellar ataxia _____

10. chronograph _____

11. circumrenal _____

12. chondrocostal _____

13. costalgia _____

14. decimeter _____

15. dentin _____

16. dorsodynia _____

17. extrahepatic _____

18. fibromyalgia _____

19. fistulatome _____

20. hemic calculus _____

21. homophobia _____

22. infracostal _____

23. insulinemia _____

24. interauricular _____

25. internalize _____

26. intracranial _____

27. myeloradiculodysplasia _____

28. nasogastric _____

29. nontoxic _____

30. occipital _____

31. parasynovitis _____

32. perivisceritis _____

33. pertussoid _____

34. polyblennia _____

35. posticteric _____

36. prenarcosis _____

37. purulent synovitis _____

38. renogram _____

39. retromorphosis _____

40. sanguineous _____

41. sincipital _____

42. sonometer _____

43. supervirulent _____

44. supradiaphragmatic _____

45. synovectomy _____

46. trigastric _____

47. tuborrhea _____

48. vaccinotherapeutics _____

49. virusemia _____

50. viscerotonia _____

LATIN VERBS

I would have given the name insectology *to that part of natural history which has insects as its object: that of* entomology *... would undoubtedly have been more suitable...but its barbarous sound terrify'd me.*

[Bennet's *Contemporary Natural History*, London 1776]

Earache and disorders of the ear are cured by the urine of a wild boar that has been kept in a glass jar, or by the gall of a wild boar or of a pig or an ox with equal portions of citrus and rose oil added. But the best cure of all is warm gall of a bull with leek juice. If there are suppurations, honey should be added, and if there is a foul odor the gall should be warmed with the rind of a pomegranate.

[Pliny, *Natural History* 28.48.173]

Most Latin verbs have four principal parts, as illustrated by *secō, secāre, secuī, sectus* (to cut).

Principal Part	Example	Meaning
1st: Present Active Indicative	*secō*	I cut
2nd: Present Active Infinitive	*secāre*	to cut
3rd: Perfect Active Indicative	*secuī*	I cut, have cut
4th: Perfect Passive Participle	*sectus*	having been cut

Latin verbs are divided into four classes, or groups, called **conjugations**. This classification is based on the stem vowel of the present infinitive, the second principal part of the verb. The ending of the present infinitive in the first conjugation is *-āre*, in the second it is *-ēre*, in the third, *-ere*, and in the fourth, *-īre*.

Latin verbs have three stems on which the various tenses are formed: the present, the perfect active, and the perfect passive. Only the first and third of these have been fruitful in furnishing English derivatives, and these are the only ones considered here. The first stem is that of the infinitive and the third is that of the perfect passive

participle, which is an adjective of the first and second declension, with the endings *-us*, *-a*, or *-um*, indicating masculine, feminine, or neuter gender, respectively. In this manual, the perfect passive participle is given with the ending *-us*, the form in which all such adjectives are cited here.

Thus, Latin verbs have two combining forms; the first is formed by dropping the ending of the infinitive and the second by dropping the *-us* of the perfect passive participle. The verb *dūcere, ductus* (lead, bring) has two combining forms, DUC- and DUCT-, giving the stem of such English derivatives as **induce**, **reduce**, **induction**, and **reduction**. As with Greek verbs, Latin verbs are customarily cited in Latin dictionaries and grammars in the form of the first person singular (*duco*, I lead; *cado*, I fall). English dictionaries usually cite Latin verbs in the form of the present infinitive, and that is how they are cited in this manual.

Some verbs appear only in the passive form but with active meanings. These are known as **deponent** verbs. The infinitives of the four conjugations of deponent verbs end in *-ārī*, *-ērī*, *-ī*, and *-īrī*. The combining form is found by dropping these endings. The deponent verb *patior, patī,*

Conjugation	Present Indicative	Present Infinitive	Perfect Indicative	Perfect Passive Participle
1st	*secō* (cut)	*secāre*	*secuī*	*sectus*
2nd	*habeō* (have)	*habēre*	*habuī*	*habitus*
3rd	*fundō* (pour)	*fundere*	*fūdī*	*fūsus*
4th	*sciō* (know)	*scīre*	*scīvī*	*scītus*

passus (endure, suffer) gives us such words as **patient**, **patience**, and **passion**.

SUFFIXES

Many suffixes are added only to the stems of verbs. Latin suffixes often undergo some changes in English words and are presented here in the form in which they appear in English.

-able: forms adjectives: capable of (being), able to:

ten-**able**   dur-**able**

-ation: forms nouns indicating an action or process: the act of (being), the result of (being), something that is:

gest-**ation**   form-**ation**

-ce: forms nouns: the act of (being), the state of (being):

patien-**ce**   innocen-**ce**

-cy: forms nouns: the act of (being), the state of (being):

constan-**cy**   hesitan-**cy**

-ible: forms adjectives: capable of (being):

aud-**ible**   divis-**ible**

-id: forms adjectives: in a state or condition of:

flu-**id**   tep-**id**

-ile: forms adjectives: capable of (being), like:

fac-**ile**   infant-**ile**

-ion: forms nouns: the act of:

tens-**ion**   correct-**ion**

-ive: forms adjectives: pertaining to:

act-**ive**   nat-**ive**

-ment: forms nouns: agent or instrument:

liga-**ment**   instru-**ment**

-or: forms nouns: agent or instrument:

abduct-**or**   invent-**or**

-orium: * forms nouns: place for something:

audit-**orium**   script-**orium**

-ory: * **(1)** forms adjectives: pertaining to:

exposit-**ory**   compuls-**ory**

(2) forms nouns: place for something:

dormit-**ory**   laborat-**ory**

-ure, -ura: form nouns: result of an action:

fiss-**ure**, fiss-**ura**   script-**ure**

ENGLISH SUFFIX -E

Note the use of the English suffix **-e** to form verbs from Latin infinitives: **reduce** (*dūcere*, lead), **excite** (*excitāre*, rouse), **inspire** (*spirāre*, breathe), and so forth.

PRESENT PARTICIPLES

The Latin present participle is a third-declension adjective that is formed on the stem of the present infinitive. The forms of the nominative and genitive singular are *-āns*, *-antis* for the first conjugation; *ēns*, *-entis* for the second and third; and *-iēns*, *-ientis* for some of the third and for the fourth conjugation. The combining form of participles is found by dropping the *-is* ending of the genitive case. In some instances this combining form becomes an English adjective translated with -ing added to the meaning of the verb, as in the following:

sonant (*sonāre*, sound)	sounding
latent (*latēre*, lie hidden)	lying hidden
cadent (*cadere*, fall)	falling
incipient (*incipere*, begin)	beginning
sentient (*sentīre*, feel)	feeling

In other instances, this combining form becomes an English noun meaning a person or thing that does something, as in the following:

inhabitant (*inhabitāre*, inhabit)	a person who inhabits
somnifacient (*somnus*, sleep and *facere*, make)	a drug that produces sleep

Most English derivatives of Latin present participles are abstract nouns ending in -ce or -cy. These endings repre-

---

* The suffixes -arium and -ary, with the same meaning as -orium and -ory, are usually found with nouns: sanitarium (*sānitās*, health), library (*liber*, book).

sent the -*t* of the present participle stem plus the abstract noun-forming suffix -*ia*; the resultant -*tia* becomes either -ce or -cy in English. These noun-forming suffixes mean the act of (being) or the state of (being), as in the following:

redundancy (*redundāre*, be superfluous)	the state of being redundant or superfluous
reverence (*reverēri*, revere)	the state of being revered
sequence (*sequī*, follow)	the act of following
science (*scīre*, know)	the state of knowing

Sometimes words have been formed in English as if from Latin present participles, although such verbs did not exist in Latin. Some of these words have been formed from Greek nouns and verbs: **intoxicant** (and **intoxicate**, as if from a Latin verb *intoxicāre*, *intoxicātus*). Note that intoxicant, as well as other similar formations, although structurally adjectives, are now used as nouns.

INCEPTIVE VERBS

The letters -**sc**- inserted between the stem and the ending of the Latin infinitive denote the beginning of an action. Example: *valere*, be well, *valescere*, begin to get well. The present participles of inceptive verbs give us many English derivatives. English: **convalescent**, beginning to get well.

VOWEL WEAKENING

During the prehistoric period in the development of the Latin language, there seems to have been a strong stress accent on the first syllable of words; as a result of this, vowels in internal syllables became weakened, both quantitatively and qualitatively. The effects of this can be seen in both nouns and verbs. The -*u*- of *caput* (head) becomes weakened to -*i*- in cases other than the nominative singular: *caput*, *capitis*. *Virgō* (maiden) loses the final -*n*- of the nominative singular, and the long -*o*- of the final syllable is reduced to short -*i*-: *virgō (n)*, *virginis*; *pater* (father), and *mater* (mother) drop the -*e*- of the final syllable: *patris*, *matris*.

This phenomenon is most apparent with verbs, especially when prefixes are added: *caedere*, *caesus* (cut): *incīdere*, *incīsus*, *dēcīdere*, *dēcīsus*; *capere*, *captus* (seize): *incipere*, *inceptus*, *recipere*, *receptus*; *facere*, *factus* (make): *efficere*, *effectus*, *inficere*, *infectus*. Sometimes the perfect passive participle was not affected by this change: cadere, *cāsus*, fall: *incidere*, *incāsus*. In the vocabularies in this manual, the verbal stems that undergo these changes are indicated by a dash before the stem in question: *facere*, *factus*, make: FAC-, FIC-, -FECT, and so forth.

Latin verbs often took on new and different meanings when compounded with prefixes. The verb *capere*, *captus*, meant to take; the compound verb *incipere*, *inceptus*, meant to take in hand, to undertake, and thus, to begin. The word incipient is from the present participle of this verb.

The Latin compound verb *inficere*, *infectus*, meaning to stain, dye, spoil, corrupt, gives rise to the word **infection**.

VOCABULARY

Note: Latin combining forms appear in ***bold italics***.

Latin	Combining Form(s)	Meaning	Example
anterior	*ANTER-*	front, in front	**anter**-ior
brāchium (Fig. 9–1)	*BRACHI-*	(upper) arm	**brachi**-um
caedere, *caesus*	*-CID-*, *-CIS-*	cut, kill	in-**cis**-or
capere, *captus*	*-CIP-*, *-CEPT-*	take	in-**cept**-ion
crescere, *crētus*	*CRESC-*, *-CRET-*	(begin to) grow	ex-**cresc**-ence
digitus	*DIGIT-*	finger, toe	**digit**-al
dūcere, *ductus*	*DUC-*, *DUCT-*	lead, bring, conduct	ab-**duct**
facere, *factus*	*FAC-*, *-FIC-*, *-FECT*	make	petri-**fac**-tion
faciēs	*FACI-*, *-FICI-*, *FACIES*	face, appearance, surface	super-**fici**-al
febris	*FEBR-*, *FEBRIS*	fever	**febr**-ile
ferre, *lātus*	*FER-*, *LAT-*	carry, bear	odori-**fer**-ous
flectere, *flexus*	*FLECT-*, *FLEX-*	bend	re-**flex**
fungus	*FUNG-*	[mushroom] fungus	**fung**-al
fundere, *fūsus*	*FUS-**	pour	dif-**fus**-e
gignere, *genitus*	*GENIT-*	bring forth, give birth	**genit**-al
gerere, *gestus*	*GER-*, *GEST-*	carry, bear	di-**gest**

Latin	Combining Form(s)	Meaning	Example
immūnis	*IMMUN(I)-*	[exempt] safe, protected	**immun**-ologist
inferior	*INFERIOR-*	below	**inferior**-ity
lābī, lapsus	*LAB-, LAPS-*	slide, slip	re-**laps**-e
latus, lateris	*LATER-*	side	**later**-al
ōs, ōris	*OR-, OS*	mouth, opening	**or**-al
ossa	*OSS-*	bone	**oss**-ify
pediculus	*PEDICUL-*	louse	**pedicul**-osis
posterior	*POSTER-, -POSTERIOR*	behind, in back	**poster**-olateral
secāre, sectus	*SECT-*	cut	re-**sect**
somnus	*SOMN-*	sleep	**somn**-olence
stabilis	*STABIL-, STABL-*	stable, fixed	**stabil**-e
superior	*SUPERIOR-*	above	**superior**-ity
tūmēre	*TUM(E)-*	be swollen	**tum**-or

*Both principal parts of Latin verbs are not always productive of English derivatives.

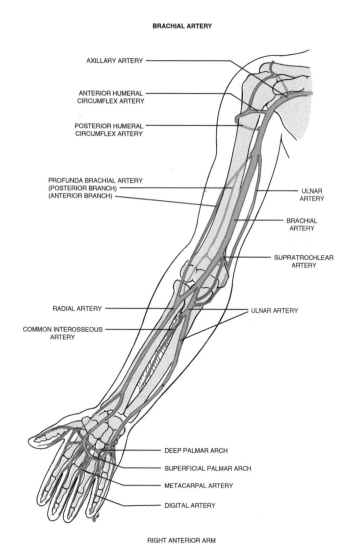

BRACHIAL ARTERY

AXILLARY ARTERY

ANTERIOR HUMERAL
CIRCUMFLEX ARTERY

POSTERIOR HUMERAL
CIRCUMFLEX ARTERY

PROFUNDA BRACHIAL ARTERY
(POSTERIOR BRANCH)
(ANTERIOR BRANCH)

ULNAR
ARTERY

BRACHIAL
ARTERY

SUPRATROCHLEAR
ARTERY

RADIAL ARTERY

ULNAR ARTERY

COMMON INTEROSSEOUS
ARTERY

DEEP PALMAR ARCH

SUPERFICIAL PALMAR ARCH

METACARPAL ARTERY

DIGITAL ARTERY

RIGHT ANTERIOR ARM

Figure 9–1. Brachial artery. (From Taber's Cyclopedic Medical Dictionary, ed 19. F. A. Davis, Philadelphia, 2001, p 271, with permission.)

COMBINING FORM -FY-

The combining form -FY- (make) is found in many English verbs. This is an adaptation in English of the French -fier, from Latin verbs in -ficāre, a first-conjugation form of *facere* found in compound verbs: *magnificāre*, make great; **magnify**; *sanctificare*, make holy, **sanctify**.

GENIT-

Many words containing **genit**-, often with the adjectival suffix **-al**, refer to the organs of the reproductive system: **genitoplasty**, **hypergenitalism**, and so forth.

PLANES OF THE BODY

A plane (Latin *plānum*) of the body is a flat surface formed by making an imaginary cut through the body. Planes are used as points of reference by which positions of parts of the body are indicated (Fig. 9–2). There are three principal planes of the body, all based on the assumption that the body is in an upright position:

midsagittal plane (Latin *sagitta*, arrow), also called the **sagittal** or **median** plane: a vertical plane dividing the body into two equal and symmetrical right and left halves

frontal plane (Latin *frons, frontis*, front), also called the **coronal** plane (Latin *corōna*, crown, borrowed from the Greek, *korōnē*): a vertical plane at right angles to the midsagittal plane dividing the body into anterior and posterior portions

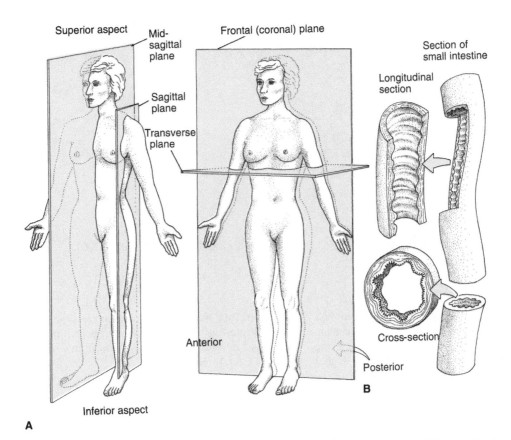

Figure 9–2. Body planes and sections. (From Scanlon, VC, and Sanders, T: Essentials of Anatomy and Physiology, ed 4. F. A. Davis, Philadelphia, 2003, p 14, top, with permission.)

transverse plane (Latin *trans-*, across, *versus*, turned), also called the **horizontal plane**: a horizontal plane across the center of the body and at right angles to the midsagittal and frontal planes dividing the body into upper and lower portions

Abduction of a limb is movement away from the median plane of the body, and **adduction** is movement toward the median plane (Fig. 9–3). An **abductor** is a muscle that on contraction draws a part away from the median plane, and an **adductor** is a muscle that draws a part toward the median plane.

ETYMOLOGICAL NOTES

Aristotle and Pliny discuss insects.

There are creatures called insects, as their name (*entoma*) indicates. They have incisions either on their upper or lower parts, or on both. They have neither separate bony parts (*ostōdes*) nor fleshy parts (*sarkōdes*) but consist of something intermediate, as their bodies, both inside and outside, are uniformly hard (*skleron*). [Aristotle, *History of Animals* 4.523b 13–18].

There are living creatures (*animalia*) of immeasurable minuteness which some people maintain do not breathe and are actually bloodless. There are great numbers and many kinds of these, some living on land and some in the air, some winged—bees, for example—some lacking wings—centipedes, for example—and some having the characteristics of both—ants, for example—and some lacking both wings and feet. All of these are correctly named insects (*insecta*), because of the incisions which encircle the necks of some, the chests or stomachs of oth-

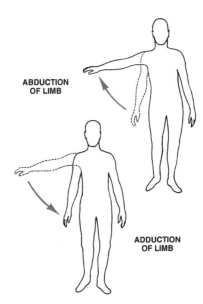

Figure 9–3. Abduction and adduction of limbs. (From Taber's Cyclopedic Medical Dictionary, ed 19. F. A. Davis, Philadelphia, 2001, p 5, with permission.)

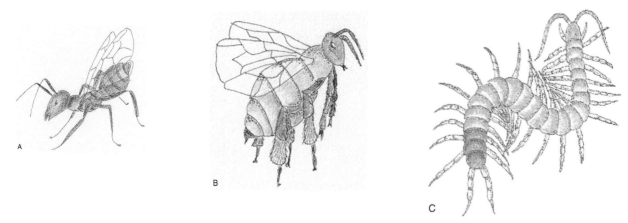

Figure 9–4. Insects. (*A*) Ant. (*B*) Bee. (*C*) Centipede. (Drawings by Laine McCarthy, 2001.)

ers, and, in others, which separate their limbs from their bodies, these being connected by a slender tube (*fistula*). With some of these the incision does not encircle the entire body, but lies like a wrinkle on the belly or higher up. They have vertebrae that are flexible like gutter-tiles, displaying nature's craftsmanship in a more remarkable fashion than anywhere else. [Pliny, *Natural History* 11.1.1.1] (Fig. 9–4)

Exercise 1: Analyze and Define

Analyze and define each of the following words. In this and in succeeding exercises, analysis should consist of separating the words into prefixes (if any), combining forms, and suffixes or suffix forms (if any) and giving the meaning of each. Be certain to differentiate between nouns and adjectives in your definitions. Consult a medical dictionary for the current meanings of these words.

1. abduct _____

2. ablation _____

3. adduct _____

4. afferent _____

5. antebrachium _____

6. anterolateral _____

7. areflexia _____

8. bisection _____

9. calcification _____

10. calorific _____

11. contralateral _____

12. decalcify _____

13. dentigerous _____

14. detoxify _____

15. digestion _____

16. digiti _____

17. dorsiflect _____

18. ductile _____

19. excrescence _____

20. frigolabile _____

21. fungi (pronounced funj'eye) _____

22. fungistasis _____

23. genitalia _____

24. gestosis _____

25. helminthicide _____

26. immunogenic _____

27. inception _____

28. incipient _____

29. incisor _____

30. ingestant _____

31. introflexion _____

32. intumesce _____

33. labile _____

34. orad _____

35. orifice _____

36. ossification _____

37. pediculus _____

38. posteroexternal _____

39. prolapsus _____

40. reflex _____

41. relapse _____

42. section _____

43. somnifacient _____

44. somnolent _____

45. stabile (pronounced stay'bile) _____

46. subfebrile _____

47. superficial _____

48. tumefaction _____

49. tumescence _____

50. virucidal _____

Exercise 2: Word Derivations

Give the word derived from Greek and/or Latin elements that matches each of the following. Verify your answers in a medical dictionary. **Note that the wording of the dictionary definition may vary from the wording below.**

1. (Passing from) front to rear _____

2. (Located) behind and above (a part) _____

3. Pertaining to the arm _____

4. Paralysis (of the muscles) on one side of the face (two words) _____

5. To cut out _____

6. Agent that destroys a virus _____

7. (Occurring) after a fever _____

8. Carrying away from (a central organ or section) _____

9. Containing calcium _____

10. (Prolonged or abnormal) inability to sleep _____

11. Agent that kills fungi _____

12. Surrounding the mouth _____

13. Capable of being cut _____

14. Infestation with lice _____

15. Pertaining to the nose and mouth _____

16. Incapable of being destroyed by low temperature _____

17. Pertaining to the teeth and face _____

18. (Opposite to or) away from the mouth _____

19. On the same side _____

20. To turn into bone _____

Exercise 3: Drill and Review

The meaning of each of the following words can be determined from its etymology. Determine the meaning of each word. Verify your answer in a medical dictionary.

1. aborad _____

2. adoral _____

3. afebrile _____

4. brachialgia _____

5. calcemia _____

6. concrescence _____

7. cyanhidrosis _____

8. cystigerous _____

9. cytocidal _____

10. decalcification _____

11. deossification _____

12. digitate _____

13. dorsiduction _____

14. ductule _____

15. excision _____

16. exsanguination _____

17. facial _____

18. faciobrachial _____

19. febrifacient _____

20. flexor _____

21. fungoid (pronounced fung'oid) _____

22. fungistatic _____

23. genitoplasty _____

24. hemifacial _____

25. hypergenitalism _____

26. immunology _____

27. incise _____

28. indigestible _____

29. ingestion _____

30. lateroflexion _____

31. leptophonia _____

32. leukocidin _____

33. melaniferous _____

34. microbicide _____

35. microgenitalism _____

36. ossific _____

37. pediculicide _____

38. pediculophobia _____

39. posterointernal _____

40. prolapse _____

41. prosopospasm _____

42. reflexogenic _____

43. resectable _____

44. sanguinopurulent _____

45. schizophrenia _____

46. somniferous _____

47. thermostabile _____

48. transection _____

49. tumefacient _____

50. viscerosomatic _____

BODY SYSTEMS

CARDIOVASCULAR SYSTEM

RESPIRATORY SYSTEM

DIGESTIVE SYSTEM

OPTIC SYSTEM

FEMALE REPRODUCTIVE SYSTEM

URINARY TRACT SYSTEM

10

CARDIOVASCULAR SYSTEM

If you kill a living animal by severing its great arteries, you will find that the veins become empty at the same time as the arteries. This could never happen unless there were anastomoses between them.

[Galen, *On the Natural Faculties* 3.15]

Advances were made in the field of medicine at the great institutions of learning in Alexandria, the Museum and the Library. Both were established in the early 3rd century BC by Ptolemy I, a former Macedonian general of Alexander the Great and the founder of the Ptolemaic dynasty in Egypt. The medical school there (as well as the other institutes) became the focal point for men of learning for many centuries. In the middle of the 2nd century AD, the physician Galen went there after studying at the Asclepium, the famed medical school in his native city of Pergamum in Asia Minor. Galen's theory of the movement of the blood in the human body influenced and even ruled medical thinking up to the 17th century, when William Harvey discovered that blood circulates. Harvey found that all blood that leaves the heart, after passing to the organs and parts of the body, returns to its point of departure, and then begins the process all over again. This discovery revolutionized medical thought and formed the basis for modern scientific medicine.

Galen believed that food was converted in the intestines into a fluid that he called chyle (Greek *chylos*, juice) [*On the Use of the Parts* 4.3], which was then carried to the liver, where it was transformed into blood and charged with a vapor or spirit. Unaware of the circulatory movement of the blood, he thought that this supercharged blood was then carried from the liver through the veins to the various parts of the body in a forward and backward movement. One part of Galen's theory on the movement of the blood is of special interest. He believed that some of the blood that was carried by the veins to the right ventricle of the heart, instead of flowing back through the veins to the liver, passed through the septum into the left ventricle by means of small passages between the right and left heart.

> The thinnest portion of the blood is drawn from the right cavity (*koilia*) of the heart into the left through passages in the septum (*diaphragma*) between these parts. These passages can be seen for the most part of their length; they are like pits with wide openings, but they keep getting narrower and it is not possible to see the end of them because of both their small size and the fact that the animal being dead, all of its parts are cold and shrunken [Galen, *On the Natural Faculties* 3.15].

Rigid adherence to the theory that blood passed directly through the septum from the right to the left ventricle prevented the realization of the true nature of the circulation of the blood for 15 centuries.

However, one man, the theologian Michael Servetus, dared to challenge the theories of Galen concerning the nature of the movement of the blood. Servetus was born in

1511 in Spain, studied theology at Toulouse in France, and then went to Paris to study medicine. This was early in the period of the Reformation, and Servetus held views that were considered almost heretical by both Catholics and Protestants. Along with his religious tracts, he wrote a work on physiology, the content of which, however, was clothed in the title *Christianismi restitutio* (Restitution of Christianity). The work was published in 1553; in it, Servetus challenged Galen's theory regarding the presence of a certain natural spirit that entered the blood in the liver. In addition, he maintained that the blood did not pass through the septum from the right to the left ventricle but rather that it passed from the right ventricle to the lungs, where it was purified by inspired air and then, lighter in color, was conveyed to the left ventricle. Servetus was arrested, tried for heresy, found guilty, and burned alive at Geneva on October 27, 1553. Although Servetus' book was burned with its writer, a few copies survived, and his theories undoubtedly exerted influence on later scientists. It took three quarters of a century before the actual circulation of the blood in the human body was perceived and made known.

In 1628, William Harvey, a fellow of the Royal College of Physicians in London, published his great work. It was written in Latin and was called *Exercitatio anatomica de motu cordis et sanguinis* (An Anatomical Treatise on the Motion of the Heart and Blood). Harvey's work was flawless as far as it went. It stopped short of completion only because in his time the microscope was not yet capable of revealing a clear image at high power. Harvey did not realize how the arterial blood passed into the veins via the capillaries. Marcello Malpighi's microscopic examination of the circulatory system of the frog revealed the action of the network of capillaries in joining the arterioles to the venules. His work, *De Pulmonibus* (On the Lungs), was published at Bologna in 1661.

CIRCULATION OF BLOOD

Blood commences its journey through the body as it is pumped from the upper end of the left ventricle into the great artery, the aorta (Figs. 10–1, 10–2). The aortic valve prevents the blood from flowing back into the ventricle (**aortic regurgitation**). Blood can flow in only one direction, away from the heart, the direction in which the entire arterial network carries the blood. As the blood moves away from the heart, it enters the many branches of the arteries, of which two (the **coronary arteries**) supply blood to the muscle of the heart. **Myocardial infarction** (MI) is the loss of living heart muscle as a result of **coronary artery occlusion**. MI usually occurs when an atheromatous plaque in a coronary artery ruptures and the resulting clot obstructs the injured blood vessel. Perfusion of the muscular tissue that lies downstream from the blocked artery is lost. If blood flow is not restored within a few hours, the heart muscle dies.

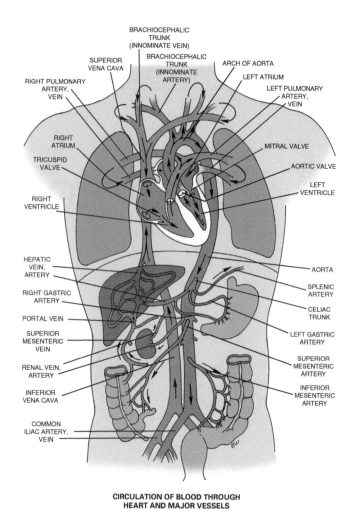

CIRCULATION OF BLOOD THROUGH HEART AND MAJOR VESSELS

Figure 10–1. Circulation of blood through heart and major vessels. (From Taber's Cyclopedic Medical Dictionary, ed 19. F. A. Davis, Philadelphia, 2001, p 407, with permission.)

As the arteries branch, they become increasingly smaller and are called arterioles, until they unite in a network of tiny vessels, the capillaries. Here the oxygenated blood from the left side of the heart delivers needed oxygen to the tissues of the body. From these microscopically small vessels, blood passes into the venules, small veins, and then into the venous system. The blood finally enters the right atrium through the two venae cavae. The superior vena cava returns blood from the organs and parts above the diaphragm (except the lungs), and the inferior vena cava returns blood from organs and tissues below the diaphragm.

From the right atrium, the blood passes through the tricuspid valve into the right ventricle. Here the blood begins another journey, the pulmonary or lesser circulation. Deoxygenated blood from the venous system returns to the heart and flows through the pulmonary circulation, where it is oxygenated in the capillary networks of the lung. The deoxygenated blood passes into the pulmonary artery, which branches out in the lungs, becoming smaller

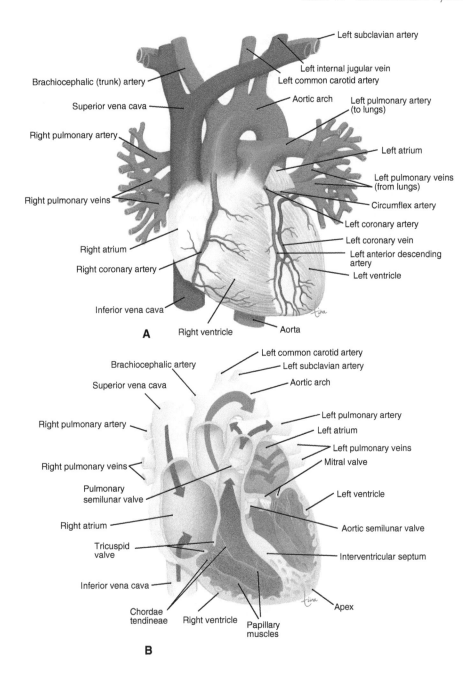

Figure 10–2. The heart. (*A*) Anterior view. (*B*) Frontal section. (From Scanlon, VC, and Sanders, T: Essentials of Anatomy and Physiology, ed 4. F. A. Davis, Philadelphia, 2003, p 262, with permission.)

and smaller. The arterioles unite with capillaries, which in turn unite with the pulmonary venules, which carry blood into the left atrium through the left superior and inferior pulmonary veins. From the left atrium, the blood enters the left ventricle through the mitral or bicuspid valve to start its journey all over again. The contractions of the cardiac muscle, which pumps about four quarts of blood per minute, are governed by the vagus nerve, which slows the muscular action, and the sympathetic nervous system,

which accelerates it. Regulation is achieved with a pacemaker, the sinoatrial node. If this natural pacemaker is defective, an electrical device called an artificial or electrical pacemaker can be installed either externally or internally to control the heartbeat through rhythmic electrical discharges. Defects and malfunctions, either congenital or acquired, along this complicated network of vessels and valves can cause numerous potentially fatal disorders that we call heart disease.

VOCABULARY

Life is short, the Art lasting, opportunity elusive, experiment perilous, judgment difficult. The physician must be ready not only to do what is necessary, but to see to it that his patient, the attendants, and all external arrangements are ready.[Hippocrates, Aphorisms 1.1]

Note: In the table below and throughout this text, Latin combining forms are shown in **bold italics**.

Greek or Latin	Combining Form(s)	Meaning	Example
amylon	**AMYL-**	starch	**amyl**-ase
angina	***ANGIN-***	choking pain, angina pectoris	**angin**-a
aortē	**AORT-**	aorta	**aort**-osclerosis
arctāre, arctātus	***ARCT(AT)-***	compress	aort-**arct**-ia
athērē	**ATHER-**	[soup] fatty deposit	**ather**-oma
ātrium	***ATRI-***	[entrance hall] atrium	**atri**-otome
bolē	**BOL-**	a throwing	em-**bol**-us
capillus	***CAPILL***	[hair] capillary	**capill**-ary
kirsos	**CIRS-**	dilated and twisted vein, varix	**cirs**-omphalos
claudere, clausus	***-CLUD-, -CLUS-***	close	oc-**clus**-ion
cor, cordis	***COR, CORD-***	heart	**cord**-ate
corōna	***CORON-***	crown	**coron**-al
cuspis, cuspidis	***CUSP, -CUSPID***	point	bi-**cuspid**
dexter	***DEXTR-***	right (side)	ambi-**dextr**-ous
forma	***-FORM***	shape	coli-**form**
gurgitāre, gurgitātus	***GURGIT-, GURGITAT-***	flood, flow	re-**gurgit**-ant
pectus, pectoris	***PECTOR-***	breast, chest	**pector**-al
phleps, phlebos	**PHLEB-**	vein	**phleb**-otomy
pulmō, pulmōnis	***PULM(ON)-***	lung, pulmonary artery	**pulmon**-itis
rhythmos	**RHYTHM-**	[steady motion] heartbeat	ar-**rhythm**-ic
saeptum	***SEPT-***	wall, partition	**sept**-um
sinus	***SIN-, SINUS-***	[curve, hollow] sinus	**sinus**-itis
sinister	***SINISTR-***	left (side)	**sinistr**-ocerebral
sphygmos	**SPHYGM-**	pulse	**sphygm**-oid
stellein	**STAL-, STOL-**	send, contraction	sy-**stol**-ic
tendere, tensus	***TENS(I)-***	stretch	hyper-**tens**-ive
thrombos	**THROMB-**	blood clot	**thromb**-osis
topos	**TOP-**	place	**top**-ical
vagus	***VAG-***	[wandering] the vagus nerve	vaso-**vag**-al
varix, varicis	***VARIC-, VARIX***	dilated and twisted vein, varix	**varic**-es
vās	***VAS-***	(blood) vessel; vas deferens	**vas**-ectomy
vēna	***VEN-***	vein	**ven**-ostat
venter, ventris	***VENTR-***	belly, abdomen, abdominal cavity	**ventr**-ose

ETYMOLOGICAL NOTES

I swear by Apollo the healer, by Asclepius, by Hygieia, by Panacea and by all the gods and goddesses as witnesses, that I will fulfill this oath and this covenant.[The beginning of the *Hippocratic Oath*]

Among Apollo's many attributes was the ability to heal the sick as well as to bring down destruction and death upon the wicked. After the time of Homer, Apollo was often called Paean, whom Homer calls the physician of the gods. As a healer, Apollo was outstripped by his son Asclepius, born to the nymph Coronis. Asclepius, who received his medical education from the famed centaur Chiron, became so skilled that not only was he able to heal the sick, he also acquired the ability to bring the dead back to life. This unusual talent was said to have angered Hades, the ruler of the Home of the Dead, and he complained to his brother Zeus that his realms were becoming depopulated. Zeus struck Asclepius dead with one of his lightning bolts.

Once, when Asclepius was pondering how to restore Glaucus, son of King Minos of Crete, to life, a snake coiled around his staff. He struck the creature and killed it. Later, a second snake came along carrying a leaf in its jaws and placed it upon the head of the dead snake. The serpent came to life, and Asclepius used the same medicament to restore Glaucus. And so a snake curled around the staff of Asclepius became the symbol of this great healer. It is now the symbol of the American Medical Association. (Fig. 10–3).

The words **systole** and **diastole** are from the Greek verb *stellein* (send). Systole refers to the period of contraction of the heart when the blood is sent through the aorta and the pulmonary artery. Diastole is the period of expansion when the heart dilates and the atria and ventricles fill with blood from the venae cavae and the pulmonary vein. Blood pressure is taken by means of an inflatable cloth cuff known as a **sphygmomanometer** (Greek *manos*, occurring at intervals), which is placed around the upper arm. Air is pumped into the sphygmomanometer (commonly referred to as a blood pressure cuff) by compressing a bulb, and the cuff expands, compressing the patient's arm. This compression causes a column of mercury to rise, indicating the pressure within the cuff. Once the pressure is sufficient to stop the flow of blood through the brachial artery, which is detected by listening to the heartbeat through a stethoscope pressed against the patient's arm, the pressure is released. When the heartbeat is once again audible, the level of the column of mercury indicates the systolic pressure. As more air is let out of the cuff, the pulse fades for a moment. The level of the mercury at this point indicates the diastolic pressure.

The **mitral** valve of the heart lies between the left atrium and the left ventricle and allows passage of blood from the atrium into the ventricle. It is a one-way valve, and a

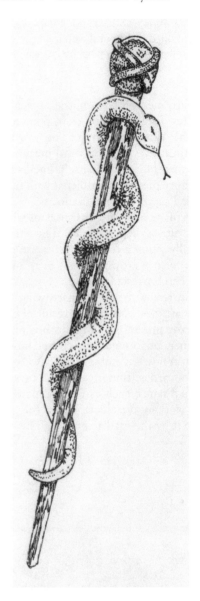

Figure 10–3. The Staff of Asclepius. (Drawing by Laine McCarthy, 2002.)

mitral defect can cause **mitral regurgitation**, a backflowing of the blood. It is also called the bicuspid valve because of its two cusps. The Latin word *mitral* comes originally from the Greek word *mitra*, referring to a type of turban worn by certain people of Asia Minor. In Virgil's *Aeneid*, the Moorish king Iarbas was scorned by Dido, a Phoenician princess who had recently settled in North Africa. On hearing that Dido and Aeneas, a wanderer from Troy, were openly flaunting their love, Iarbas prayed to Jupiter for vengeance, referring contemptuously to Aeneas as another Paris:

et nunc ille Paris cum semiviro comitatu,
Maeonia mentum mitra crinemque madentem
subnixus, rapto potitur.

And now that Paris with his band of half-men,
his chin and oiled hair bound with a
Maeonian miter, possesses what he has stolen.

[*Aeneid* 4.215–217]

The modern medical term mitral comes directly from the word miter or mitre, a tall, cleft, pointed hat worn by bishops of the Western church. The word valve comes from the Latin *valvae*, a plural word meaning a particular kind of door that folded within itself. **Facies mitralis** is the facial appearance of a person afflicted with mitral malfunction: distended capillaries and cyanosis.

There are many and various causes of what is referred to as a heart attack or as a stroke. The site of the initial attack is usually either a coronary artery, so called because these vessels form a crown (*corōna*) over and around the heart, or the cerebrovascular system (Fig. 10–4). Coronary artery disease results from the narrowing or closing of the coronary arteries, usually as a result of either **atherosclerosis** or the presence of a **thrombus** or an **embolus**. An embolus may be formed from clotted blood and thus is a form of thrombus. An embolus can also be formed from a portion of a cardiac tumor, such as a myxoma, or from any foreign substance such as fibrous matter, fat, or gas. The artery is then unable to carry the blood that is pumped into it by the cardiac muscle. The resulting con-dition, called **coronary occlusion** or **coronary thrombosis**, can and often does lead to **ischemia**, which can be the cause of **myocardial infarction**, cardiac arrest, and sudden death.

An **aneurysm** (Greek *ana-*, up, *eurys*, wide, *-m(a)*, noun-forming suffix) is the local distention of the wall of a blood vessel, usually an artery, and often the aorta (Fig. 10–5). The dilation is caused by a weakening of the vascular wall, often as a result of arteriosclerosis coupled with hypertension. Aneurysms of the aorta may occur anywhere along this great artery. They often occur in the abdominal region (abdominal aortic aneurysm [AAA]) or in the area of the pulmonary arteries (thoracic aortic aneurysm [TAA]). Rupture of an aneurysm with subsequent massive hemorrhage is a frequent cause of death.

Cerebral **apoplexy**, or stroke, is caused by intracerebral hemorrhage (often resulting from an aneurysm) or by thrombosis, embolism, or a reduction in or loss of the blood supply to the brain (vascular insufficiency).

Digitalis (Latin *digitus*, finger), a heart stimulant that acts by increasing the force of muscular contractions, is made of the dried leaves of the plant *Digitalis purpurea*, so called because of the fingerlike shape of its corolla.

The Greek verb *ballein* (throw) has many derivatives. The science of projectiles is **ballistics**. But it is in the form BOL-, from the noun *bolē* (a throwing), that it is most pro-

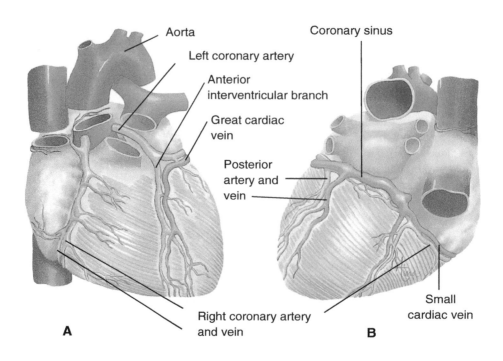

Figure 10–4. Coronary arteries. (*A*) Anterior (*B*) Posterior. (From Scanlon, VC, and Sanders, T: Essentials of Anatomy and Physiology, ed 4. F. A. Davis, Philadelphia, 2003, p 263, with permission.)

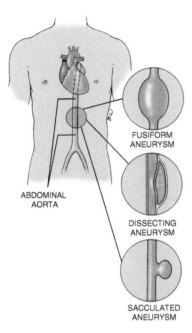

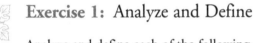

FUSIFORM
ANEURYSM

ABDOMINAL
AORTA

DISSECTING
ANEURYSM

SACCULATED
ANEURYSM

AORTIC ANEURYSMS

Figure 10–5. Aortic aneurysms. (From Taber's Cyclopedic Medical Dictionary, ed 19. F. A. Davis, Philadelphia, 2001, p 110, with permission.)

ductive. An **embolism** is the blockage of a blood vessel by any mass of nondissolved matter, a blood clot, or an air bubble. **Metabolism** is the sum of the processes of **anabolism**, the process by which the blood supplies the material for growth and repair of tissues, and **catabolism**, the process by which complex compounds are reduced to simpler ones, usually accompanied by the release of energy.

The verb *diaballein*, meaning throw across, had a secondary meaning of slander, make a false accusation. From this verb the noun *diabolē* (slander) was formed. The noun *diabolos* meant one who slanders, an evil person. This word is found in the Septuagint (I *Chron.*, 21.1) meaning the enemy, or Satan. Matthew (4.1) writes, "At that time Jesus was led into the wilderness by the Spirit, and there he was tempted by the devil (*diabolos*)."* When the Scriptures were translated into Old English, the Latin *diabolus* of the Vulgate was translated as *deofol* (devil). *Diabolos* remains in English in the word **diabolic** (devilish).

Exercise 1: Analyze and Define

Analyze and define each of the following words. In this and in succeeding exercises, analysis should consist of separating the words into prefixes (if any), combining forms, and suffixes or suffix forms (if any) and giving the meaning of each. Be certain to differentiate between nouns and adjectives in your definitions. Consult a medical dictionary for the current meanings of these words.

1. amylase _____

2. amylolysis _____

3. anginoid _____

4. aortoclasia _____

5. arctation _____

6. atheroma _____

7. atheronecrosis _____

8. atriotome _____

9. capillarectasia _____

10. cirsomphalos _____

11. cirsotome _____

12. coliform _____

13. corona dentis _____

14. coroner _____

15. cusp _____

16. dextrocardia _____

17. ectopia cordis _____

18. endaortitis _____

19. entopic _____

20. expectoration _____

21. extravasation _____

22. formation _____

23. hypertension _____

24. hypotensive _____

25. nasoseptitis _____

26. nonseptate _____

27. occlude _____

28. pectorophony _____

29. phlebectopia _____

30. phlebomyomatosis _____

31. pulmometry _____

32. regurgitant _____

33. sinistrocerebral _____

34. sinogram _____

35. systole _____

36. tachyarrhythmia _____

37. tensiometer _____

38. thrombectomy _____

39. thromboclasis _____

40. topagnosis _____

41. toponarcosis _____

42. vagotropism _____

43. vagus _____

44. varices _____

45. vascular _____

46. vasectomy _____

47. vasovagal _____

48. venostasis _____

49. ventricle _____

50. ventroscopy _____

Exercise 2: Word Derivations

Give the word derived from Greek and/or Latin elements that matches each of the following. Verify your answer in a medical dictionary. **Note that the wording of the dictionary definition may vary from the wording below.**

1. Production of starch _____

2. Irregularity or loss of rhythm, especially of the heart _____

3. Capillary disorder or disease _____

4. Excision (of a portion) of a (varicose) vein _____

5. Shaped like a heart _____

6. Toward the right (side) _____

7. Having the stomach on the right side of the body _____

8. Within the lungs _____

9. Pain in the chest _____

10. Formation of stones in the veins _____

11. Having better hearing with the left ear _____

12. Resembling a sinus _____

13. Shaped like a crown _____

14. Instrument for measuring the pulse _____

15. Process or act of stretching _____

16. Producing a blood clot _____

17. Fear of being in a (particular) place _____

18. Having three points _____

19. Small varix _____

20. Incision into the abdominal cavity _____

Exercise 3: Drill and Review

The meaning of each of the following words can be determined from its etymology. Determine the meaning of each word and verify your answer in a medical dictionary.

1. amylophagia _____

2. anginophobia _____

3. aortarctia _____

4. asystolia _____

5. atheromatosis _____

6. bradyarrhythmia _____

7. capillaroscopy _____

8. cirsotomy _____

9. cordiform _____

10. coronavirus _____

11. dentoid _____

12. dextral _____

13. dolichofacial _____

14. dysrhythmia _____

15. ectopia renis _____

16. febrifacient _____

17. frigorific _____

18. homogeneous _____

19. immunobiology _____

20. indentation _____

21. interatrial _____

22. kleptomaniac _____

23. meningovascular _____

24. mesodiastolic _____

25. nyctophilia _____

26. osteothrombosis _____

27. pectoral _____

28. peristaltic _____

29. phlebolith _____

30. polysinusitis _____

31. prediastolic _____

32. protospasm _____

33. pulmonologist _____

34. sanguiferous _____

35. septotome _____

36. sinistral _____

37. sphygmogram _____

38. stereognosis _____

39. subpulmonary _____

40. systolic _____

41. thromboendocarditis _____

42. toponeurosis _____

43. tracheloschisis _____

44. vagitis _____

45. varicophlebitis _____

46. vasculitis _____

47. vasorrhaphy _____

48. venectasia _____

49. venosclerosis _____

50. ventricular _____

RESPIRATORY SYSTEM

It is through the veins that we take in most of our breath, for they are the vents of the body, taking in the air and bringing it to the smaller vessels where it is cooled and then released.

[Hippocrates, *The Sacred Disease* 7]

All organs, parts, tissues, and cells of the body require oxygen to function. The purpose of the respiratory system is to provide the blood with air in order for the blood to carry oxygen to all parts of the body. In all cells of the body, oxygen is exchanged for carbon dioxide, which is carried in the bloodstream to the lungs to be discharged into the atmosphere. The process of the inspiration (breathing or inhaling) of oxygen and expiration (breathing out or exhaling) of carbon dioxide is called **respiration.** This is one of the vital processes of life. (Fig.11-1).

Air enters the body through the nose and mouth and travels downward through the pharynx and larynx, past the vocal cords, and into the trachea or windpipe. The trachea branches into two tubes, the right and the left bronchi, which enter the lungs (Fig. 11–2). After these bronchial tubes enter the lungs, they branch off into increasingly smaller tubes called bronchioles until they finally reach a dead end. The inner surface of the lungs is lined with innumerable tiny sacs called alveoli, which become filled with air at each inspiration (Fig. 11–3). The pulmonary arteries from the heart branch off into arterioles in the lungs and then into capillaries. Blood in the capillaries receives the oxygen from the alveoli as the hemoglobin molecules in the blood become saturated with oxygen from the alveoli. Hemoglobin saturated with oxygen is called **oxyhemoglobin.** As the blood becomes oxygenated, it discharges carbon dioxide, which passes to the alveoli and is then exhaled. The oxygenated blood passes from the capillaries into the pulmonary veins to be carried back to the heart and pumped to all parts of the body to exchange oxygen for carbon dioxide, and the process commences all over again. This exchange, the crucial part of the process of respiration, normally takes place about 18 times per minute in the human body, from the moment of birth to the instant of death. Of anatomic note, the pulmonary vein is the only vein in the body that carries oxygenated blood, whereas the pulmonary artery is the only artery that carries deoxygenated blood.

Each lung is enclosed within a sac called the pleura, which has two layers: the inner or visceral, and the outer or parietal (pronounced par-eye′-et-al, Latin *pariēs, pariētis,* wall). Normally, there is no space within these two layers except for a thin film of lubricating fluid. In certain lung diseases, however, a space may be forced between these layers by the accumulation of fluid, **hydrothorax**; by the accumulation of blood, **hemothorax**, which is caused by the rupture of small blood vessels in pulmonary disorders; or by the accumulation of air, **pneumothorax**, which is caused by perforation of the pleura that allows air to enter and fill this pleural space.

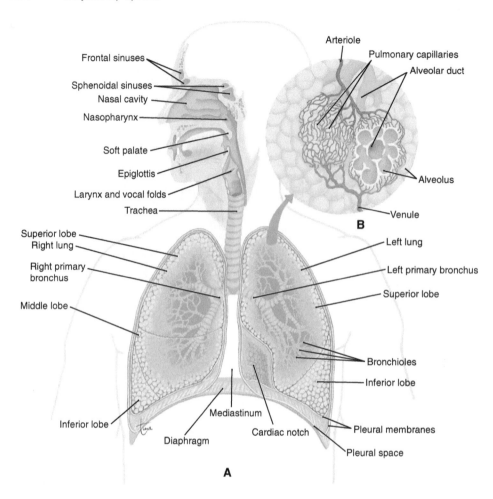

Figure 11–1. Respiratory system. (*A*) Anterior view. (*B*) Alveoli and pulmonary capillaries. (From Taber's Cyclopedic Medical Dictionary, ed 19. F. A. Davis, Philadelphia, 2001, p 2036, with permission.)

The lungs, with their pleural sacs, are separated from one another by a cavity called the **mediastinum**. The word mediastinum is a New Latin formation meaning in the middle, from Medieval Latin *mediastanus* (intermedial), from Latin *medius* (middle). Beneath the lungs lies a muscular membrane, the diaphragm, which flattens and contracts during inspiration, allowing air to be drawn into the lungs and expelling air from the lungs. The entire area between the diaphragm and the base of the neck is called the thorax. The thoracic cavity contains the heart, the lungs, and the origins of the great blood vessels.

Any interference with the flow of air into and out of the lungs is a potential cause of pulmonary disease, and any interference with the exchange of oxygen and carbon dioxide is a potential cause of respiratory failure. Interference with the process of respiration can result from disorders of the central nervous system; chemical changes in the blood; bacterial and viral invasion; and physical changes in the respiratory organs caused by inhaling irritating material, such as asbestos.

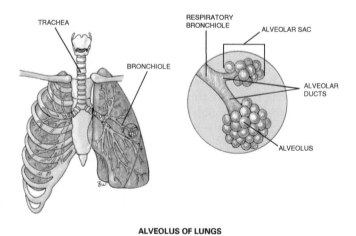

ALVEOLUS OF LUNGS

Figure 11–2. Lungs. Anterior view of (*A*) upper and lower respiratory tracts and (*B*) alveoli and pulmonary capillaries. (From Scanlon, VC, and Sanders, T: Essentials of Anatomy and Physiology, ed 4. F. A. Davis, Philadelphia, 2003, p 330, with permission.)

VOCABULARY

I especially approve of a physician who in the acute diseases, those which are fatal to the majority of the people, shows a certain amount of superiority over the others.

These acute diseases are those which the ancients have named pleurisy, pneumonia, phrenitis, intense fever, and other diseases in which fever is generally unremitting [Hippocrates, Regimen in Acute Diseases 5].

Note: Latin combining forms are shown in ***bold italics***.

Greek or Latin	Combining Form(s)	Meaning	Example
alveus	***ALVE-****	hollow, cavity	**alve**-us
amygdalē	**AMYGDAL-**	[almond] tonsil	**amygdal**-ine
anthrax, anthrakos	**ANTHRAX, ANTHRAC-**	coal; anthrax	**anthrac**-oid
auxein	**AUX-, -AUXE,† -AUXIS**	grow, increase	**aux**-in
baktērion‡	**BACTER(I)-**	[small staff] bacterium	**bacteri**-a
bronchos	**BRONCH(I)-§**	[windpipe] bronchus	**bronchi**-al
kapnos	**CAPN-**	[smoke] carbon dioxide	hypo-**capn**-ia
kokkos	**COCC-, -COCCUS**	[berry] coccus (a type of spherical bacterium)	strepto-**coccus**
konis	**CONI-, KONI-**	dust	**coni**-ofibrosis
labium	***LABI-***	lip	**labi**-onasal
larynx, laryngos	**LARYNX, LARYNG-**	larynx	**laryng**-itis
paresis¶	**PARESIS**	slackening of strength, paralysis	vaso-**paresis**
pharynx, pharyngos	**PHARYNX, PHARYNG-**	[throat] pharynx	**pharyng**-eal
physa	**PHYS-**	air, gas	**phys**-ometra
pleura	**PLEUR-**	[side] pleura	**pleur**-itis
pnein	**PNE-**	breathe	a-**pne**-a
pneuma, pneumatos	**PNEUM(AT)-**	[breath] air, gas	**pneum**-arthrosis
pneumōn	**PNEUM(ON)-**	lung	**pneumon**-ia
sidēros	**SIDER-**	iron	**sider**-ocyte
spīrāre, spīrātus	***SPIR(AT)-***	breathe	a-**spirat**-or
staphylē	**STAPHYL-**	[bunch of grapes] uvula, palate; staphylococci (microorganisms that cluster together like a bunch of grapes)	**staphyl**-oderma
sternon	**STERN-**	chest, breast, breastbone	**stern**-ocostal
stēthos	**STETH-**	chest, breast	**steth**-oscope
streptos	**STREPT-**	[twisted] streptococci (microorganisms that form twisted chains)	**strept**-icemia
sūdor	***SUD(OR)-***	sweat, fluid	tran-**sud**-ate
thōrax, thōrakos	**THORAX, THORAC-**	chest cavity, pleural cavity, thorax	pneumo-**thorax**
trachys	**TRACH(E)-, TRACHY-**	[rough] trachea	**trache**-ostomy

*Words containing the diminutive form alveol- refer to alveoli of the lungs or to dental alveoli.
†These forms of aux-, auxe-, and -auxin indicate nouns meaning increase in size, abnormal growth of a part.
‡*bacterium* (plural, *bacteria*) is the Latinized form of this word.
§Words beginning with, ending with, or containing bronchi- are from *bronchia*, the bronchial tubes.
¶The Greek noun *paresis* is formed from the preposition *para* and the verb *hienai* (send, throw). The compound verb *parienai* meant to let fall, and thus the noun *paresis* meant falling or slackening (of strength).

ETYMOLOGICAL NOTES

In the winter occur pleurisy, pneumonia, colds, sore throat, coughs, pains in the side, chest, and hip, headache, dizziness, and apoplexy. [Hippocrates, *Aphorisms* 23]
Those with hemorrhoids do not get pleurisy or pneumonia [Hippocrates, *Humors* 20].

Diphtheria (Greek *diphthera*, leather) takes its name from a leatherlike false membrane composed of pus and dead cells that forms on the mucous surfaces of the air passages, a characteristic manifestation of this disease. It is caused by the diphtheria bacterium *Corynebacterium diphtheriae*, named from the Greek *korynē*, club, from the clublike shape of these bacteria), which lodges in the throat and trachea, producing exotoxins that are lethal to the cells of the adjacent tissues. As the disease progresses, this leatherlike false membrane causes difficulty in swallowing. If the air passages become sufficiently swollen, **tracheostomy** or **intubation** may be necessary to provide a respiratory passage. The word **trachea** is from Greek *tracheia*, the feminine form of this adjective, originally modifying the feminine noun *artēria* (artery). The ancient Greek anatomists thought that the arteries carried air (*aēr*, air, *tērein*, guard); the windpipe, or trachea, was called the "rough artery" because of the rings of cartilage that surround it.

Emphysema, a condition that results most often from cigarette smoking or exposure to other pollutants, takes its name from the Greek *emphysēma*, meaning a swelling or inflation, from the verb *emphysan* (inflate). Emphysema is a form of chronic obstructive pulmonary disease (COPD), which affects millions of smokers. The significance of the name is that the disease is characterized by an increase in the size of the terminal air spaces, which causes an excess of air in the lungs (hyperinflation) and destruction of the alveolar walls. The lung loses its normal elasticity, and inspiration and expiration require muscular effort. **Hypoventilation** then results in impaired gas exchange, leading to **hypoxia** and **hypercapnia**. Cardiac function may become disturbed and death may occur.

Influenza, or grippe, is a contagious respiratory viral infection; symptoms are coryza (inflammation of the nasal mucous membrane with profuse discharge from the nostrils, commonly called a cold), cough, sore throat, myalgia, and general weakness. It takes its name from the Italian *influenza*, influence (literally, a flowing upon). In the 16th century and later, the name was applied to various epidemic diseases afflicting the people of Italy, which were thought to descend from the heavens. In 1743, it was applied specifically to the disease that we know as influenza, then called *la grippe*, which was ravaging Western Europe.

Pneumonia is an inflammation of the lungs usually resulting from infections caused by bacteria, viruses, or other pathogenic organisms. The most common of the bacterial agents are **streptococci, staphylococci**, and certain atypical bacteria. Pneumococcal or lobar pneumonia

(caused by **pneumococci**) usually invades one or more entire lobes of the lungs. Signs of pneumococcal pneumonia include chill, cough, chest pain, expectoration of rust-colored sputum, and, as the disease progresses, tachypnea, tachycardia, and cyanosis. Prompt treatment with appropriate antibiotics generally ensures early recovery. Although pneumococci used to be uniformly sensitive to treatment with penicillins, drug-resistant strains are exceptionally common, making the choice of antibiotic therapy increasingly difficult. Pneumonias in immunocompromised patients are sometimes caused by *Pneumocystis carinii* (*P. carinii*) or by fungal species such as *Aspergillus* or *Candida*. *P. carinii*, also known as PCP, has been a common cause of death in patients with acquired immunodeficiency syndrome (AIDS). The development of active antiretroviral drug cocktails has restored immune function to AIDS patients and reduced the incidence of PCP.

Sir Alexander Fleming (1881–1955), the British bacteriologist, applied the term **penicillin** to a culture of certain molds that he observed inhibiting the growth of bacteria. These molds were two of the genus *Penicillium*, named from the Latin *pēnicillum* (brush), because of the brushlike or broomlike appearance of the mold under microscopy. The Latin *pēnicillum* is a diminutive of *pēnis*, the original meaning of which was tail.

Anthrax is a highly infectious disease caused by the spore-forming bacteria *Bacillus anthracis*. Anthrax commonly attacks hoofed animals, particularly goats, horses, sheep, and cattle. Humans can acquire anthrax from exposure to infected animals or their hair and wool, hide, or waste matter. One manifestation of the disease in humans is cutaneous anthrax (Latin *cutis*, skin). This is characterized by the eruption of reddish carbuncles (Latin *carbunculus*, diminutive of *carbō*, *carbōnis*, coal) called anthrax boils, accompanied by localized erythema of the skin. The disease gets its name from the color of this inflammation, which looks like burning coal or charcoal. Another form of this disease is inhalation anthrax, which attacks the mediastinum, causing hemorrhage and pulmonary edema, and may also involve the gastrointestinal tract. Inhalation anthrax is also called **woolsorter's disease** and **ragsorter's disease**.

Anthrax is a potential agent for use in **biological warfare** or bioterrorism. Most bioterrorism experts have concluded that it is technologically difficult to use anthrax effectively as a weapon on a large scale because anthrax cannot be spread from person to person.

There are a number of respiratory diseases caused by exposure to occupational pulmonary irritants. These usually lead to a fibrotic interstitial lung disease such as **anthracosis**, also known as black lung, a disease often suffered by coal miners. Anthracosis is characterized by carbon deposits within the lungs due to inhalation of smoke or coal dust. **Byssinosis** affects those who work in cotton mills. **Silicosis** affects those who work in granite and sandstone industries. Bronchial carcinoma can result from **asbestosis** in those who are exposed for any length of time to the fibers of asbestos. **Siderosis** affects iron and steel workers and welders. **Silo filler's disease**, which affects those who work in grain silos, is caused by exposure to nitrogen dioxide and is characterized by irritation of the eyes and pharynx and damage to the lungs.

Tuberculosis (TB) is a disease caused by *Mycobacterium tuberculosis*. It usually affects the respiratory system, but may attack other body systems. In pulmonary TB, the most common form of this disease, early signs are the development of lesions of the lung tissues. These lesions, collections of giant cells, are called **tubercles** (little swellings), from which the disease gets its name. Pulmonary TB is also known as **consumption**. It has been called "the great imitator" because of its various clinical presentations and the multiplicity of organs affected. Pulmonary TB was known to the ancient Greek physicians as *phthisis* (a wasting illness).

> In the case of those who are afflicted with phthisis, if the sputum that is coughed up has an offensive smell when poured upon hot coals, and if the hair falls from the head, the disease will be fatal [Hippocrates, *Aphorisms* 5.11].

The incidence of TB declined steadily from the 1950s until about 1990, when the AIDS epidemic, an increase in the homeless population, an increase in immigrants from endemic areas, and a decrease in public surveillance caused a resurgence of the disease. Populations at greatest risk for TB include patients infected with human immunodeficiency virus (HIV), Asian and other refugees, the urban homeless, alcoholics and other substance abusers, people incarcerated in prisons or psychiatric facilities, nursing home residents, patients taking immunosuppressive drugs (as is the case with organ transplant recipients), and people with chronic respiratory disorders, diabetes mellitus, renal failure, or malnutrition. People from these risk groups should be assessed for TB if they develop pneumonia; all health-care workers should be tested annually.

Pertussis, commonly known as whooping cough, is caused by the bacillus *Bordetella pertussis*, first isolated and identified by Jules Bordet, a Belgian physician and bacteriologist (1870–1961), and Octave Gengou, a French bacteriologist, and named after Bordet. Routine immunization beginning at 2 months of age prevents this disease.

The Greek word *sphygmos* (pulse) had an alternate form *sphyxis*, most commonly found in the word **asphyxia**, lack of a pulse. This word has now come to mean a condition caused by insufficient intake of oxygen. Its adjectival form, **asphyctic**, means either pertaining to, affected with asphyxia, or without a pulse. Modern derivatives of Greek *asphyxia* include **asphyxiate**, **asphyxiated**, and **asphyxiation**, all having to do with suffocation, the lack of oxygen.

Exercise 1: Analyze and Define

Analyze and define each of the following words. In this and in succeeding exercises, analysis should consist of separating the words into prefixes (if any), combining forms, and suffixes or suffix forms (if any) and giving the meaning of each. Be certain to differentiate between nouns and adjectives in your definitions. Consult a medical dictionary for the current meanings of these words.

1. alveolar _____

2. amygdalopathy _____

3. anthracosis _____

4. anthrax _____

5. antisudorific _____

6. apnea _____

7. aspiration _____

8. auxin _____

9. bacteriolysin _____

10. bacteriophage _____

11. bronchiolectasis _____

12. coccobacilli _____

13. coniosis _____

14. dermatoconiosis _____

15. diplococcemia _____

16. dyspnea _____

17. hemilaryngectomy _____

18. hydropneumothorax _____

19. hypocapnia _____

20. koniometer _____

21. labiomycosis _____

22. laryngismus _____

23. meningococcemia _____

24. mycobacterium _____

25. myxadenitis labialis _____

26. oligopnea _____

27. oropharynx _____

28. otorhinolaryngology _____

29. paresis _____

30. peripleuritis _____

31. pharyngismus _____

32. pneumatosis _____

33. pneumocephalus _____

34. pneumolith _____

35. pneumonolysis _____

36. pyohemothorax _____

37. respiration _____

38. siderofibrosis _____

39. spirogram _____

40. staphylococcus _____

41. staphylolysin _____

42. sternotracheal _____

43. stethoscope _____

44. streptococcolysin _____

45. sudor _____

46. thoracic _____

47. thoracoceloschisis _____

48. tracheocele _____

49. trichobacteria _____

50. vasoparesis _____

Exercise 2: Word Derivation

Give the word derived from Greek and/or Latin elements that matches each of the following. Verify your answer in a medical dictionary. **Note that the wording of the dictionary definition may vary from the wording below.**

1. Resembling a bacterium _____

2. Any fungal infection of the bronchi or bronchial tubes _____

3. Bronchial hemorrhage _____

4. Study of dust (and its effects) _____

5. Pertaining to both the teeth and lips _____

6. Increased carbon dioxide (in the blood) _____

7. (Abnormal) enlargement of the spinal cord _____

8. Specialist in the study of the ear, (nose), and larynx _____

9. Hernia through the pharyngeal wall _____

10. Surgical puncture of a lung _____

11. Producing or forming iron _____

12. Presence of staphylococci in the blood _____

13. Split or cleft sternum _____

14. Hernia of the pleura or lungs _____

15. Inflammation of the muscles of the chest _____

16. Secreting or promoting the secretion of sweat _____

17. Suture of a lung _____

18. Any disease of the thorax _____

19. Instrument used to open the trachea _____

20. Across the thorax _____

Exercise 3: Drill and Review

The meaning of each of the following words can be determined from its etymology. Determine the meaning of each word. Verify your answer in a medical dictionary.

1. abrachia _____

2. acapnia _____

3. alveolitis _____

4. amygdalolith _____

5. antifungal _____

6. antistaphylococcic _____

7. bacteriostatic _____

8. blennorrhagia _____

9. bradypnea _____

10. coccoid _____

11. coniofibrosis _____

12. diaphoretic _____

13. digitiform _____

14. dromomania _____

15. dysmorphic _____

16. echocardiogram _____

17. esthesioscopy _____

18. fungitoxic _____

19. hemiparesis _____

20. hemosiderosis _____

21. hydrotherapy _____

22. hypocalcemia _____

23. inspiration _____

24. kinesioneurosis _____

25. laparohepatotomy _____

26. laryngocentesis _____

27. meatoplasty _____

28. odontatrophy _____

29. orexogen _____

30. pachypleuritis _____

31. pedorthist _____

32. peribronchiolitis _____

33. photophilic _____

34. pneumohypoderma _____

35. polyneuropathy _____

36. presbyacusia _____

37. prostatorrhea _____

38. rhinopharyngeal _____

39. schistothorax _____

40. sideropenia _____

41. spirometry _____

42. staphyloncus _____

43. sternopericardial _____

44. stethospasm _____

45. streptococci _____

46. sudoresis _____

47. thoracomyodynia _____

48. trachyphonia _____

49. trichomycosis _____

50. xanthophose _____

12

DIGESTIVE SYSTEM

There is but one entrance, the mouth, for the various kinds of food. But what is nourished is not one single part, but many, and they are widely separated. And so, do not be surprised at the great number of organs which Nature has created for the purpose of nutrition.

[Galen, *On the Natural Faculties* 1.10.23]

Every part of the body needs nutrition to maintain its ability to function and to repair and replace damaged cellular tissue. Cells receive their nutrition from the circulating blood, which carries the usable material from digested food in the intestine to all parts of the body. When the cells receive this digested food, it is changed into other compounds for use by the body. This is called **metabolism** and involves two processes: **anabolism** and **catabolism**. **Anabolism**, the constructive phase of metabolism, is the process by which simple substances are converted into complex substances and then into protoplasm—that is, the conversion of nonliving material into living cellular material. **Catabolism**, the destructive phase of metabolism, is the process by which complex substances are converted into simpler substances; it is usually accompanied by the release of energy. The sum of anabolism and catabolism maintains, builds up, and repairs the cellular structure of the body and provides energy for the body to function properly. All of this depends on nutrition.

Nutrition is achieved in the body through the various processes of ingestion, digestion, absorption, and metabolism (Fig. 12–1). The first three of these processes take place in the alimentary tract. This passage begins at the mouth and ends at the anus, where undigested, unabsorbed, and unused wastes are eliminated from the body. Ingested food is softened by mastication and by the addition of saliva. Three pairs of glands secrete and supply saliva: the parotid, the submandibular, and the sublingual. The masticated, moistened, and softened food, called a bolus, is swallowed (a process called **deglutition**) and passes through the pharynx into the esophagus. A thin structure of membranous cartilage called the epiglottis folds over the larynx during deglutition to prevent food from entering the larynx and moving into the respiratory passage.

The esophagus is a tube about 10 inches long; its only function is to convey food to the stomach. At the juncture of the esophagus and the stomach is a muscle called the cardiac sphincter (also known as the lower esophageal sphincter). It lies at the entrance to the upper orifice of the stomach, called the cardia (Greek, *kardia*, heart) because of its proximity to the heart. This sphincter muscle prevents the reflux of food and acid from the stomach into the esophagus. If the cardiac sphincter malfunctions and food and acid regurgitate into the esophagus, there is an irritation to the esophageal mucosa from the gastric acid called gastroesophageal reflux disease (GERD), which causes heartburn or **pyrosis**. Damage to the esophageal mucosa caused by long-term reflux of gastric acid is called Barrett's esophagus, named for British surgeon Norman Barrett (1903–1979).

Most of the organs of the alimentary tract lie in the area known as the abdominopelvic cavity, which is lined with a

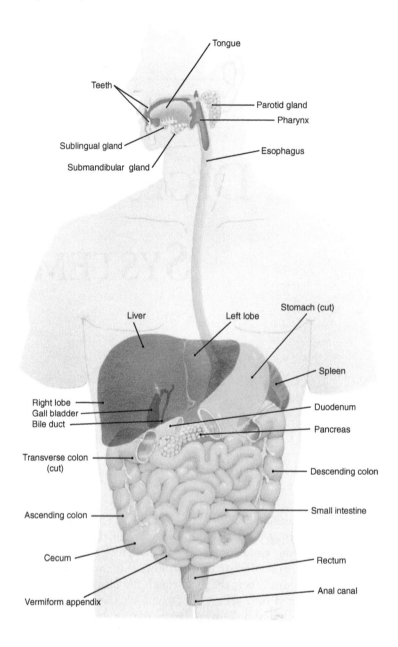

Figure 12–1. The digestive system. (From Scanlon, VC, and Sanders, T: Essentials of Anatomy and Physiology, ed 4. F. A. Davis, Philadelphia, 2003, p 351, with permission.)

serous membrane called the **peritoneum**. The outer surface of this membrane is called the **parietal** (Latin *paries, parietis*, wall) peritoneum, and the inner surface covering the visceral organs is called the **visceral** peritoneum. Inflammation of this membrane is the condition known as **peritonitis**, which can originate from inflammation or infection of any of the peritoneal organs. Each portion of the alimentary canal lying within the enclosure of the peritoneum is attached to the posterior wall of the body by a double fold of peritoneal membrane known as the **mesentery**. Individual mesenteries are named for the specific organ to which each is attached, for example, the **mesogastrium**, the **mesoduodenum**, and so forth. Two other double folds of the peritoneum, called the **omenta** (plural

of omentum), lie between the stomach and two other abdominal viscera; one, the greater or gastrocolic omentum, is attached to the colon; and the other, the lesser or gastrohepatic omentum, is attached to the liver. Organs of the abdominal cavity that are not held in position by mesenteries, but lie behind the peritoneum, are called retroperitoneal organs. The kidneys are retroperitoneal organs.

Food, still undigested, enters the stomach through the cardiac sphincter (Fig. 12–2). Here proteins are digested by pepsin, the chief enzyme of gastric juice, and hydrochloric acid. The mass of digesting food, called chyme, is propelled forward to the lower end of the stomach, the pylorus. The force that propels food through the

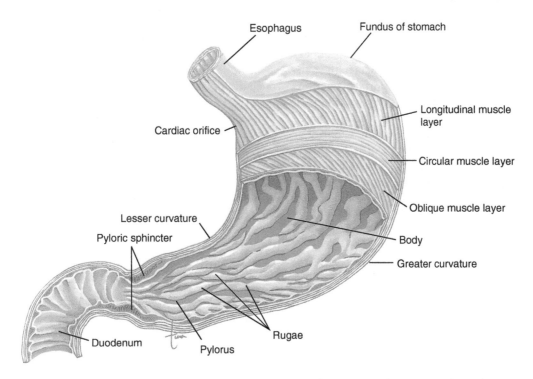

Figure 12–2. The stomach, anterior view, sectioned. (From Scanlon, VC, and Sanders, T: Essentials of Anatomy and Physiology, ed 4. F. A. Davis, Philadelphia, 2003, p 357, part *A*, with permission.)

digestive tract from the esophagus to the anus is **peristalsis**, an involuntary wavelike series of contracting and relaxing motions of the walls of the organs through which the digesting and digested food pass. At the juncture of the stomach and the duodenum is the pyloric sphincter, which is normally closed but relaxes and opens to allow partially digested food to pass into the duodenum.

The **duodenum** is the first of three divisions of the small intestine. It is followed by the **jejunum** and the **ileum**. The process of digestion is completed here. When fats enter the duodenum, the gallbladder sends bile through the bile duct to emulsify the fat. Bile is manufactured in the liver and sent through the hepatic duct to the gallbladder to be stored until fatty substances enter the duodenum, stimulating its release. Bile and other juices, including pancreatic juice and juice from the intestine itself, *succus entericus*, complete the process of digestion. The nutrients of digested food pass into the bloodstream in the small intestine. The mucous lining of the small intestine contains thousands of minutely small projections called villi (plural of villus); these contain a network of capillaries that carry the nutrients from the digested food to the arterial capillaries, which then unite with the venous capillaries to join the venules and venous system.

The residue of the digested food passes through the ileocecal sphincter into the large intestine, which consists of the **cecum**, **colon**, and **rectum**. The rectum ends at the anal opening (Fig. 12–3). The colon itself consists of four segments: the ascending colon, the transverse colon, the descending colon, and the sigmoid colon. In addition to these organs is the appendix, a dead-end tube that extends from the cecum. It has no apparent function and makes itself known only when it becomes inflamed, a condition called appendicitis. The large intestine forms fecal matter from the waste food after digestion, lubricates it with mucus, absorbs water from it, and carries the waste to the colon and the anal area for defecation. There are two anal

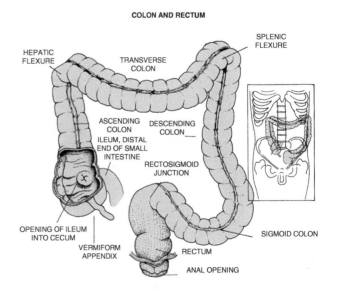

Figure 12–3. The colon and rectum.

sphincters: the first, or internal, is involuntary; the second, or external, is voluntary.

The **liver**, one of the vital organs of the body, produces **bile**, which is carried through the hepatic ducts to the gallbladder for storage (Fig. 12–4). Other important functions of the liver include elimination of toxins, production of proteins, storage of glucose, and production of blood-clotting factors. Bile is not only stored in the gallbladder but becomes concentrated by absorption of water. If the bile becomes too concentrated, minerals or cholesterol in the bile may precipitate and form gallstones. If one or more of these stones is carried into the common bile duct and obstructs that passageway, the condition known as **choledocholithiasis** occurs and can result in **jaundice** (see Lesson 3 for the etymology of this word).

Bile is carried from the liver by the left and the right hepatic ducts, which unite to form the common hepatic duct. This duct branches off into the cystic duct, which carries bile to the gallbladder to be concentrated and stored until needed for digestion. Inflammation of the left or right hepatic ducts or the cystic duct is known as **cholangitis**. Radiographic examination of any of these ducts, a procedure known as **cholangiography**, has been replaced by **ultrasonography**. Surgery to remove stones

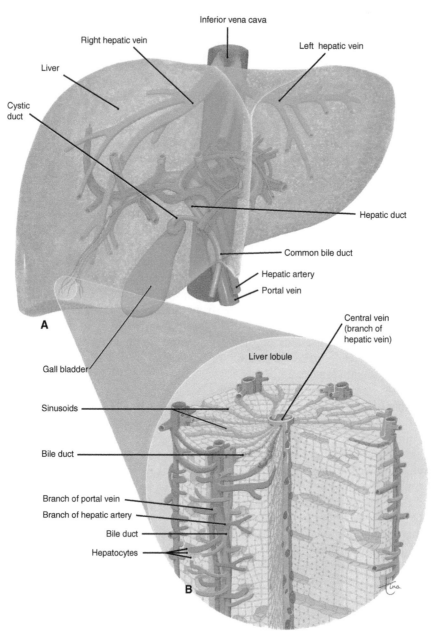

Figure 12–4. The liver. (*A*) Liver and gallbladder. (*B*) Lobule. (From Scanlon, VC, and Sanders, T: Essentials of Anatomy and Physiology, ed 4. F. A. Davis, Philadelphia, 2003, p 360, with permission.)

in the gallbladder or common bile duct (**cholangiotomy**) can sometimes be performed laparoscopically.

Bile leaving the gallbladder enters the hepatic duct; as it descends into the duodenum, this vessel is now called the common bile duct, and the Greek word *dochos* (receptacle) is used in naming it. Thus, inflammation of the common bile duct is called **choledochitis**. As this duct is about to enter the duodenum, it is joined by the pancreatic duct carrying pancreatic digestive enzymes. Control over the entry of bile and the pancreatic juices is exercised by a muscle called the sphincter of Oddi, named after Ruggero Oddi, a 19th-century Italian physician. If concretions (gallstones) form in the gallbladder, the condition is known as **cholelithiasis**. If it becomes necessary to create a passage between the common bile duct and the small intestine, a surgical procedure called **choledochoenterostomy** is used.

The entire alimentary, or gastrointestinal (GI) tract is lined with a mucus-secreting membrane called the mucosa. Inflammation or erosion of the gastric mucosa causes the condition known as **gastritis**. Gastric ulcers are defined as mucosal destruction that extends through the muscularis mucosæ, the muscular layer of the GI tract. The term peptic ulcer disease (PUD) refers to ulcerations of the stomach, duodenum, or both, but ulcerations can occur in any portion of the GI tract. Zollinger-Ellison syndrome (named for American surgeons Robert M. Zollinger, 1903–1992, and Edwin H. Ellison, 1918–1970) is caused by neuroendocrine tumors, usually in the pancreas, which stimulate the stomach to secrete excessive amounts of hydrochloric acid and pepsin. This condition, called a hypersecretory state, can cause PUD.

Treatment of peptic ulcer disease has evolved from dietary management and use of antacids to gastric acid suppression with H_2 blockers (H_2-receptor antagonists) and proton (Greek *protos*, first) pump inhibitors, and now to eradication of *Helicobacter pylori*. This is a gram-negative bacterium that is etiologically related to most peptic ulcers and also to gastritis. The eradication of *H. pylori* requires antibiotics as well as therapy to suppress gastric acid secretion.

VOCABULARY

When the more lax intestine, which is named the colon, tends to be painful, and when the pain is nothing more than flatulence, one should endeavor to promote digestion by reading aloud and other exercises. Hot baths and hot food and drinks are helpful, but all cold foods, all manner of cold, all sweets, all kinds of beans and whatever else contributes to flatulence should be avoided. [Celsus, De Medicina 1.6.7]

Note: Latin combining forms are shown in ***bold italics***.

Greek or Latin	Combining Form(s)	Meaning	Example
bīlis	***BILI-***	bile	**bili**-rubin
kardia*	**CARDI-**	cardia (upper orifice of the stomach)	**cardi**-oesophageal
caecus	***CEC-***	[blind] cecum	**cec**-um
klyzein	**CLY(S)-**	rinse out, inject fluid	**cly**-sis
kopros	**COPR-**	excrement, fecal matter	**copr**-olith
kreas, kreatos	**CREAT-**	flesh	pan-**creat**-ic
dochos	**-DOCH-**	duct	chole-**doch**-al
duodēnī	***DUODEN-***	[12] duodenum	**duoden**-um
oisophagos	**ESOPHAG-**	esophagus	**esophag**-ismus
faex, faecis	***FEC-***	[sediment] excrement, fecal matter	**fec**-es
geuein	**GEUS(T)-**	taste	oxy-**geus**-ia
gingīva	***GINGIV-***	gum (of the mouth)	**gingiv**-itis
glōssa	**GLOSS-**	tongue	**gloss**-olabial
īleum	**ILE-**	ileum	**ile**-um
jējūnus	***JEJUN-***	[empty] jejunum	**jejun**-um
līen (pronounced in two syllables: lie′-en)	***LIEN-***	spleen	**lien**-ocele
lingua	***LINGU-***	tongue	**lingu**-al

Greek or Latin	Combining Form(s)	Meaning	Example
osmē	**OSM-**	sense of smell; odor	dys-**osm**-ia
osphrēsis	**OSPHR-**	sense of smell	**osphr**-esis
peptein	**PEPS-**, **PEPT-**	digest	dys-**peps**-ia
proktos	**PROCT-**	anus	**proct**-oscopy
pylē	**PYLE-**	[gate] portal vein	**pyle**-thrombosis
pylōros	**PYLOR-**	[gatekeeper] pylorus	**pylor**-ic
rectus	*RECT-*	[straight] rectum	**rect**-al
skōr, skatos	**SCAT-**	excrement, fecal matter	**scat**-ology
sialon	**SIAL-**	saliva, salivary duct	**sial**-osyrinx
sigma	**SIGM-**	[sigma, the Greek letter s] sigmoid colon	**sigm**-oid
sphinctēr	**SPHINCTER-**	sphincter muscle	**sphincter** ani
splanchnon	**SPLANCHN-**	internal organ, viscus	**splanchn**-a
typhlos	**TYPHL-**	[blind] cecum	**typhl**-opexy
zymē	**ZYM-**	[leaven] ferment, enzyme, fermentation	en-**zym**-e

kardia is the Greek word for heart; it is also used to designate the upper orifice of the stomach connecting with the esophagus. It is so named because of its proximity to the heart.

ETYMOLOGICAL NOTES

Celsus, the 1st-century AD Roman physician, was aware of the shape, size, and position of the internal organs, knowledge that he acquired, seemingly, by dissection. In his discussion of these organs, after a description of the liver, he turns his attention to the digestive tract.

These are the locations of the visceral organs. The gullet (*stomachus*), which is the beginning of the intestines, is sinewy and begins at the seventh vertebra of the spine. It joins the stomach (*ventriculum*) in the region of the precordia. The stomach, which is the receptacle of food, is comprised of two coats, and it is located between the spleen and the liver, with both of these organs overlapping it a little. There are also thin membranes by which the stomach, the spleen, and the liver are connected, and they are joined to that membrane which I have described above as the transverse septum.

The lowest part of the stomach turns a little to the right and narrows as it enters the top of the intestine. This entry is called by the Greeks *pylorus* because, like a gateway, it allows through to the lower parts whatever is to be excreted.

From this point begins the *jejunum intestinum,* which is not folded upon itself as much. It is called the empty intestine because it does not retain what it has received, but immediately passes it along to the lower parts.

After that comes the thinner intestine, folded into many loops, which are connected to the more internal parts with membranes. These loops are turned toward the right, ending in the region of the hip, occupying, however, mostly the upper parts.

Then this intestine joins crosswise with another, which, beginning on the right side, is long, and on the left it is pervious but on the right it is not and so it is called *caecum intestinum.*

But that one which is pervious . . . bending backward and to the right, descends straight downwards to the place of excretion, and for this reason is called the *rectum intestinum.*

The omentum, which lies over all these organs, is smooth and compact at its lower part, but at the top is softer. It produces fat, which, like the brain and bone marrow, is without feeling. [*De Medicina* 4.1.6–10]

The duodenum is so named because it is about the length of 12 fingerwidths. Actually, it varies in length from 8 to 11 inches, the average being 10 inches.

Salmonella is a form of gastroenteritis that is produced by the ingestion of food containing one or more of the *Salmonella* organisms. The disease was named after the American pathologist Daniel E. Salmon (1850–1914), who first isolated the genus of these organisms.

Diverticula (Latin *di-*, apart, aside, *vertere*, turn, and *-cula*, the plural of *-culum*, the diminutive suffix) are small pouches or sacs formed by herniation of the wall of a canal or organ, occurring most frequently in the colon (Fig. 12–5). This condition is known as **diverticulosis**, a condition more commonly found in patients over the age of 40, and may present no complications. However, these pouches can become filled with digested wastes and inflamed, a condition called **diverticulitis**, which is often accompanied by abdominal pain (usually in the left lower quadrant of the abdomen) and fever. If treatment (usually with antibiotics) does not alleviate the condition, especially if the inflammation spreads, surgery may be necessary to remove the effected area of the intestine, and may sometimes result in a **colostomy**, an incision into the intestine to create an opening to the surface of the abdomen through which fecal matter can be eliminated.

The pancreas gland was so named because it is entirely constituted of flesh without muscular tissues. John Banister (1540–1610), in *The History of Man* (London, John Daye, 1578), wrote of the pancreas: "This body is called Panchreas, that is, all carnous or fleshy, for that it is made and contexted of Glandulous flesh." Both Aristotle and Galen used the word *pankreas* to refer to this organ.

The word hiatus means an opening. A hernia is the protrusion of an organ or part of the organ through the wall of the canal or cavity in which it is normally contained. A **hiatal hernia** is the protrusion of any organ, usually the stomach, upward through the esophageal hiatus of the diaphragm, that is, the opening of the diaphragm through which the esophagus passes. More common types of hernia are umbilical and inguinal.

The Greek noun *zymē* meant leaven (Latin *levāre*, raise), any substance that causes fermentation in bread dough, fruit juice, and so forth. Words containing *zym-* refer to fermentation or to the presence of enzymes. **Enzymes**, complex proteins, are catalysts (Greek *kata-*, down, *lyein*, break), agents that induce chemical changes in other substances without being altered themselves. Enzymes are found in digestive juices and act on the mass of ingested food as it passes along the alimentary tract, breaking it down into simpler compounds. Each enzyme has a more or less specific function: **ptyalin**, secreted in the salivary glands, hydrolyzes starch; **pepsin** and **rennin**, in the gastric juice, act on protein; and **steapsin**, an enzyme

present in pancreatic juice, hydrolyzes fat. Thus, ptyalin is an amylase, or amylolytic enzyme, and steapsin is a lipase, or lipolytic enzyme. A list of the principal enzymes can be found in your medical dictionary.

A **zymogen** is a substance that develops into an enzyme or ferment. **Zymology** is the science of fermentation; **azymic** denotes the absence of an enzyme or of fermentation, and **zymolysis** refers to the changes produced by an enzyme. Biblical scriptures refer to the festival of Passover and Unleavened Bread. In the Septuagint (the Greek translation of the Old Testament), reference is made in Exodus 29.2 to loaves of unleavened bread, *artous* (accusative plural of *artos*, bread) *azymous*, and unleavened cakes, *lagana* (plural of *laganon*, a thin broad cake) *azyma*.

The Greek noun *sphinctēr*, from which the sphincter muscles take their name, is related to the verb *sphingein* (bind tight). Also related to this verb is the noun *sphinx* (strangler, destroyer). In Greek mythology, a dreadful calamity befell the kingdom of Thebes. A monster, the Sphinx, was sent by Hera, queen of the gods, to ravage the land. Apollodorus, the mythographer and author of *The Library*, described the Sphinx: She had the face of a woman; the breast, feet, and tail of a lion; and the wings of a bird. She posed a riddle to the Thebans (which she had learned from the Muses): What has one voice and becomes four-footed, two-footed, and three-footed? While the Thebans were pondering the riddle, she snatched them one by one and devoured them. Finally, Oedipus came along and found the answer, declaring that man as an infant is four-footed, as an adult is two-footed, and as an old man gains a third foot in a staff. The Sphinx killed herself, and Oedipus was asked to wed the late king's widow, Jocasta, and become the ruler of the land. Although it was unknown to both at the time, Jocasta was his mother. And so begins the tragic tale of Oedipus the King.

The portal vein, which carries blood to the liver, is formed by the union of several veins of the visceral area. It enters the liver at the porta hepatis, a fissure on the undersurface of the liver where the hepatic artery also enters this organ and where the right and left hepatic ducts leave it. In medical terminology, the portal vein is referred to by the Greek word *pylē* (gate or entrance). Thus, **pylemphraxis**, a term not frequently used in medical literature, means an occlusion of the portal vein. More specifically, **pylethrombosis**, commonly known as portal vein thrombosis, is a condition that can lead to massive gastrointestinal bleeding. The word *pylē* is generally found in the plural form *pylai* in Greek; in this form, it meant the gates of a city or the entrance to an area. Perhaps the most famous of these gates in Greek history was a narrow mountain pass in the northern part of Greece, Thermopylae, the "hot gate" (*thermos*, hot), so called because of the hot sulphur springs there. Thermopylae was thought to be the northern entry into Greece, and it was here that a famous battle was fought in 480 BC. The Greek forces, after holding the pass for 2 days against the huge Persian army that was invading Greece from the north, were forced to abandon their posi-

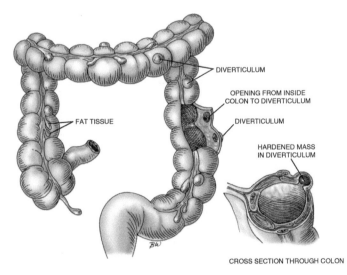

DIVERTICULUM

OPENING FROM INSIDE
COLON TO DIVERTICULUM

FAT TISSUE

DIVERTICULUM

HARDENED MASS
IN DIVERTICULUM

CROSS SECTION THROUGH COLON

MULTIPLE DIVERTICULA OF THE COLON

Figure 12–5. Multiple diverticula of the colon. (From Taber's Cyclopedic Medical Dictionary, ed 19. Philadelphia: F. A. Davis, 2001, p 600, with permission.)

tion when a Greek traitor showed Xerxes, the Persian king, a way around the pass. Leonidas, the Spartan king, and 300 of his men, together with 700 Thespians, are said to have perished here while making a symbolic stand against the barbarian army.

Botulism, a form of food poisoning caused by eating foods contaminated with *Clostridium botulinum*, especially prevalent in preserved meats, takes its name from the Latin word for preserved meat, *botulus* (stuffed intestine or sausage).

Exercise 1: Analyze and Define

Analyze and define each of the following words. In this and in succeeding exercises, analysis should consist of separating the words into prefixes (if any), combining forms, and suffixes or suffix forms (if any) and giving the meaning of each. Be certain to differentiate between nouns and adjectives in your definitions. Consult a medical dictionary for the current meanings of these words.

1. ateloglossia _____

2. azymia _____

3. biliary _____

4. cardiospasm _____

5. cecopexy _____

6. cecoptosis _____

7. choledochal _____

8. clysis _____

9. colorectostomy _____

10. coprolith _____

11. creatorrhea _____

12. defecation _____

13. dolichosigmoid _____

14. duodenohepatic _____

15. esophagismus _____

16. eupepsia _____

17. fecaloid _____

18. gingivoglossitis _____

19. hypodermoclysis _____

20. ileocecal sphincter _____

21. ileocolic _____

22. ileocolostomy _____

23. jejunostomy _____

24. labioglossopharyngeal _____

25. laparotyphlotomy _____

26. lienomalacia _____

27. lingula _____

28. melanoglossia _____

29. orolingual _____

30. osmodysphoria _____

31. oxygeusia _____

32. pancreatic _____

33. parosmia _____

34. parosphresia _____

35. pepsin _____

36. periesophagitis _____

37. peripylephlebitis _____

38. proctoclysis _____

39. protoduodenum _____

40. pseudosmia _____

41. pylethrombosis _____

42. pyloroduodenitis _____

43. rectostenosis _____

44. retrolingual _____

45. scatology _____

46. sigmoiditis _____

47. sigmoidopexy _____

48. typhloempyema _____

49. zymogen _____

50. zymolysis _____

Exercise 2: Word Derivation

Give the word derived from Latin and/or Greek elements that matches each of the following. Verify your answer in a medical dictionary. **Note that the wording of the dictionary definition may vary from the wording below.**

1. Absence of (the sense of) taste _____

2. Pertaining to bile _____

3. Suturing (of the severed ends) of the common bile duct _____

4. Vomiting of fecal material _____

5. Formation of a passage between the duodenum and the intestine _____

6. Hernia of the esophagus _____

7. Pertaining to the tongue and lips _____

8. Burning sensation of the tongue _____

9. Formation of a passage between two parts of the jejunum _____

10. (Abdominal) incision into the ileum _____

11. Relating to the spleen and pancreas _____

12. Branch of medicine dealing with diseases and disorders of the organs of smell _____

13. Suture or attachment of the rectum to some other part _____

14. Abnormal narrowing of the pyloric orifice _____

15. An incision of the bladder through the rectum _____

16. Behind or pertaining to the area posterior to the cecum _____

17. Tumor of a salivary gland _____

18. Obstruction of any internal organ _____

19. Concerning the area beneath the tongue _____

20. Distortion of normal smell perception _____

Exercise 3: Drill and Review

The meaning of each of the following words can be determined from the word's etymology. Determine the meaning of each word. Verify your answers in a medical dictionary.

1. acanthoma _____

2. adenectopia _____

3. allolalia _____

4. ankyloproctia _____

5. biligenesis _____

6. binaural _____

7. calorifacient _____

8. capnophilic _____

9. cardiopyloric _____

10. cecostomy _____

11. coprolalia _____

12. dearterialization _____

13. dromotropic _____

14. duodenojejunostomy _____

15. dyspeptic _____

16. gingivalgia _____

17. hemianosmia _____

18. heterogeusia _____

19. hyperimmune _____

20. hypoglossal _____

21. ileoproctostomy _____

22. immunotherapy _____

23. intraduodenal _____

24. lateroabdominal _____

25. mesenteriopexy _____

26. mesojejunum _____

27. nasopharyngography _____

28. onychauxis _____

29. osmidrosis _____

30. osteophlebitis _____

31. oxypathia _____

32. pachyglossia _____

33. pancreatoncus _____

34. paratyphlitis _____

35. peptogenic _____

36. pleuroclysis _____

37. presphygmic _____

38. prosopodiplegia _____

39. rectorrhaphy _____

40. resectoscope _____

41. retroesophageal _____

42. scatoscopy _____

43. sialoschesis _____

44. somatocrinin _____

45. sphincterismus _____

46. streptodermatitis _____

47. trachelopexy _____

48. ultramicrobe _____

49. vascularize _____

50. vasitis _____

OPTIC SYSTEM

There is a certain weakness of the eyes in which people see well in the daytime but not at all at night. This condition does not exist in women whose menstruation is regular. Those who suffer with this disability should anoint their eyeballs with the drippings from a liver while it is roasting—preferably that of a he-goat; if that is not possible, one from a she-goat; and the liver itself should be eaten.

[Celsus, *De Medicina* 6.6.38]

The globe of the eye is surrounded by three layers of tissue (Fig. 13–1). Portions of each layer have different names as described in the following sentences. The outermost layer, or **sclera**, is a tough, fibrous coat that forms a protective covering for the delicate nerves and membranes beneath. The anterior, visible, and transparent portion of the sclera is called the **cornea**. The sclera and the cornea form one continuous coat. The anterior portion of the sclera is covered with a transparent mucous membrane, the **conjunctiva**, an extension of the lining of the eyelids. The portion of the conjunctiva that lines the eyelids is called the **palpebral conjunctiva** (Latin *palpebra*, eyelid) and the membrane covering the sclera is the **bulbar conjunctiva**; the loose fold connecting the two is the **fornix conjunctivae** (Latin *fornix*, arch).

The exterior surface of the sclera is covered with a thin layer of tissue called the episclera, which contains blood vessels to nourish the sclera. A common disease of the sclera is **episcleritis**. Its cause is unknown, and the inflammation usually subsides after a few days of treatment.

The cornea is subject to bacterial, viral, and fungal infection as well as to injury by foreign bodies. Ulceration and abrasion of the cornea are common and usually resolve with application of ophthalmic medications. *Streptococcus pneumoniae* is a common cause of bacterial corneal ulcers called **keratitis**. The most common viral cause of corneal ulcers is herpes simplex virus (HSV); this condition is known as **herpetic keratitis**. Herpes corneae, an inflam-

mation of the cornea, is also caused by herpes virus. Herpes virus is the most common corneal cause of blindness in the United States. Infectious mononucleosis is another viral cause of keratitis. **Hypopyon keratitis**, a serpentlike ulcer with pus in the anterior chamber of the eye, can be a complication of both bacterial and viral ulceration. Other causes of keratitis can include drying of the cornea, found in Bell's palsy and as a side effect of certain drugs. Fungal corneal ulcers, once seen primarily in agricultural workers, are now seen more frequently because of the introduction of corticosteroid drugs for use in ophthalmology. Local (or topical) use of steroids increases susceptibility to all infections. Corneal ulceration can also be caused by avitaminosis A, the lack of vitamin A, as a result of either dietary deficiency or impaired absorption and utilization from the gastrointestinal tract. Avitaminosis A can cause a hardening and drying of the epithelium throughout the body, a condition known as **xerosis**. Xerosis of the conjunctiva and cornea is called **xerophthalmia**. Corneal ulceration caused by avitaminosis A is characterized by a softening of the cornea called **keratomalacia**, and often by necrosis, leading to perforation.

The middle layer of the eye, or vascular layer, is a dark brown tissue called the **uvea** because of its resemblance to a grape (Latin *ūva*). The uveal tract is composed of the iris, the ciliary body, and the choroid. The uveal tract contributes blood supply to the retina and is protected by the outer layer, the cornea, and the sclera. The choroid is the

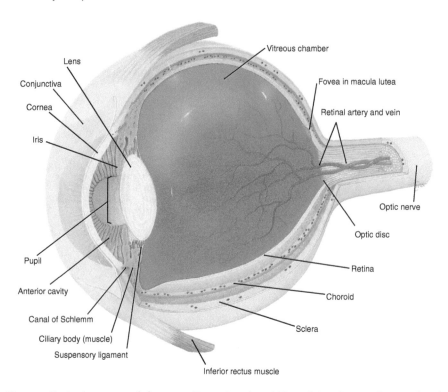

Figure 13–1. Anatomy of the eye. (From Scanlon, VC and Sanders, T: Essentials of Anatomy and Physiology, ed 4. F. A. Davis, Philadelphia, 2003, p 194.)

posterior portion extending to the point opposite the lens; the ciliary body is a thickened triangular structure; and the iris is the anterior extension of the ciliary body.

The ciliary body secretes a fluid called the aqueous humor into the posterior chamber of the eye, the area behind the iris and in front of the vitreous body. The aqueous humor flows from the posterior chamber into the anterior chamber through the pupil and leaves the eye through the trabecular (diminutive of Latin *trabs, trabis*, a beam of wood) meshwork and a canal, called Schlemm's canal after Friedrich Schlemm, a German anatomist (1795–1858). Schlemm's canal opens at the inner corner of the anterior chamber between the cornea and the iris. Approximately 30 collector channels leading from Schlemm's canal carry the aqueous humor into the venous system. Intraocular pressure is controlled by the rate at which the aqueous humor leaves the eye through Schlemm's canal.

When, for any reason, the aqueous humor fails to drain normally, intraocular pressure increases and gradually damages nerve fibers at the optic disc. If this is allowed to go unchecked, blindness can occur. This condition is called **glaucoma**. Infection or inflammation can cause blockage of Schlemm's canal, but more often normal drainage is impaired without infection or inflammation. Glaucoma is categorized by whether or not the angle between the posterior cornea and anterior iris is open or not. Two common forms of glaucoma are primary open-angle glaucoma (POAG) and closed-angle glaucoma. Glaucoma can be detected by the use of an instrument

called a **tonometer**, which measures intraocular pressure, and can be treated with drugs and/or surgery. Extremely high pressure can cause blindness in a short time by damaging the optic nerve or by compressing the blood vessels of the retina to the point where the supply of blood is cut off.

The **retina**, an outgrowth of the optic nerve, is the innermost layer of the globe of the eye. It is a thin, semi-transparent sheet of neural tissue that lines the inner aspect of the posterior two-thirds of the globe. The retina receives visual images through the lens and transmits these images through the optic nerve to the proper receptors in the brain. The retina is composed of 10 layers of cells. The first of these, the inner coating, consists of pigmented epithelial cells. The second layer consists of rods and cones, nerve receptors that respond to light. The rods control night vision (**scotopia**), and their function depends on a supply of vitamin A. Thus, deficiency in this vitamin can cause night blindness (**nyctalopia**).

The cones of the retina are sensitive to color, and any interference with their normal transmission of visual images can result in one or more forms of color blindness. There are three types of cones, each sensitive to a different portion (color) of the light spectrum. Light has three primary colors: red, green, and blue. If there is a lack of sensitivity in the cones that are sensitive to red, the person is said to have protanopia (Greek, *prōtos*, first) because red is the first of the primary colors. Green blindness is called **deuteranopia** (Greek, *deuteros*, second). Color blindness in which blue and yellow appear gray is called **tritanopia**

(Greek, *tritos*, third). The opposite of these conditions, an oversensitivity in the cones, is thought to be the cause of visual defects in which the person sees everything either through a red haze (**erythropia**), a green haze (**chloropia**), or a blue haze (**cyanopia**). When all objects appear yellow, the condition is called **xanthopsia**. Color vision defects are usually hereditary. Age-related macular (Latin, *macula*, spot) degeneration (ARMD) is the most frequent cause of central visual field blindness in the United States. The pathogenesis of this disease remains unclear.

The condition known as detached retina occurs when the rod and cone layer (the sensory layer) of the retina becomes partially separated from the pigmented epithelial layer of the retina (Fig. 13–2). The upper exterior portion of the retina is the area most commonly affected, but any part may become detached. Among the causes of detachment of the retina are choroiditis, retinitis, trauma, and malignant melanoma of the choroid. Most retinal detachments are caused by degeneration of the vitreous humor, the jellylike semifluid that fills the eyeball. Some cases of retinal detachment are idiopathic, without apparent cause. This condition can usually be corrected by microscopic vitreous surgery. This may involve severing and removing tissue, diathermy, and laser photocoagulation.

The lens of the eye is held in place by bands of ligament (zonula ciliaris) connecting it to the ciliary body on either side. It lies between the aqueous humor in front and the vitreous humor behind. The purpose of the lens is to focus the light rays on the retina at the fovea centralis retinae, commonly called the **fovea**, by refracting them to the proper degree. When focusing is normal, the condition is called **emmetropia**, and no refractive errors are present.

There are three fairly common abnormalities that interfere with normal focusing: **hyperopia** (hypermetropia), **myopia**, and **astigmatism** (Fig. 13–3).

Myopia, or nearsightedness, is caused by a larger than normal eye that causes light rays to focus in front of the retina. This condition is corrected by the use of eyeglasses or concave contact lenses.

Hyperopia, or farsightedness, results from the failure of light rays to focus directly on the retina. Hyperopic eyes tend to be small, with a shallow anterior chamber. Parallel rays of light entering the eye are focused behind the retina instead of on the retina. Hyperopia can be corrected by the use of eyeglasses or convex contact lenses.

Astigmatism results when the lens or the cornea is egg shaped rather than spherical, causing some of the light rays to focus behind the retina and some to focus in front of it. The condition is so named because those who suffer from it have difficulty in focusing their sight on a point (Greek *stigma*).

Surgery using lasers to correct these three common focusing conditions is called LASIK. The acronym stands for laser in situ keratomileusis (*in situ*, Latin, in the natural or normal place; *keratos*, Greek, cornea; *mileusis*, Greek, shaping). As the name suggests, the procedure involves using a laser to reshape the cornea into the proper configuration.*

-OMA
In the terminology of ophthalmology, many words ending in **-oma** do not designate tumors, but various abnormalities.

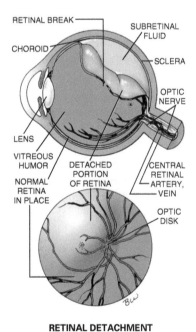

RETINAL DETACHMENT

Figure 13–2. Retinal detachment. (From Taber's Cyclopedic Medical Dictionary, ed 19. Philadelphia: F. A. Davis, 2001, p 1798.)

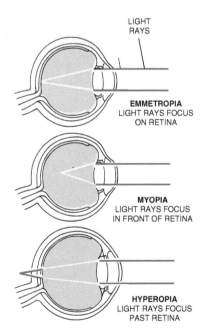

Figure 13–3. Emmetropia, myopia, and hyperopia.

*Information on LASIK is from the LASIK Institute (*www.LASIKInstitute.org*).

VOCABULARY

It is a bad sign if hiccough and redness of the eyes follow vomiting.[Hippocrates, Aphorisms 7.2]

Note: Latin combining forms are shown in ***bold italics***.

Greek or Latin	Combining Form(s)	Meaning	Example
blepharon	**BLEPHAR-**	eyelid	**blephar**-ostat
chorioeidēs	**CHOROID-**	[skinlike] choroid	**choroid**-itis
korē	**COR(E)-**	[girl] pupil (of the eye)	**core**-oplasty
kyklos	**CYCL-**	circle; the ciliary body	**cycl**-oplegia
dakryon	**DACRY-**	tear; lacrimal sac or duct	**dacry**-elcosis
herpēs, herpētos	**HERPES, HERPET-**	[shingles] herpes, a creeping skin disease	**herpet**-iform
iris, iridos	**IR(ID)-**	[rainbow] iris	**irid**-ectomy
jungere, junctus	***JUNCT-***	join	con-**junct**-ivitis
keras, keratos	**KERAT-**	[horn] cornea	**kerat**-itis
lacrima	***LACRIM-***	tear	**lacrim**-al
myein	**MY-**	close, shut	**my**-opia
oculus	***OCUL-***	eye	**ocul**-ar
ōps	**OP(S)-**	vision	dys-**ops**-ia
ophthalmos	**OPHTHALM-**	eye	**ophthalm**-ia
optos	**OPT-**	[seen] vision; eye	**opt**-ical
phakos	**PHAC-, PHAK-**	[lentil] lens	a-**phak**-ia
rēte, rētis	***RET-, RETIN-***	[net] retina; network, plexus	**retin**-a
stigma, stigmatos	**STIGM-, STIGMAT-**	point, mark, spot	a-**stigmat**-ism
xēros	**XER-**	dry	**xer**-oma

ETYMOLOGICAL NOTES

If the winter is dry and the winds are from the north, and if the spring is rainy and the winds are from the south, the summer will be laden with fever and will cause oph-thalmia and dysenteries. [Hippocrates, Airs, Waters, and Places 10]

The word *glaukōma* (Greek *glaukos*, gleaming, gray) was used by Aristotle, Galen, and others to indicate the condition of opacity of the lens of the eye called a cataract. The earliest examples of the word glaucoma in English mean cataract. It was not until 1705 that the difference between a true glaucoma and ordinary cataract was recognized in dissection by the French physician Pierre Brisseau. The term **glaucoma**, as now used, refers to the condition of increased intraocular pressure. As intraocular pressure increases, the optic disk (the area of the retina where the optic nerve enters) atrophies and changes color from its natural pink to a light gray color. It is this progressive atro-phy of the optic disk that causes blindness in absolute glau-coma, the final stage of this disease.

The ultimate etymology of the medical term **cataract** is uncertain. The Greek *kataraktēs*, found in Latin as *catarac-*

ta, meant a waterfall, particularly a cataract of the Nile or Euphrates river. Later it came to mean a floodgate, as in the description of the flood in Genesis 7.11:

In the six hundredth year of Noah's life, in the second month, the seventeenth day of the month, the same day were all the fountains of the great deep broken up, and the windows [or floodgates] of heaven were opened. [*Bible*, King James version].

The Hebrew word for the "windows of heaven" is *àrubot*, which was translated in the Septuagint by *kataraktai*, and in the Vulgate by *cataractae*. *àrubot* are also the "windows from on high" in Isaiah 24.18:

And it shall come to pass, that he who fleeth from the noise of the fear shall fall into the pit; and he that cometh up out of the midst of the pit shall be taken in the snare: for the windows from on high are open, and the founda-tions of the earth do shake. [*Bible*, King James version]

It is uncertain whether the Greek *kataraktēs* is from *katarassein* (dash down) or from *katarrhēgnynai* (break in pieces). The first use of the word in its modern medical sense seems to have been by the French physician Ambroïse Paré (1510–1590) in a treatise in which he refers to a *cataracte* of the eye. Perhaps Paré had the idea that a cataract was a sort of gate that shut out the light. The modern surgical method for treatment of cataract by removal of the lens was introduced by the French surgeon Jacques Daviel (1696–1762). His method was explained in an article in the Annals of the Royal Academy of Surgery (Paris), *Sur une nouvelle méthode de guérir la cataracte par l'extraction du cristallin*, in 1753.

The herpes virus takes its name from the Greek *herpēs* (shingles), an acute inflammatory eruption of the skin or mucous membrane, a term that was used by Hippocrates in this sense. The noun *herpēs* is derived from the verb *herpein* (move slowly, creep), probably from the slow advance of the inflammation on the body. Pliny, in writing of ulcers and their treatment, says, "There is an animal which the Greeks call *herpes* by means of which all creeping ulcers are healed" [*Natural History* 30. 39.116]. It is not known what Pliny was referring to here because the Greek word meant only the inflammatory disease. He may have meant some sort of snake because the Latin noun *serpēns, serpentis* (Latin, *serpere*, creep) meant a serpent or snake. The etymological identity between the Latin and Greek verbs *serpere* and *herpein*, both meaning creep, would not have been lost on Pliny. Cognate* words in Latin and Greek, if they show an initial *s-* in Latin, show an initial "h" sound (the so-called rough breathing)† in Greek; compare Latin *sēmi-* and Greek *hēmi-* (half); Latin *sex* and Greek *hex* (six); Latin *sūdor* (sweat), and Greek *hydor* (water), and so forth. The name for the acute infectious skin disease herpes zoster comes from the Greek noun *herpēs*, plus the Greek *zōstēr* (belt). Herpes zoster is more commonly called shingles, from the Latin verb *cingere* (gird) with a noun *cingulum* (belt), formed from the verb. The word entered English through Old French *chengle*, with the alternate forms *cengle* and *sangle*. This skin infection was named by the ancient Greek physician Hippocrates because of the serpentlike scaly eruption and inflammation that generally encircles the trunk of the body. The virus that causes herpes zoster is a parasite and can affect one at any age, although it generally makes its unwelcome appearance in adulthood. It is a refractory disease, that is, one that is resistant to treatment.

There would seem to be no relationship between the trachea and trachoma, the eye disease that has blinded millions of people, particularly in Asia and Africa; but both terms are from the Greek adjective *trachys* (rough). The trachea is so named because of the rings of cartilage that surround it, giving that organ its characteristic rough surface. Trachoma is caused by the microorganism *Chlamydia trachomatis* (Greek *chlamys*, cloak) and is a form of conjunctivitis. It manifests itself by the presence of follicles

(diminutive of Latin *follis*, bag), small secretory sacs, which become hypertrophic and cause scarring of the palpebral conjunctiva. Ulceration of the cornea often ensues from secondary bacterial infection, which ultimately causes blindness.

Myopia, nearsightedness, does not take its name from Greek *mys*, muscle (with the combining form MY-), but from the verb *myein* meaning close or shut, from the characteristic squinting of those affected with myopia in an attempt to see more clearly.

The pupil of the eye was so called by the ancient Romans because the reflection seen by one looking at the pupil of another's eye appeared like a little dot (Latin *pūpilla*). The Greek word *korē* (girl, doll) was used by both Hippocrates and Galen to name the pupil of the eye. The combining form CORE-, coreometry, coreoplasty, is from *korē*.

Galen used the word iris to refer to the iris of the eye; Pliny used it to refer to a precious stone. But to the ancient Greeks and Romans, Iris was the many-hued goddess of the rainbow, who acted as a special messenger for both the king and the queen of the gods (Fig. 13–4). We meet her in Virgil's *Aeneid* at the end of the fourth book. The Phoenician queen Dido, exiled from her homeland, founded the city of Carthage in North Africa. In despair because her lover, Aeneas, deserted her after a year of intimacy, Dido attempted to take her own life by falling upon her sword. But her spirit would not leave her because Proserpina, the queen of the Underworld, had not taken a

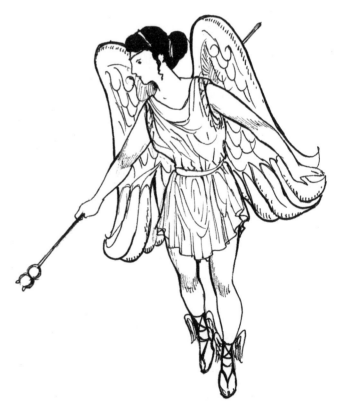

Figure 13–4. Iris.

---

*Just as the vocabularies of modern French, Spanish, Italian, and the other Romance languages are derived from Latin, so the vocabularies of Latin, ancient Greek, Sanskrit, and other related ancient languages were derived from an earlier parent language, which we call Indo-European. Words in two (or more) Indo-European languages, each derived from the same presumed Indo-European word, are called cognates.

†See Lesson 1 for a discussion of rough breathing.

lock of hair from her head in order to permit her to enter the realms of the dead, because she was a suicide. Juno, the queen of the immortals, took pity on her and sent Iris to release her struggling soul from her body.

Ergo Iris croceis per caelum roscida pinnis,
mille trahens varios adverso sole colores,
devolat et supra caput adstitit. "Hunc ego Diti
sacrum iussa fero teque isto corpore solvo":
sic ait et dextra crinem secat; omnis et una
dilapsus calor atque in ventos vita recessit.

And Iris, all covered with dew, flew down
from heaven on saffron wings, trailing
a thousand colors reflected in the
rays of the sun, and stood above her head.
"As I have been ordered, I take this offering sacred to Dis*
and free you
from your body." So Iris spoke, and
with her hand cut the lock of hair.
All of a sudden the warmth left her,
and life faded into the winds.

(*Aeneid* 4.700–705)

Exercise 1: Analyze and Define

Analyze and define each of the following words. In this and in succeeding exercises, analysis should consist of separating the words into prefixes (if any), combining forms, and suffixes or suffix forms (if any) and giving the meaning of each. Be certain to differentiate between nouns and adjectives in your definitions. Consult a medical dictionary for the current meanings of these words.

1. achromatopsia _____

2. amblyopia _____

3. anisometropia _____

4. anisopia _____

5. ankyloblepharon _____

6. binocular _____

7. blepharism _____

8. blepharostat _____

9. chloropia _____

10. choroid _____

11. corestenoma _____

12. cyclokeratitis _____

*Dis is another name for Hades or Pluto, king of the underworld.

13. dacryohemorrhea _____

14. enophthalmos _____

15. herpes facialis _____

16. heterochromia iridis _____

17. hydrophthalmos _____

18. hypermetropia _____

19. hypometropia _____

20. iralgia _____

21. iridadenosis _____

22. iridocyclectomy _____

23. isocoria _____

24. keratorrhexis _____

25. lacrimation _____

26. macropsia _____

27. microphakia _____

28. micropsia _____

29. myopia _____

30. nasolacrimal _____

31. nyctamblyopia _____

32. ophthalmia neonatorum _____

33. optometrist _____

34. orthoptic _____

35. oxyopia _____

36. palinopsia _____

37. phacolysis _____

38. photopia _____

39. polycoria _____

40. presbyopia _____

41. pseudopsia _____

42. purulent conjunctivitis _____

43. retinodialysis _____

44. schizoblepharia _____

45. sinistrocular _____

46. stigmatism _____

47. suppurative choroiditis _____

48. varicoblepharon _____

49. xanthopsia _____

50. xeroma _____

Exercise 2: Word Derivation

Give the word derived from Greek or Latin elements that matches each of the following. Verify your answer in a medical dictionary. **Note that the wording of a dictionary definition may vary from the wording below.**

1. (Congenital) absence of all or part of the iris _____

2. Discharge from the eyelid _____

3. Inflammation of the conjunctiva _____

4. Pain in a lacrimal gland _____

5. Measurement of the pupil _____

6. Vision in which all objects appear to be blue _____

7. Paralysis of the ciliary muscle _____

8. Agent that stimulates the secretion of tears _____

9. Having a double pupil in the eye _____

10. Pertaining to herpes _____

11. Excision of a portion of the cornea _____

12. Incision of the lacrimal duct _____

13. Concerning or affecting one eye _____

14. Any fungal disease of the eye _____

15. Paralysis of the eye (muscles) _____

16. Dryness of the lips _____

17. Instrument for observing (change of curvature of) the lens _____

18. Pertaining to the retina and choroid _____

19. Dry mouth _____

20. Ulceration of the lacrimal apparatus _____

Exercise 3: Drill and Review

The meaning of each of the following words can be determined from its etymology. Determine the meaning of each word. Verify your answer in a medical dictionary.

1. abdominocystic _____

2. allophasis _____

3. anerythropsia _____

4. antigen _____

5. astigmatism _____

6. blepharodiastasis _____

7. brachia _____

8. capnography _____

9. chondroplasty _____

10. choroidoretinitis _____

11. conjunctivoplasty _____

12. corectopia _____

13. coremorphosis _____

14. cryptesthesia _____

15. cyclectomy _____

16. dentoalveolitis _____

17. ergophobia _____

18. flexile _____

19. herpes labialis _____

20. herpetiform _____

21. hypergeusesthesia _____

22. immunotoxin _____

23. infusion _____

24. intubation _____

25. intumescent _____

26. iridotasis _____

27. keratocele _____

28. macrolabia _____

29. megalophthalmus _____

30. monobrachius _____

31. myope _____

32. oculonasal _____

33. ophthalmatrophy _____

34. optometry _____

35. osmesthesia _____

36. pancreatolith _____

37. pediculosis capitis _____

38. phacoanaphylaxis _____

39. posterolateral _____

40. prostatomegaly _____

41. protanopia _____

42. retinopathy _____

43. septulum _____

44. somnolentia _____

45. sonic _____

46. stereo-ophthalmoscope _____

47. sternocostal _____

48. tachypnea _____

49. thyrotropin _____

50. variciform _____

FEMALE REPRODUCTIVE SYSTEM

It is not easy for large creatures, whether animal or anything else, to reach full development in a short time. For this reason horses and similar animals, although their life span is shorter than that of humans, have a longer period of gestation. The birth of horses occurs after a year; but in humans it is about ten months. For the same reason, birth takes a long time in elephants, whose gestation period is two years because of their great size.

[Aristotle, *Generation of Animals* 777b]

GYNECOLOGY

The principal organs of the female reproductive system are the **ovaries, fallopian tubes**, **uterus**, and **vagina**. The ovaries are two almond-shaped glands lying on either side of the cavity of the pelvis. The ovaries produce ova (Latin, plural of *ōvum*, egg) and hormones. These hormones, among which are estrogen and progesterone, are responsible for the development and maintenance of female secondary sexual characteristics and the regulation of the menstrual cycle. Within each ovary are hundreds of thousands of structures called **follicles** (*Latin folliculus*, diminutive of *follis*, bag), each consisting of epithelial cells surrounding a primitive ovum, the oogonium, which develops into an oocyte, and then into an ovum (Fig. 14–1). During the normal sexual life of a woman, on an average of once every 28 days, a single ovum matures and is released from the ovaries. This process, called **ovulation**, occurs approximately 14 days before the next menstrual period begins. The mature ovum enters the fallopian tube and is transported toward the uterus. If sperm are present, it may become fertilized; if not, the ovum

degenerates and is passed out of the body with the next period of menstruation. Shortly after the follicle expels its ovum, the mass of cells of the follicle changes into a yellowish body called the **corpus luteum** (Latin *corpus*, body, and *lūteus*, yellow). The corpus luteum grows for about a week after ovulation. If the ovum is not fertilized, the corpus luteum degenerates. If fertilization takes place, the corpus luteum continues to grow for the next several weeks and then is gradually replaced by connective tissue.

The two fallopian tubes, also called **oviducts** (often with the combining form OOPHOR- or SALPING-, from Greek *salpinx*, tube), extend from the uterus to each ovary. Their purpose is to transport the mature ovum each month from the ovary to the uterus and spermatozoa from the uterus toward the ovary. The union of the ovum and sperm, fertilization, normally occurs in the fallopian tube. The fertilized ovum, or **zygote** (Greek *zygōtos*, yoked, from *zygon*, yoke), then implants in the uterus and develops there into the embryo. Occasionally, the zygote remains in the fallopian tube, resulting in tubal, or ectopic, pregnancy.

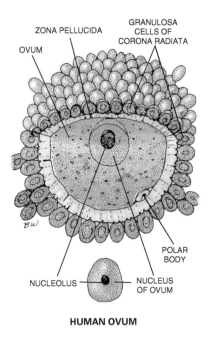

ZONA PELLUCIDA

GRANULOSA
CELLS OF
CORONA RADIATA

OVUM

POLAR
BODY

NUCLEOLUS

NUCLEUS
OF OVUM

HUMAN OVUM

Figure 14–1. Human ovum. (From Taber's Cyclopedic Medical Dictionary, ed 19. F.A. Davis, Philadelphia, 2001, p 1477, with permission.)

The uterus, or womb, is a hollow, muscular, pear-shaped and pear-sized organ that lies in the true pelvis between the bladder and rectum (Fig. 14–2). It consists of three parts: the **fundus** (Latin *fundus*, base, foundation) or uppermost portion; the **corpus** (Latin *corpus*, body), or central area; and the **endocervix**, the lowermost portion of the uterus, which opens into the vagina. The mucous membrane lining the inner surface of the uterus is called the endometrium (Greek *mētra*, uterus); the muscular wall of the endometrium forming its main mass is called the myometrium. During a woman's childbearing years, from the beginning of menstruation (menarche) to the end (menopause), the uterine endometrium passes through the cyclic changes of menstruation each month.

The menstrual cycle consists of four phases: the menses, the proliferative phase, the ovulatory phase, and the secretory phase. During the proliferative phase, the endometrial lining proliferates, or thickens, in response to the main hormone of this phase, estrogen. During the ovulatory phase, the proliferative endometrium is transformed into the secretory endometrium at the time of ovulation. During the secretory phase, the endometrium is stabilized and prepared for implantation of the fertilized embryo. If the ovum is not fertilized and implantation

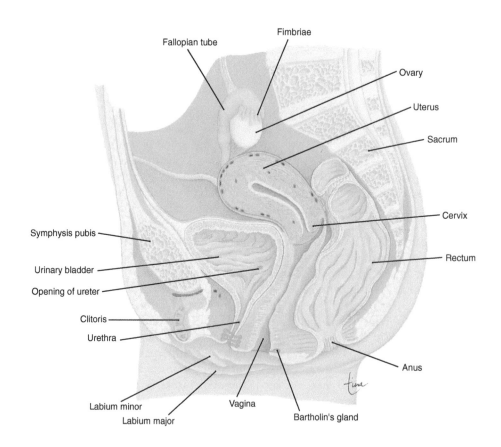

Fallopian tube

Fimbriae

Ovary

Uterus

Sacrum

Cervix

Rectum

Symphysis pubis

Urinary bladder

Opening of ureter

Clitoris

Urethra

Anus

Labium minor

Vagina

Bartholin's gland

Labium major

Figure 14–2. Female genital organs. Midsagittal section. (From Scanlon, VC, and Sanders, T: Essentials of Anatomy and Physiology, ed 4. F. A. Davis, Philadelphia, 2003, p 441, with permission.)

does not occur, the lining of the endometrial cavity is sloughed through the endocervix and vagina (i.e., menstruation).

At birth the inner lining of the endometrium, the decidua (Latin *deciduus*, falling down, from *cadere*, fall) is shed. During pregnancy, the decidua basilis (New Latin, from Greek *basis*, base), the portion of the endometrium lying between the chorionic membrane enclosing the fetus and the myometrium, develops into the maternal portion of the placenta. Contractions of the uterine myometrium assist in expelling the fetus, placenta, and membranes.

The vagina (Greek *kolpos*, *koleon*, or *elytron*) is a muscular, membranous sheath extending from the cervix uteri to the vulva, the external genitalia. It serves as a passage for the entrance of the penis in coitus, for receiving semen,

and for the discharge of the menstrual flow. It is the passageway, or birth canal, through which the fetus passes during labor and delivery.

The uterine cervix is the most inferior portion of the uterus, and opens into the vagina. The **ectocervix** is the portion of the cervix visible through the vagina during gynecologic examination. **Dysplasia** of the cells of the ectocervix, if left untreated, can progress to cervical cancer. Human papillomavirus (HPV) infection is a known cause of cervical dysplasia. The **Papanicolaou test** (named for the Greek-born American scientist Nicholas Papanicolaou (1883–1962), commonly called a Pap test or Pap smear, is used to screen for the presence of cervical dysplasia. **Colposcopy** is a procedure used to evaluate abnormalities of the ectocervix.

VOCABULARY

If a woman is going to have a male child her complexion will be good; if a female child, her complexion will be bad. [Hippocrates, Aphorisms 42]

The embryo of a male child is usually on the right and that of a female usually on the left. [Hippocrates, Aphorisms 48]

Note: Latin combining forms are in ***bold italics***.

Greek or Latin	Combining Form(s)	Meaning	Example
agōgos	**AGOG-**	leading, drawing forth	lact-**agog**-ue
archē	**ARCH-, -ARCHE**	beginning, origin	men-**arche**
cervix, cervīcis	***CERVIC-, CERVIX***	neck (of the uterus), cervix uteri	**cervic**-al
kolpos	**COLP-**	vagina	**colp**-oscopy
kyein	**CYE-**	be pregnant	**cye**-sis
eurynein	**EURY(N)-**	widen, dilate	metr-**euryn**-ter
gala, galaktos	**GAL-, GALACT-**	milk	**galact**-orrhea
(g)nascī, nātus	***-GN-, NAT-***	be born	pre-**nat**-al
*gonad**	**GONAD-**	sex glands, sex organs	**gonad**-otropin
gravidus†	***GRAVID-***	pregnant	primi-**gravid**-a
hymēn	**HYMEN-**	membrane; hymen	**hymen**-otomy
hystera	**HYSTER-**	uterus	**hyster**-ectomy
lac, lactis	***LACT-***	milk	**lact**-ation
mamma	***MAMM-***	breast	**mamm**-ography
mastos	**MAST-, MAZ-‡**	breast	**mast**-ectomy
mēn	**MEN-**	[month] menstruation	**men**-opause
mētra	**METR-, -METRA**	uterus	**metr**-algia
oophoron§	**OOPHOR-**	ovary	**oophor**-ectomy
ōvārium¶	***OVARI-***	ovary	**ovari**-an
ōvum	***OV-***	egg	**ov**-iduct
parere, partus	***PART-, -PARA***	give birth¶	primi-**para**

*The word *gonad* did not exist in either Greek or Latin; it is a modern formation as if from a Greek *gonas, gonados*, probably derived from the noun *gonē* (birth).
†The adjective *gravidus*, in the feminine singular form, *gravida*, was used as a noun to mean a pregnant woman.
‡In Greek *mazos* was an alternate form of the word *mastos*: micromazia.
§The compound word *oophoron* did not exist in Greek. It is a modern formation from Greek (*ōon*, egg, and *phor-*, from *pherein*, bear, carry).
¶The word *ōvārium* did not exist in Latin, although there is a rare word, *ōvārius*, found only in an inscription, meaning an egg-keeper, that is, one who takes charge of newly laid eggs (Latin *ōvum*). The Latin suffix *-arium* meant "a place (for something)"; thus, *ōvārium*, "a place for the ovum," is a valid formation. Such formations are called New Latin.
¶Words ending in -para indicate a woman who has given birth: primipara (Latin *prīmus*, first); nullipara (Latin *nullus*, none).

Greek or Latin	Combining Form(s)	Meaning	Example
pelvis	**PELV-**	[basin] pelvis	**pelv**-ic
pūbēs	**PUB-**	[signs of manhood] pubic hair, pubic bone, pubic region, pubis	**pub**-ic
pūbertās	**PUBER(T)-**	[manhood] puberty	**puber**-al
salpinx, salpingos	**SALPING-, -SALPINX**	[war trumpet] fallopian tube	**salping**-ography
syrinx, syringos	**SYRING-, -SYRINX**	[pipe] fistula, cavity, oviduct, sweat glands, syringe	**syring**-e
thēlē	**THEL(E)-**	nipple	**thel**-ium
tokos	**TOC-**	childbirth, labor	**toc**-ophobia
uterus	**UTER-**	womb, belly, uterus	**uter**-ine
vāgīna	**VAGIN-**	[sheath] vagina	**vagin**-itis

Noun-Forming Suffix	Meaning	Examples
-ter	instrument, device	metreuryn-**ter**, rhineuryn-**ter**

ETYMOLOGICAL NOTES

The Amazons, legendary warrior women of Asia Minor, were said to have one breast removed so as not to interfere with the use of the bow; thus their name: *a-mazon*. The Amazon River was discovered in 1500 by the Spanish explorer Vincente Pinzón, who named it *Rio Santa Maria de la Mar Dulce*. The first descent of the river from the Andes mountains to the sea was made in 1541 by Francisco de Orellano, who renamed it the *Amazonas* from a battle that he and his followers had with a fierce tribe whose women fought alongside the men. De Orellano may have thought that these were indeed the Amazons described by the Greek writers.

The word *hymen* meant any of a variety of membranes; various writers used it to designate the pericardium, the peritoneum, the membrane that enclosed the brain, the nictitating (Late Latin* *nictitāre, nictitātus*, blink, wink) membrane (a third eyelid present in birds and some reptiles), parchment, and so forth. The ancients seem not to have used the word hymen in its modern anatomical meaning.

In Greek mythology, Hymen was the god of marriage and weddings, often invoked in a wedding song, *Hymenaeus*, the Hymeneal. In his great poem, the *Metamorphoses*, Ovid recites the story of a wedding that was attended by the god Hymen, but one to which he failed to bring his customary auspices. The bridegroom and bride were Orpheus and Eurydice (Fig. 14–3). Ovid tells us that the wedding torches of Hymen sputtered and smoked, but however much they were swung about, they failed to blaze. In further witness of this ill-starred wedding, as Eurydice was crossing the lawn, she was bitten on the ankle by a poisonous serpent and perished on the spot. As is well known, Orpheus went to the underworld and sang so persuasively to Hades and Proserpina, the rulers there, that he was permitted to lead his bride back to the upper world. But, at the last moment, he failed to observe his instructions and looked back to make certain that she was following him. She was, indeed, but no sooner had he looked back than she turned and retraced her steps to the world of the dead.

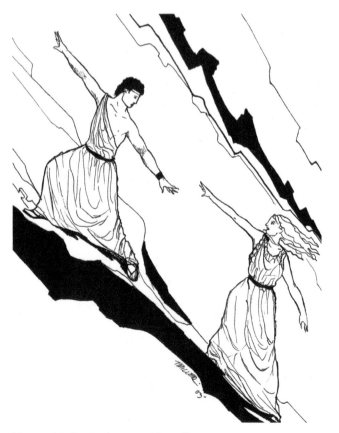

Figure 14–3. Orpheus and Eurydice.

*Latin of the 3rd and 4th centuries AD is usually called Late Latin.

Bracchiaque intendens prendique et prendere certans
nil nisi cedentes infelix arripit auras.
Iamque iterum moriens non est de coniuge quicquam
questa suo (quid enim nisi se quereretur amatam?).
Supremumque "vale," quod iam vix auribus ille
acciperet, dixit revolutaque rursus eodem est.

Stretching out his arms to embrace her and to feel
her embrace he, unhappy one, grasped nothing
but the empty air. And now, again dying, she had
no complaint against her husband (for what could
she complain of except that she had been loved?).
Uttering a last *vale,* which he could scarcely hear
she slipped back to that place she had just left.

[Ovid, *Metamorphoses* 10.58–63]

The ancient Greeks believed that women were especially susceptible to emotional disorders and that these
disorders arose from the womb. Galen used the word *hys-
terikos* (hysterical), and seems to have used it to refer to
suffering in the womb and the emotional upheaval caused
by this distress. Hippocrates says, "When a woman suffers
from hysterics or difficult labor, it is a good thing to
sneeze" [*Aphorisms*, 5.35].

The two oviducts serve to convey the ovum from the
ovary to the uterus. These tubes are called the fallopian
tubes, named for Gabriele Falloppio (1523–1562), the
Italian anatomist who discovered the existence and the
purpose of the ovaries and the tubes that bear his name.
Like his teacher, Andreas Vesalius (1514–1564), the most
important figure in European medicine after Galen and
before Harvey, he was accused of vivisection of humans in
his enthusiasm for research.

Another name for the fallopian tubes is the salpingian
tubes, a term that is also used for the eustachian tubes of
the ear (named for the 16th-century Italian anatomist
Bartolommeo Eustachio). These two sets of tubes are
named salpingian from the Greek word *salpinx, salpingos*
(war trumpet) because of their shape. The common medical terminology for a complete hysterectomy, or removal
of the uterus, fallopian tubes, and ovaries, is total abdominal hysterectomy bilateral salpingo-oophorectomy (TAH
BSO).

The combining forms *syring-* and *-syrinx* have varied
meanings in medicine, but usually refer to a cavity or hollow area, a fistula, or some other tubelike passage.
Syringomyelia is a disease of the spinal cord characterized
by the development of cavities in the surrounding tissues.
A **sialosyrinx** is a fistula into the salivary glands or a tube
for draining these glands. **Syringosystrophy** (Greek *stro-
phē*, turning, twisting) is a twisted condition of the oviduct.
A **syringe** is an instrument for injecting fluids into body
cavities, tissue, and vessels.

In Greek, the *syrinx* was the shepherd's pipe, or pipes of
Pan. Ovid, in the *Metamorphoses*, tells how the pipes of Pan
came into existence (Fig. 14–4). Once upon a time there
lived on the mountain slopes of Arcadia in Greece a young,
beautiful woodland nymph named Syrinx. One day, Pan,
that rustic divinity, saw Syrinx and pursued her. Pan almost

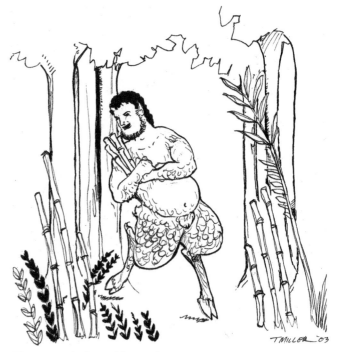

Figure 14–4. Pan with panpipes.

caught the unwilling nymph when she prayed to her sisters
for help. Pan caught her; but when he clutched her in his
arms, he found that he held only a bunch of reeds. While
Pan sighed over his disappointment, his breath blowing
through the reeds made a pleasing sound. He bound a
number of the reeds of unequal length together and called
them the syrinx, the pipes of Pan.

"Hoc mihi concilium tecum" dixisse "manebit,"
atque ita disparibus calamis conpagine cerae
inter se iunctis nomen tenuisse puellae.

"This union with you, at least, will remain,"
he said. And so pipes made of unequal
lengths of reeds joined together with wax
still keep the name of the nymph, *Syrinx.*

[Ovid, *Metamorphoses* 1.710-712]

Forms ending in **-agogue** entered English in the 14th
century in words borrowed from Old French. Some of
these words, like pedagogue and synagogue, had existed in
Latin (*paedagōgous* and *synagōga*) and both were borrowed
from Greek (*paidagōgos*, a slave who took children to
school or who taught them at home, and *synagōgē*, a place
for gathering). The Greek words *agōgos* and *agōgē* are ultimately derived from the verb *agein* (lead, drive), which is
cognate with the Latin verb *agere, actus*, with the same
meanings. Words ending in -agogue usually refer to agents
used to promote the flow or secretion of fluids within the
body. A **sialagogue** is an agent that increases the flow of
saliva.

The word **dyspareunia**, painful intercourse, has an
interesting etymology. It is derived from an adjective *dys-
pareunos* (*dys-*, unpleasant, painful, and *pareunos*, a lying
with or beside, from *para-*, alongside, and *eunazesthai*, go

to bed) that meant "ill- or badly mated." This adjective is found in Greek literature in a passage describing a bed.

In Sophocles' tragedy *Trachiniae* (*Women of Trachis*, lines 794ff), Hyllus, the son of the great Heracles, has come to the city of Trachis to report to Deianira, wife of Heracles, that her husband is dying just outside of the city. Heracles' flesh has been burned away by a magic cloak that Deianira has sent to him in ignorance of its dread powers. This cloak had been given to Deianira many years before by the centaur Nessus, whom Heracles had killed after he had attempted violence on Deianira, then Heracles' bride. The centaur, dying, gave his cloak to the young bride and told her to give it to Heracles if she ever felt that his affections were fading. Now, many years later, Heracles has been away on a foreign conquest. It is reported to Deianira that he is on the outskirts of the city and has requested a cloak to wear when offering sacrifices to the gods for a successful campaign. He has brought back with him as his prize the beautiful Iole, an oriental princess.

Deianira sent him the cloak that Nessus had given her, mindful of his advice. The cloak burned into the hero's flesh and, as he lay dying in the greatest agony, he cursed his "ill-mated" wedding bed (*dyspareunon lektron*) and Deianira herself. Zeus, at length, rescued him from his suffering and brought him up to Mount Olympus as a god, with Hebe, the daughter of Zeus and Hera, as his companion for eternity.

Epithelium (Greek *epi-*, over, *thēlē*, nipple) is the layer of cells that forms the epidermis of the skin and the surface of mucous and serous membranes. It was first discovered by the German histologist Jacob Henle (1809–1885). It is not clear why this type of tissue was named "membrane over the nipple" except for the obvious fact that epithelial tissue does cover the nipple of the breast. **Endothelium**, the layer of cells that lines the vessels and organs of the cardiovascular system, was named by the Swiss physician Wilhelm His (1831–1904).

Exercise 1: Analyze and Define

Analyze and define each of the following words. In this and in succeeding exercises, analysis should consist of separating the words into prefixes (if any), combining forms, and suffixes or suffix forms (if any) and giving the meaning of each. Be certain to differentiate between nouns and adjectives in your definitions. Consult a medical dictionary for the current meanings of these words.

1. anisomastia _____

2. antepartum _____

3. antenatal _____

4. archigaster _____

5. celiohysterectomy _____

6. cervicovaginitis _____

7. colpocystocele _____

8. endometrium _____

9. extrauterine _____

10. galactostasis _____

11. gonadal dysgenesis _____

12. gravida macromastia _____

13. hematosalpinx _____

14. hydrocolpos _____

15. hymenorrhaphy_____

16. hyperemesis gravidarum _____

17. hyperlactation _____

18. hysterosalpingography _____

19. inframammary _____

20. intrauterine _____

21. laparohystero-oophorectomy _____

22. mammogram _____

23. mastomenia _____

24. mazoplasia _____

25. menarche _____

26. menostaxis _____

27. metreurynter _____

28. micromazia _____

29. multigravida _____

30. neonatology _____

31. oligomenorrhea _____

32. oophorocystosis _____

33. ovariocyesis _____

34. pelvicephalography _____

35. perisalpingoovaritis _____

36. pneumogalactocele _____

37. polythelia _____

38. prepubescent _____

39. prosopotocia _____

40. pubarche _____

41. puberty _____

42. pyosalpinx _____

43. salpingosalpingostomy _____

44. sialosyrinx _____

45. syringoencephalomyelia _____

46. syringoma _____

47. theloncus _____

48. tocophobia _____

49. uterotubal _____

50. vaginismus _____

Exercise 2: Word Derivation

Give the word derived from Greek and/or Latin elements that means each of the following. Verify your answer in a medical dictionary. **Note that the wording of a dictionary definition may vary from the wording below.**

1. Inflammation of the cervix uteri _____

2. Pain in the vagina _____

3. Dilation of a (nonpregnant) uterus _____

4. Milk production _____

5. Any disease of the sexual organs _____

6. Inflammation of a membrane _____

7. Fixation of the uterus to the gastric wall _____

8. Substance that stimulates milk production _____

9. Mammary gland inflammation _____

10. Newborn (infant) _____

11. Incision (or removal) of an ovary _____

12. Inflammation (of the region) around the vagina _____

13. (Occurring) after childbirth _____

14. Having a wide head _____

15. Tumor of the sweat glands _____

16. Plastic surgery of the nipple _____

17. Pregnancy _____

18. Period after puberty _____

19. Concerning the uterus and rectum _____

20. Dry labor _____

Exercise 3: Drill and Review

The meaning of each of the following words can be determined from its etymology. Determine the meaning of each word. Verify your answer in a medical dictionary.

1. amenorrhea _____

2. archenteron _____

3. astigmometer _____

4. cheirognostic _____

5. colpomicroscope _____

6. cyanomycosis _____

7. dacryocyst _____

8. digitus _____

9. dysthanasia _____

10. endometriosis _____

11. expiration _____

12. gonadotropin _____

13. heterokeratoplasty _____

14. hydrometra _____

15. hyperthyroidism _____

16. hysterolith _____

17. ileocystoplasty _____

18. ischidrosis _____

19. lacrimotome _____

20. lactation _____

21. mammography _____

22. mastochondroma _____

23. melanin _____

24. metrectopia _____

25. osmesis _____

26. oviduct _____

27. oxytocin _____

28. panhysterocolpectomy _____

29. pelvitherm _____

30. phacohymenitis _____

31. poliovirus _____

32. prenatal _____

33. pseudocyesis _____

34. psychopharmacology _____

35. pubalgia _____

36. quadriceps _____

37. rectocele _____

38. retrocervical _____

39. salpingocyesis _____

40. sarcoadenoma _____

41. sclero-oophoritis _____

42. sialagogue _____

43. splanchnoptosis _____

44. stethoparalysis _____

45. syringocarcinoma _____

46. thelarche _____

47. uterine _____

48. vaginogenic _____

49. xanthocyanopia _____

50. xeroderma _____

15

GENITOURINARY SYSTEM

If a carbuncle forms on the penis, it should first be bathed with water through a syringe. Then it should be burned with a salve made of copper ore mixed with boiled honey, or with fried sheep's dung mixed with honey. When the carbuncle falls off, use the same salve for ulcers in the mouth.

[Celsus, *De Medicina* 6.18.5]

MALE REPRODUCTIVE SYSTEM

The principal organs of the male reproductive system are the **testes** (plural of testis) or **testicles**, the **epididymides** (plural of epididymis),* the **duct system**, the **penis**, and **accessory glands** (Fig. 15–1). The function of the male reproductive system is to manufacture sperm cells, or spermatozoa, and to convey these to the reproductive organs of the female through copulation. The two testes, the male gonads, are ovoid glands located in the scrotum that produce spermatozoa and the male hormone testosterone. Each testis is divided into numerous lobules, each containing one to three seminiferous tubules within which **spermatogenesis** takes place (Fig. 15–2).

The epididymis is a small structure located on the posterior surface of each testicle. It consists of a coiled mass of ducts enclosed within the tunica vaginalis. Spermatozoa are stored within the epididymides until they are released during ejaculation. From the epididymis, the sperm pass into the vas deferens, sometimes called the ductus deferens. The two seminal vesicles, located on either side of the prostate, secrete a mucoid substance that empties into the vas deferens at ejaculation. The prostate gland secretes a

*From Greek *epi-*, upon, and *didymos*, testis.

thin, opalescent, alkaline fluid that is also added to the spermatozoa at ejaculation. The thick, viscid fluid containing the spermatozoa and the mixed product of the accessory glands, the prostate, and the seminal vesicles, is called **semen**. During ejaculation, semen passes into the ejaculatory duct, a short, narrow tube formed by the union of the vas deferens and the excretory duct of the seminal vesicles. From there it travels into the **urethra**, a canal that extends from the bladder to the tip of the penis and serves as the passage for both urine and semen.

The epithelium of the seminiferous tubules of the testes can be destroyed through damage or disease. Inflammation of the testes, bilateral **orchitis**, from mumps may cause sufficient degeneration to result in sterility. Mumps is the most common infectious cause of orchitis; spermatogenesis is irreversibly damaged in 30 percent of cases of mumps orchitis. Other causes of orchitis include tuberculosis, syphilis, and gonorrhea.

Sterility may also be caused by exposing the testes to increased temperature, which inhibits spermatogenesis. It is thought that the testes are located outside the body in the scrotum to keep their temperature below that of the body. In addition to this, the scrotum is supplied with sweat glands that aid in keeping the testes cool in warm temperatures.

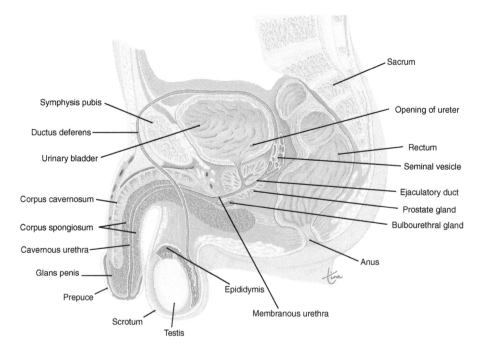

Figure 15–1. Male genital organs. Midsagittal section. (From Scanlon, VC, and Sanders, T: Essentials of Anatomy and Physiology, ed 4. F. A. Davis, Philadelphia, 2003, p 438, with permission.)

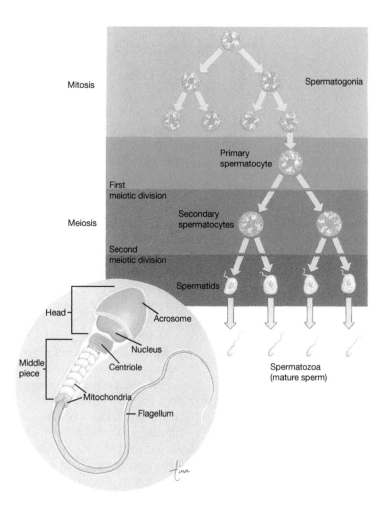

Figure 15–2. Spermatogenesis. (From Scanlon, VC, and Sanders, T: Essentials of Anatomy and Physiology, ed 4. F. A. Davis, Philadelphia, 2003, p 435, with permission.)

During the development of the male fetus, the testes are lodged within the body. Some time before birth, in the late stages of gestation, the testes descend into the scrotum. Occasionally, this descent does not take place, or occurs incompletely, so that one or both testes remain within the abdomen or somewhere along the line of descent. This is called **cryptorchidism**. Spermatogenesis is not possible in a testicle that remains within the body, perhaps because of the destruction of epithelium from body heat. Therefore, surgery is frequently performed to relocate the undescended testicle into the scrotum. Such an operation (suturing the testicle to the tissue of the scrotum) is called **orchidopexy** (formerly **orchiorrhaphy**). This surgery is commonly referred to as "button surgery" because of the tiny button sutured to the exterior of the scrotum, which holds the testicle in place during the healing process.

There are anywhere from 120 to over 500 million sperm in a normal amount of ejaculate (2 to 5 mL). The ejaculate must contain this large number of sperm for a single sperm to find and fertilize the ovum. Any one sperm is capable of fertilizing the ovum of the female. When male sperm count falls substantially, infertility usually results.

URINARY SYSTEM

The kidneys are a pair of organs lying on the left and right side of the upper abdominal cavity behind the peritoneum. They are, therefore, referred to as retroperitoneal organs (Fig. 15–3). The kidneys filter wastes from the blood and maintain its proper acid-alkaline balance. End products of metabolism include the following: (1) those from proteins,

mostly nitrogenous substances, such as urea and uric acid; (2) detoxified material from the liver, such as drugs, antibiotics, alcohol, and other toxins; (3) all substances in the circulating blood that are present in amounts greater than needed, such as sugar, alkalines, and acids; and (4) excess water.

On the medial side of each kidney is an indentation called the hilus. Three important structures enter each kidney at the hilus: the renal artery, the renal vein, and the ureter. After entering the hilus, the renal artery branches into smaller arteries that, in turn, branch into arterioles. These arterioles enter the nephrons, the functional unit of the kidney. Each kidney contains about one million nephrons. Within each nephron is a cluster of capillaries called the **glomerulus**. The walls of these glomeruli comprise, collectively, what is called the glomerular membrane. Blood plasma passes through this membrane, with blood cells and most of the protein excluded. The fluid that passes through the glomerular membrane is called the glomerular filtrate.

This filtrate contains the metabolic wastes and other substances in excess of amounts needed by the body for proper functioning. The glomerular filtrate also contains substances the body needs, such as the small amount of protein that is not filtered out by the glomerular membrane, as well as glucose and certain salts and acids. These substances must be returned to the circulating blood. Within the nephron, the glomerular filtrate passes through a series of passages called tubules. All but a small portion of the glomerular filtrate is reabsorbed into the blood, first through the capillaries of the nephron, and then into the venous system and the renal vein. The portion of glomerular filtrate that does not re-enter the

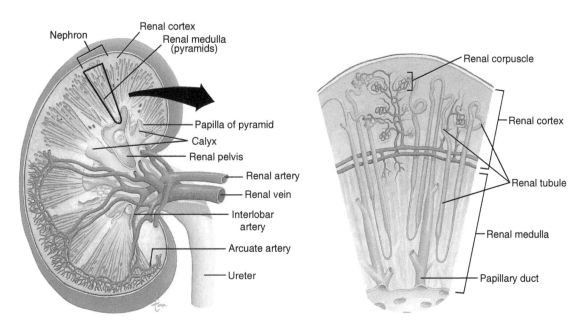

Figure 15–3. Kidney, frontal section. (Reproduced from Scanlon, VC, and Sanders, T: Essentials of Anatomy and Physiology, ed 4. F. A. Davis, Philadelphia, 2003, p 401, with permission.)

circulating blood is made up of waste material. These wastes enter the large end of a funnel-shaped cavity in the hilus of the kidney called the renal pelvis. This fluid is now urine, and it passes out of the renal pelvis into the ureter to be carried to the bladder.

> Two veins, white in color, lead from the kidneys into the vesica; they are called by the Greeks ureters because they think that it is through them that the urine descends and flows into the vesica. [Celsus, *De Medicina* 4.1.10]

One ureter exits from each kidney. As the urine enters the ureters, it is forced along by peristaltic contractions that occur at varying intervals from a few seconds to a few minutes. The urine enters the bladder through the ureteric orifices, which open to allow passage of the urine, and then close to prevent a reflux. **Nephrolithiasis** (kidney stones) is a common renal disorder. The most common type of renal calculus, or stone, contains calcium oxalate. Factors known to precipitate stone formation include **hypercalciuria**, **hyperoxaluria**, low urine volumes, and infections. Renal calculi may occur in any location along the urinary tract.

Urine is stored in the bladder until the volume reaches a certain amount. Then the internal and external urethral sphincters open to allow it to pass through the urethra. Emptying of the bladder by the passage of urine through the urethra is called **micturition** (Latin *micturīre*, *micturītus*, urinate).

DISORDERS OF KIDNEY FUNCTION

Any kind of damage to the kidney that impairs its ability to filter the blood of metabolic wastes and toxins results in abnormal kidney function, or renal insufficiency. Some disorders are congenital. Table 15–1 summarizes several causes of acute renal failure (ARF). **Bilateral renal agenesis**, the failure of both kidneys to form during gestation, results in death within a few days after birth. Unilateral

Table 15–1. Causes of Acute Renal Failure

Where	What's Responsible	Examples
Prerenal	Inadequate blood flow to the kidney	Severe dehydration; prolonged hypotension; renal ischemia or emboli; septic or cardiogenic shock
Renal	Injury to kidney glomeruli or tubules	Glomerulonephritis; toxic injury to the kidneys (e.g., by drugs or poisons)
Postrenal	Obstruction to urinary outflow	Prostatic hyperplasia; bladder outlet obstruction

Source: From *Taber's Cyclopedic Medical Dictionary*, ed 19. FA Davis, Philadelphia, 2001, p 1777, with permission.

agenesis is not necessarily fatal because one kidney is sufficient to sustain life.

Complete loss of function, or ARF, often results immediately after kidney damage from a number of causes: (1) parenchymal damage to the kidney caused by toxins, such as contrast dye, or from infectious etiologies, such as glomerulonephritis; (2) certain drugs, such as cyclosporines, angiotensin-converting enzyme (ACE) inhibitors for the treatment of hypertension, or nonsteroidal anti-inflammatory drugs (NSAIDs), all of which cause functional impairment; (3) decreased blood flow to the kidneys resulting in renal ischemia secondary to shock or dehydration; and (4) obstruction of the urinary outflow tract.

The immediate result of ARF is a rapid concentration of urea, uric acid, potassium, and other undesirable substances in the blood. Failure to excrete nitrogenous wastes in the urea and uric acid causes the condition known as **uremia**, or **azotemia**. Failure to excrete potassium causes the condition called **hyperkalemia**. **Oliguria** usually accompanies ARF and is present when the daily urine volume is insufficient to remove the solute loads that are the end products of metabolism.

Streptococcal infection, particularly in the respiratory tract, can result in acute glomerular nephritis, or **glomerulonephritis**. It is not the infection itself that causes damage to the kidneys; rather, the glomeruli become inflamed in a reaction to the antibodies that are formed to combat the infection. This causes malfunction of the nephrons in varying degrees, sometimes resulting in ARF. Usual symptoms of glomerulonephritis include **hematuria**, **proteinuria**, **albuminuria**, **oliguria**, red blood cell casts, pruritus, nausea, constipation, hypertension, and **edema**. Treatment with immunosuppressive drugs may reverse the lesions caused by glomerulonephritis in patients with ARF.

Rhabdomyolysis is a potentially fatal disease in which the by-products of skeletal muscle destruction accumulate in renal tubules, causing ARF. Rhabdomyolysis may result from crush injuries, toxic effects on skeletal muscles produced by drugs or chemicals, extremes of exertion, shock, sepsis, and severe hyponatremia (Greek, *hypo-*, deficient, New Latin, *natrium*, sodium, Greek, *haima*, blood), or can result from a decreased concentration of sodium in the blood. Life-threatening hyperkalemia and metabolic acidosis may result from untreated rhabdomyolysis.

Inflammation of the renal pelvis is called **pyelitis**, but the disease invariably extends into the body of the kidney itself, the renal parenchyma. The proper term for the disease when it affects both the pelvis and the body of the kidney is **pyelonephritis**. Almost any pyogenic bacterium can cause this disease, although in most cases *Escherichia coli* is the responsible microbe. Prompt therapy with antibiotics is effective in treating this disease. Sometimes it is desirable to obtain an x-ray view of the movement of blood through the renal veins. This procedure, called an **intravenous pyelogram** (IVP), involves injecting a radiopaque substance through the renal vein and taking a series of x-ray films to observe its progress. An IVP may reveal calculi, lesions, or deformities in the pelvic area.

Anemia is a disease associated with chronic renal insufficiency. **Erythropoietin** is a cytokine made by the kidneys that stimulates the proliferation of red blood cells. Insufficient kidney function results in insufficient erythropoietin production, with a consequent diminution in the number of erythrocytes. Synthetic erythropoetin is used to treat patients with anemia and renal failure.

RENAL DIALYSIS—THE ARTIFICIAL KIDNEY

Renal dialysis may be initiated in cases of kidney damage so severe that these organs cannot function efficiently enough to prevent fatal toxicity of the blood. Renal dialysis acts as an artificial kidney with the filtering process occurring outside the body. The functional unit of the dialysis machine is a semipermeable membrane that allows all of the blood to flow through except erythrocytes and proteins. The circulating blood is withdrawn from the body via an artery, and is pumped through the dialysis machine, where it passes through the semipermeable membrane, leaving behind red cells and proteins. Once through the membrane, the plasma passes into a liquid called the dialyzing fluid, which contains most of the constituents of normal plasma except the waste products of metabolism, principally urea. The toxic wastes in the plasma diffuse into the dialyzing fluid and remain there when the plasma, now rid of most of the waste matter, is returned through the membrane into the body. To prevent coagulation of the blood in the artificial kidney, the anticoagulant heparin is infused into the blood before it enters the dialysis machine. Major advances in the science of renal dialysis now allow other forms of dialysis, such as continuous ambulatory peritoneal dialysis (CAPD), with improved outcomes and ease of administration.

DIABETES MELLITUS

Diabetes mellitus, or sugar diabetes, is a chronic disease characterized by varying degrees of inability to metabolize carbohydrates. This is caused by inadequate production and secretion of insulin by the beta cells of the islets of Langerhans in the pancreas (named after Paul Langerhans, a German pathologist, 1847–1888). Another cause is resistance to the metabolic effects of insulin in the cells of the body. Manifestations of the disease are elevated blood sugar (**hyperglycemia**) and sugar in the urine (**glycosuria**). Symptoms include **polydipsia**, **polyuria**, loss of weight (despite **polyphagia**), and fatigue. When the course of diabetes is allowed to advance without proper treatment, diabetic ketoacidosis (DKA) and coma can result. DKA is characterized by severe nausea, vomiting, dyspnea, and delirium.

There are two types of diabetes mellitus (Table 15–2). Type 1 diabetes mellitus, also called insulin-dependent diabetes mellitus (IDDM), is caused by insufficient insulin production, and onset is usually earlier in life. Type 2 diabetes mellitus, called non–insulin-dependent diabetes mellitus (NIDDM), usually begins later in life and is characterized by resistance to the effects of insulin at the cellular level. Both types of diabetes lead to increased blood sugar levels.

In some patients with type 2 diabetes, the only treatment required is a well-balanced diet that is low in calories (1600 to 1800 calories per day). Tests for blood sugar (glucose) should be taken frequently, and if glucose concentration remains high in the blood and urine, it may be necessary to administer medications, such as the sulfonylureas (or possibly newer medications), which stimulate the pancreas to release insulin.

The isolation of insulin in 1921 by Drs. Frederick G. Banting, Charles H. Best, and James R. Macleod (for which Drs. Banting and Macleod were awarded the Nobel prize for medicine in 1923) has made it possible for diabetics to lead normal lives. Synthetic forms of insulin have

Table 15–2. Comparison of Type 1 Insulin-Dependent Diabetes Mellitus and Type 2 Non–Insulin-Dependent Diabetes Mellitus

	Type 1	Type 2
Age at onset	Usually <30	Usually >40
Symptom onset	Abrupt	Gradual
Body weight	Normal	Obese (80%)
HLA association	Positive	Negative
Family history	Common	Nearly universal
Insulin in blood	Little to none	Some usually present
Islet cell antibodies	Present at onset	Absent
Prevalence	0.2% to 0.3%	6%
Symptoms	Polyuria, polydipsia, polyphagia, weight loss, ketoacidosis	Polyuria, polydipsia, peripheral neuropathy
Control	Insulin, diet, and exercise	Diet, exercise, and often oral hypoglycemic drugs or insulin
Vascular and neural changes	Eventually develop	Usually develop
Stability of condition	Fluctuates, may be difficult to control	May be difficult to control in poorly motivated

Source: From *Taber's Cyclopedic Medical Dictionary*, ed 19. FA Davis, Philadelphia, 2001, p 557, with permission.

been created and may be administered to replace the insulin that is not produced by individuals with type 1 diabetes.

Insulin is thought to act as a stimulant for the intracellular transport of glucose into tissue cells, affecting the utilization of sugar in the cell. This is accomplished by increasing its conversion to glycogen and fat and its oxidation to carbon dioxide and water. Thus diminished production of insulin leads to decreased carbohydrate utilization, with consequent hyperglycemia. The basic cause of the failure of the beta cells of the pancreas to secrete an adequate amount of insulin is unknown, but may be inflammation of the pancreas, invasion by malignant cells, or a genetic disorder. Diabetes is the leading cause of chronic renal failure and subsequent renal dialysis in the United States.

The Greek word *diabētēs* is found in the medical writings of Galen and of Aretaeus, both of the 2nd century AD. The word *diabētēs* is from the verb *bainein* (go, walk, pass), and means "a passing through," a reference to the immoderate passage of urine affecting people who have this disease.

VESICLE

The word vesicle, as well as words beginning in vesicul-, is a modern formation (New Latin) as a diminutive of *vēsīca*; these words mean either (1) a small sac containing fluid, especially a seminal vesicle, or (2) a small, blister-like elevation on the skin containing serous fluid, as in the word vesicopustular.

ETYMOLOGICAL NOTES

The word kalium, the chemical name for the element potassium, was formed from the Arabic word *qali*, the name of the plant now known in English as saltwort, from the ashes of which potash was made. Sir Humphry Davy (1778–1829) first separated potassium from potash, which previously had been considered an element, and gave it the name potassium. The Swedish chemist Jons Jacob Berzelius (1779–1848) coined the name *kalium* and applied it to the newly isolated element. Such formations are

VOCABULARY

Note: Latin combining forms are in ***bold italics***.

Greek or Latin	Combining Form(s)	Meaning	Example
aktis, aktinos	**ACTIN-**	[ray] radiation	**actin**-ogenic
*agra**	**-AGRA**	[hunting] (sudden) pain, gout	pod-**agra**
cortex, corticis	***CORTIC-*, *CORTEX***	[bark, rind] outer layer (of an organ)	adrenal **cortex**
kry(m)os†	**CRY(M)-**	icy cold	**cry**-otherapy
glykys	**GLYC-**	sugar	hypo-**glyc**-emia
inguen, inguinis	***INGUIN-***	groin	**inguin**-al
lagneia	**-LAGNIA**	abnormal sexual excitation or gratification	algo-**lagnia**
orchis, orchios	**ORCHI(D)-,‡ ORCH(E)-**	testicle	mon-**orchid**-ism
pēnis	***PEN-***	[tail] penis	**pen**-ile
phallos	**PHALL-**	penis	**phall**-ic
pyelos	**PYEL-**	renal pelvis	**pyel**-onephritis
rhabdos	**RHABD-**	rod	**rhabd**-omyolysis
scrōtum	***SCROT-***	[bag] scrotum	**scrot**-ocele
sēmen, sēminis	***SEM-*, *SEMIN-***	seed, semen	in-**semin**-ation
sperma, spermatos	**SPERM(AT)-**	seed, sperm, semen	**sperm**-icide
ouron	**UR-**	urine, urinary tract, uric acid§	**ur**-ine
ourētēr	**URETER-**	ureter	**ureter**-ostoma
ourēthra	**URETHR-**	urethra	**urethr**-itis
vēsīca	**VESIC-**	(urinary) bladder	**vesic**-ocele
zōon	**ZO-**	animal, organism	**zo**-ophyte

*See the Etymological Notes in this lesson.
†There are two forms of this word in Greek: *kryos* and *krymos*, with the same meaning.
‡The combining form orchid- is used as if from a genitive case *orchidos*; the *-d-* dropped out of this word in the Greek language, leaving the genitive case *orchios*, with an alternate form *orcheōs*.
§Words beginning with, ending with, or containing uric- indicate the presence of uric acid, an acid that is formed as an end product of purine (protein) digestion. Uric acid in a common constituent of renal calculi and of the concretions of gout.

called New Latin. The word alkali is from the Arabic *al-qaliy*, the calcined ashes of the plant *qali*.

The Greek word *nitron* and the Latin *nitrum* were probably borrowed from the Arabic *natrun* (sodium carbonate). The origin of the word most likely took place in Egypt, where Nitriotes was the Greek name of a district where *nitron* was found in great quantities. The word is found in the Old Testament in Jeremiah 2.22 as Hebrew *nether*. In the King James version, the prophet says, "For though thou wash thee with nitre, and take thee much sope, yet thine iniquity is marked before me, saith the Lord God." The Hebrew word *nether* in the Old Testament is translated by *nitron* in the Septuagint and *nitrum* in the Vulgate.

The first use of the word nitrogen is found in 1790 as *nitrogène* in a work by the French chemist Jean Chaptal (1756–1832). Antoine Lavoisier had recognized that this gas, which had been discovered as being one of the elements of the atmosphere by the British scientist Daniel Rutherford, would not support life, and for this reason named it *azote* (from the Greek negative prefix *a-* and *zōē*, life).

The Roman writer Pliny discourses at length about *nitrum*, soda:

> In the soda-beds of Egypt ophthalmia is unknown. Ulcers on those who visit there heal quickly, but if ulcers form on those who are already there, they are slow to heal. Soda mixed with oil causes those who are rubbed with that mixture to sweat; it also softens the flesh…. Soda is good for a toothache if it is mixed with pepper in wine. If it is boiled with a leek and then cooked down to make a dentifrice, it restores the white color to blackened teeth. [*Natural History* 31.115–117].

The Greek word *agra* meant hunting or catching game; another word, *podagra*, meant a trap for animals. This word later came to mean a disease of the feet of animals, and then gout, a painful, inflamed condition of a joint, in humans. Formations in English use this word as a suffix, as in **odontagra** (toothache, especially from gout), **arthragra** (acute pain in the joints), and so forth. The term **podagra** is used today to mean gout, especially of the foot or large toe.

The word hilus, the indentation in the side of the kidney into which vessels enter, is a New Latin word formed from the Latin *hilum*, a rare word whose etymology is unknown. It forms the base of the noun *nihil*, nothing (as used in the English word nihilism, a doctrine of destruction). According to Festus, a Roman grammarian of the 2nd century AD, *hilum* meant "something that clings to the seed of a bean, from which we get the word *nihil*." There was no Latin form *hilus*, and the earliest example of this word in English is found in 1840 in an anatomical treatise in which it is used to indicate a notch or fissure in an organ into which vessels enter. In botany, the word hilum is used to designate the point of attachment of a seed to its vessel—for example, the "eye" of a bean.

Glomeruli, clusters of capillaries within the nephrons of the kidneys, take their name from the New Latin word *glomerulus*, a diminutive of Latin *glomus* (ball of yarn). There was a verb *glomerāre*, meaning wind into a ball or gather together. Virgil used this verb in the *Aeneid* to describe the souls of the dead gathered about the banks of the Styx, waiting to be ferried across to the realms of the dead by the boatman Charon:

> *quam multa in silvis autumni frigore primo*
> *lapsa cadunt folia, aut ad terram gurgite ab alto*
> *quam multae glomerantur aves, ubi frigidus annus*
> *trans pontum fugat et terris immittit apricis.*

> As many as the leaves that fall from trees
> in the first frost of the autumn, and as dense
> as the flocks of birds that gather together
> in flight when the season of cold drives them
> across the sea, sending them to sunny lands.

> [Virgil, *Aeneid* 6.309–312]

 ## Exercise 1: Analyze and Define

Analyze and define each of the following words. In this and in succeeding exercises, analysis should consist of separating the words into prefixes (if any), combining forms, and suffixes or suffix forms (if any) and giving the meaning of each. Be certain to differentiate between nouns and adjectives in your definitions. Consult a medical dictionary for the current meanings of these words.

1. abdominoscrotal _____

2. actinodermatitis _____

3. actinogenic _____

4. aglycemia _____

5. algolagnia _____

6. anuresis _____

7. azoospermia _____

8. cerebellar cortex _____

9. coprozoa _____

10. cortical _____

11. cryalgesia _____

12. crymophilic _____

13. cryptorchidism _____

14. dysuria _____

15. epizoon _____

16. euglycemia _____

17. glycopolyuria _____

18. inguinal reflex _____

19. inguinoscrotal _____

20. inosuria _____

21. insemination _____

22. melanuria _____

23. monorchid _____

24. nycturia _____

25. oligospermia _____

26. orcheoplasty _____

27. orchidoncus _____

28. paravesical _____

29. penile _____

30. penischisis _____

31. phalliform _____

32. podagra _____

33. polyorchidism _____

34. protozoology _____

35. pseudohematuria _____

36. pyelogram _____

37. pyosemia _____

38. rhabdomyolysis _____

39. scrota _____

40. scrotitis _____

41. seminiferous _____

42. spermatopoietic _____

43. ureterolithiasis _____

44. urethrostenosis _____

45. uricocholia _____

46. uroureter _____

47. vaginovesical _____

48. vesicocele _____

49. vesicula seminalis _____

50. zoophyte _____

Exercise 2: Word Derivation

Give the word derived from Greek and/or Latin elements that means each of the following. Verify your answer in a medical dictionary. **Note that the wording of a dictionary definition may vary from the wording below.**

1. Inflammation of a nerve or nerves resulting from exposure to x-rays _____

2. Fat in the urine _____

3. Outer layer of the adrenal gland (2 words) _____

4. (Congenital) absence of one or more testicles _____

5. Pertaining to the cervix uteri and bladder _____

6. Ulceration of the urinary tract _____

7. Loss of sense of cold _____

8. Study of the effect of cold on biological systems _____

9. Pertaining to (the region of) the groin _____

10. Sweet taste _____

11. Condition in which there is only one (descended) testicle _____

12. Science of animal life _____

13. Inflammation of the penis _____

14. Dilation of the renal pelvis _____

15. Suppression of the semen _____

16. Hernia in the scrotum _____

17. Resembling a rod _____

18. (Irritability or) spasm of the urethra _____

19. Yellow pigment of the urine _____

20. (Abnormal) love of animals _____

Exercise 3: Drill and Review

The meaning of each of the following words can be determined from its etymology. Determine the meaning of each word. Verify your answer in a medical dictionary.

1. acanthopelvis _____

2. actinotherapy _____

3. agnathia _____

4. antigalactic _____

5. brachygnathia _____

6. corticoadrenal _____

7. crymodynia _____

8. cryotherapy _____

9. dacryopyorrhea _____

10. dactyledema _____

11. dysthyroidism _____

12. fecaluria _____

13. hemocytozoon _____

14. homeo-osteoplasty _____

15. hydrophilism _____

16. hyperuricemia _____

17. hyposynergia _____

18. immunifacient _____

19. inguinolabial _____

20. leukocoria _____

21. mastatrophia _____

22. myonephropexy _____

23. neurocrine _____

24. nosophobia _____

25. oliguria _____

26. orchidoptosis _____

27. ovicide _____

28. paraparesis _____

29. pelvicephalometry _____

30. phalloncus _____

31. polyuria _____

32. porencephalitis _____

33. protozoa _____

34. pubescence _____

35. pyelocystostomosis _____

36. rhabdovirus _____

37. scrotoplasty _____

38. seminal _____

39. sone _____

40. spermatozoicide _____

41. stereo-orthopter _____

42. sternothyroid _____

43. synorchidism _____

44. thyroaplasia _____

45. trophocyte _____

46. ureteroureterostomy _____

47. urethrotome _____

48. vesicoclysis _____

49. ventrose _____

50. zoopsia _____

ADDITIONAL STUDY

HEMATOPOIETIC AND LYMPHATIC SYSTEMS

MUSCULOSKELETAL SYSTEM

NERVOUS SYSTEM

ENDOCRINE SYSTEM

16

HEMATOPOIETIC AND LYMPHATIC SYSTEMS

Human blood is composed of plasma (about 50% to 60%) and cells (about 40% to 50%) (Fig. 16–1). Plasma is composed mostly of water along with ions, proteins, hormones, and lipids. The cellular components are erythrocytes, the red blood cells (RBCs); leukocytes, the white blood cells (WBCs); and thrombocytes (platelets),* the elements that play an important role in the coagulation of blood, hemostasis, and blood thrombus formation. The function of blood is to carry nutrients, principally oxygen, to the cells and tissues of the body, and to carry away wastes, principally carbon dioxide, from the cells and tissues for disposal. In addition to this primary function, blood plays an important part in the regulation of body temperature, and in the body's defense mechanism against infection, especially through the phagocytic action of the leukocytes (see the section on leukocytes).

ERYTHROCYTES

Erythrocytes are mature RBCs. In adults, erythrocyte formation (called **erythropoiesis**) takes place in bone marrow, principally in the vertebrae, ribs, and sternum (breastbone); the spongy layer within the cranial bones (diploë); and the long bones of the arms and legs. Immature erythrocytes are called **erythroblasts**, and each contains a **nucleus** (Latin *nūcleus*, kernel, diminutive of *nux, nucis*, nut), the structure within a cell that contains the chromosomes and is responsible for the cell's metabolism, growth, and reproduction. When erythroblasts mature, they expel their nuclei and become fully developed erythrocytes called **akaryocytes**, cells without a nucleus.[†] Each erythrocyte has a typical cell membrane and an internal stroma, or framework, made of lipids and proteins to which more than 200 million molecules of **hemoglobin** are attached. Hemoglobin is composed of **hematin**, the iron-carrying portion of the molecule, and **globin**, a simple protein.

The primary function of erythrocytes is to carry oxygen to and carbon dioxide from the cells and tissues of the body.* Oxygen is carried in the hemoglobin of the blood. Hemoglobin combines with oxygen to form an unstable compound called **oxyhemoglobin**, which is carried through the arterial system to all parts of the body, where the oxygen is released into the tissues. The average life span of an RBC is about 4 months, after which it disintegrates. The iron in the hemoglobin is reused, and may be stored in the liver until needed for production of new RBCs in the bone marrow.

An erythrocyte from which the hemoglobin has been dissolved is called an **achromatic erythrocyte**, an RBC without color. Any excess amounts of hemoglobin in the body as a result of overdestruction of erythrocytes (**hemolysis**) are passed off in the urine and feces, a process that keeps the amount of hemoglobin in the body relatively stable. This principle of stability is called **homeostasis**. When it is applied to the circulating blood, it means that production and destruction of RBCs (erythrocytes) are mutually dependent on each other, and that the constituents and properties of the blood tend to remain stable. Any interference with this stability leads to hematologic disease.

When there is insufficient hemoglobin in the bloodstream for an adequate supply of oxygen to the cells and tissues, a substance called **erythropoietin**, which stimulates the production of erythrocytes, is released into the bloodstream. In 1906, French scientists Paul Carnot and Claude Déflandre announced their theory that the circulating blood carried a substance they called *"hémopoiétin,"*

---

*Greek *plate* (flat); -let is an English diminutive suffix derived from French.
[†]See *Taber's Cyclopedic Medical Dictionary, ed 19*. Philadelphia: F. A. Davis, 2001, entry for erythrocyte for further explanation of this process.
*For a discussion of this function of blood, see Lesson 11, The Respiratory System.

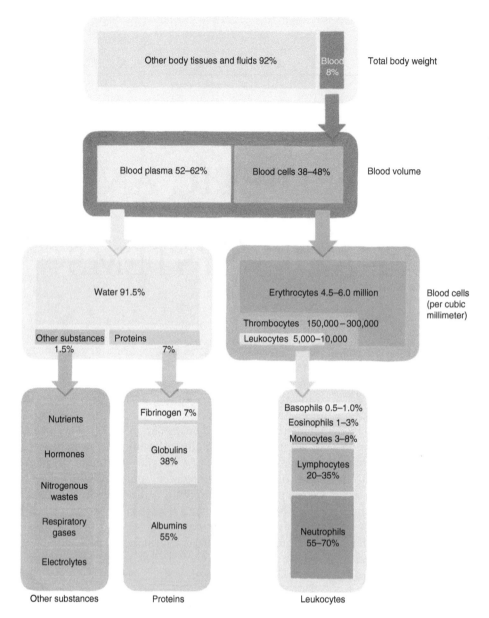

Figure 16–1. Blood composition, showing components of blood and their relationship to other body tissues. (From Scanlon, VC, and Sanders, T: Essentials of Anatomy and Physiology, ed 4. F. A. Davis, Philadelphia, 2003, p 239, with permission.)

which stimulated the production of RBCs, but their work was largely ignored.

Subsequent investigations, especially since 1950, have confirmed the presence of this substance. Erythropoietin is a cytokine (protein) produced in the kidneys that stimulates the proliferation of RBCs. Synthetic erythropoietin is used to treat anemia, especially in patients with renal or bone marrow failure.

An insufficiency of oxygen in the body, a condition called **hypoxia,*** can result from environmental exposure, disease, or toxic substances. **Altitude hypoxia** is the result of exposure to high altitudes; **anemic hypoxia** is caused by

a decrease in the concentration of hemoglobin or RBCs in the blood; and **anoxic hypoxia** is caused by malfunctioning pulmonary mechanisms, respiratory obstruction, or inadequate ventilation. Exposure to toxic substances, such as snake venoms, which enter the bloodstream and cause hemolysis, can also cause hypoxia.

The normal number of erythrocytes averages about 5,500,000 per cubic millimeter (abbreviated mm³) for males and about 4,500,000 for females. The total number in an average- size person is about 35 trillion. The volume of erythrocytes packed in a given volume of blood via the process of centrifugation, which separates the solid elements from the plasma in blood, is called the **hematocrit** (Greek *krites*, judge). The hematocrit is expressed as the

---

*Anoxia, absence of oxygen, is often used incorrectly to mean hypoxia.

percentage of total blood volume that consists of erythrocytes, or as the volume in cubic centimeters of erythrocytes packed by centrifugation. The normal average for men is about 47 percent and that for women about 42 percent. A decrease below the normal number is called **erythropenia**, and an abnormal increase in hematocrit is called **polycythemia** or **erythrocytosis**.

LEUKOCYTES

Leukocytes can be classified into two groups, both of which possess nuclei. One type, called **granulocytes**, contains **granules** (Latin *grānulum*, diminutive of *grānum*, grain, seed), minute, grainlike bodies located in the cytoplasm, the substance of a cell outside its nucleus.

Leukocytes without granules are called **agranulocytes**. Granular leukocytes, which readily accept certain kinds of dyes, are characterized and grouped according to the type of dye that will stain them. The granules of some leukocytes stain red; these cells are called **eosinophils**, or eosinophilic leukocytes, from the acid dye that stains them, **eosin**, a red dye. Other cells stain blue and are called **basophils** (Greek *basis*, base), or basophilic leukocytes, because the dye that stains them is a basic, or nonacidic—that is, alkaline—dye of a bluish color. Most leukocytes, however, take on a purplish color and are called **neutrophils**, or neutrophilic leukocytes, because they can be stained only by neutral dyes (dyes that are neither acidic

nor alkaline), which are purple. An abnormal increase in the number of eosinophils in the blood is called **eosinophilia**; a decrease is called **eosinopenia**. An abnormal increase in the number of basophils is called **basophilia**. An abnormal increase in the number of neutrophils is called **neutrophilia**, and an abnormal decrease is called **neutropenia**.

Most leukocytes, especially granulocytes, are **phagocytes**; that is, they have the ability to engulf and ingest particles of foreign substances or hostile bacteria. This is their function in the body. When hostile bacteria invade the body, the production of leukocytes is greatly increased, and an increased number of leukocytes (leukocytosis) is usually an indication of bacterial infection. When the leukocytes themselves are destroyed by invading bacteria, the dead cells collect and form the whitish mass that we call pus. If a ready outlet to the surface of the body is not found for the pus, an abscess is formed. Normally, 1 mm^3 of blood contains 5,000 to 10,000 leukocytes. A decrease in number below 5,000 is called **leukopenia** and an increase above 10,000 is called **leukocytosis**.

PLATELETS

Platelets are flat round or oval disks of microscopic size found in the blood (Fig. 16–2). They number 130,000 to 400,000 per mm^3. Sometimes called **thrombocytes**, they play an important part in the coagulation of blood, in the

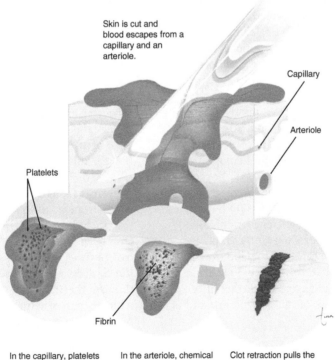

Skin is cut and blood escapes from a capillary and an arteriole.

Capillary

Arteriole

Platelets

Fibrin

In the capillary, platelets stick to the ruptured wall and form a platelet plug.

In the arteriole, chemical clotting forms a fibrin clot.

Clot retraction pulls the edges of the break together.

Figure 16–2. Platelet plug formation and clotting. (From Scanlon, VC, and Sanders, T: Essentials of Anatomy and Physiology, ed 4. F. A. Davis, Philadelphia, 2003, p 251, with permission.)

arrest of bleeding (**hemostasis**), and in **thrombus** (blood clot) formation. When there is damage to tissue, platelets adhere to each other and to the damaged parts, forming a protective mass around the injured part, thus stopping the loss of blood.

A decrease in the number of platelets is called **thrombocytopenia**. The condition known as **idiopathic thrombocytopenia purpura** (ITP) (Latin *purpura*, purple) is thrombocytopenia of unknown etiology. ITP is clinically associated with the spontaneous appearance of dark blue or purple patches on the skin and/or the mucosal surfaces of the mouth caused by hemorrhages into these areas. Such discolorations, if small, are called **macules** (Latin *macula*, spot); larger patches are called **ecchymoses**. **Thrombocytosis**, increased platelet production, occurs after loss of blood following surgery or violent injury to tissues.

CLOTTING

When blood is exposed to air, it changes into a soft, jelly-like mass called a blood clot. This process is called blood clotting or blood **coagulation**. This physical change from a liquid to a nonfluid mass is caused by a protein substance normally present in plasma, **fibrinogen**. When blood escapes from the vessels that normally contain it, a substance called **thrombin** is formed from elements present in the blood. The thrombin acts on the fibrinogen and converts it into **fibrin**, an insoluble, elastic, stringy substance that forms a network in which platelets are caught. These platelets cling together, and a clot is formed. Clotting is slowed down by cold, by a deficiency of calcium, by the presence of certain mineral salts, and by anticoagulants such as **heparin** or **coumadin**, as well as by hemolytic agents such as snake venom.

Hemophilia is a rare, hereditary blood disease that occurs almost exclusively in males. It is characterized by a prolonged coagulation time; that is, the blood fails to clot in the normal time because of a deficiency of blood-clotting proteins. There are two types of hemophilia: hemophilia A, which affects 1 in 5,000 to 10,000 boys in whom blood clotting factor VIII is either missing or defective; and hemophilia B, which affects 1 in 30,000 boys in whom blood clotting factor IX is deficient or missing. Treatment for hemophilia includes intravenous replacement of the deficient clotting factors and the addition of chemotherapeutic agents that promote clotting. Individuals with hemophilia should avoid drugs that interfere with the coagulation process (such as heparin), and must be careful to avoid trauma.

ANEMIA

Anemia is a condition in which there is a reduction in the normal number of circulating RBCs, or the quantity of hemoglobin in the blood. This loss occurs when the equilibrium (homeostasis) between production and destruction of erythrocytes is disturbed. Anemia is not a disease but rather a symptom of various diseases or conditions: excessive blood loss from disease or injury, vitamin or mineral deficiencies (especially vitamin B_{12}, folate, or iron deficiency), decreased RBC production caused by the suppression of bone marrow associated with kidney failure, or excessive cell destruction (**hemolysis**) associated with sickle cell disease. There are many types of anemia, some of which are listed here:

- **Aplastic anemia**, most common in adolescents and young adults, is caused by deficient RBC production due to bone marrow disorders resulting from exposure to chemicals, chemotherapy, or ionizing radiation. Most patients with aplastic anemia can be treated effectively with bone marrow transplants or immunosuppressive therapy.
- **Erythroblastic anemia** (also called **Cooley's anemia** after American physician Thomas Cooley, 1871–1945) is caused by an inherited trait that results in defective production of hemoglobin. This condition is also called **thalassemia major** (Greek *thalassa*, the sea) because it occurs almost exclusively among people of the Mediterranean basin.
- **Iron-deficiency anemia** results from the body's demand for more iron than can normally be supplied. It is usually caused by chronic loss of blood, as in **hypermenorrhea**, abnormal increase in menstrual flow at regular periods.
- **Pernicious anemia** (Latin *perniciosus*, destructive, from *pernicies*, destruction) usually occurs in later adult life and is characterized by **achlorhydria** (lack of hydrochloric acid in the gastric juice) as a result of reduced absorption of vitamin B_{12}.
- **Sickle cell anemia** is a hereditary hemolytic anemia characterized by large numbers of sickle-shaped erythrocytes or meniscocytes (Greek *mēniskos*, crescent) in the blood. Sickle cell anemia is caused by the presence of an abnormal type of hemoglobin (hemoglobin S), inherited from both parents, in these cells (Fig. 16–3). It occurs mainly among African-Americans, native Africans, and individuals of Mediterranean descent. Treatment for sickle cell anemia includes supportive therapy with supplemental iron and blood transfusions. Administration of hydroxyurea stimulates the production of hemoglobin S, decreases the need for blood transfusion, and reduces the incidence of painful **sickle cell crisis**, which occurs when there is a drop in the number of blood cells as a result of abnormal cell production.

LEUKEMIA

Leukemia is a class of hematologic cancers in which immature blood cells multiply at the expense of normal blood cells. As normal blood cells are depleted from the body,

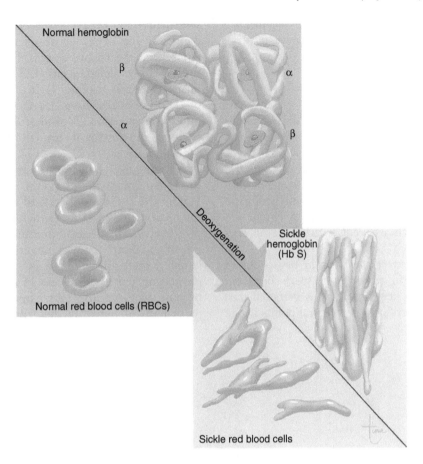

Figure 16–3. Sickle cell anemia. (From Scanlon, VC, and Sanders, T: Essentials of Anatomy and Physiology, ed 4. F. A. Davis, Philadelphia, 2003, p 55, with permission.)

anemia, infection, hemorrhage, or death can result. The leukemias are categorized as acute or chronic; by the type of cell from which they originate; and by the genetic, chromosomal, or growth factor abnormality in the malignant cells. Treatment options include chemotherapy, bone marrow transplantation, or both. New therapeutic regimens are being developed and can be tailored to treat specific illnesses.

Hairy cell leukemia is a chronic, low-grade cancer in which abnormally shaped B lymphocytes, called "hairy cells" because of their fuzzy appearance, occur. This rare disease, which generally occurs in middle-aged people, and more often in men than in women, is marked by **pancytopenia** and **splenomegaly**. Before the development of effective chemotherapeutic agents, the average survival time for patients with hairy cell leukemia was about 5 years; with chemotherapy, the survival time may be extended. Other types of leukemia include the following:

- **Acute lymphocytic leukemia,** or **ALL** (also called acute lymphoblastic leukemia) is a hematologic cancer characterized by the overgrowth of immature lymphoid cells in the bone marrow, blood, and body tissues. Although quickly fatal if left untreated, with advances in chemotherapy, nearly 80 percent of children and one third of adults with ALL are cured.
- **Acute myeloid leukemia** or **AML** (also called acute myelogenous leukemia and acute nonlymphocytic leukemia, ANLL), refers to a group of hematologic cancers in which neoplastic (Greek *neos*, new and *plassein*, form, develop) cells form in the blood and bone marrow. Treatment with cytotoxic chemotherapy and with bone marrow and stem cell transplantation currently results in complete remission for approximately 65 percent of patients with AML.
- **Chronic lymphocytic leukemia** or **CLL** is a malignancy in which abnormal lymphocytes, usually B cells, grow and infiltrate body tissues, often resulting in enlargement of lymph nodes and immune system dysfunction. Patients with early stage CLL are frequently not treated, but for patients in advanced stages of the disease, various cytotoxic chemotherapeutic regimens are available.
- **Chronic myeloid leukemia** or **CML** (also called chronic myelogenous leukemia) is a disease marked by chronic increase in the number of granulocytes, splenomegaly, and a genetic anomaly in the bone marrow called the Philadelphia chromosome, the

presence of which is used to diagnose the disease. Various chemotherapies and bone marrow transplantation are used to treat this disease.

THE LYMPHATIC SYSTEM

The lymphatic system consists of a collection of tissues and vessels concerned with the production and circulation of **lymph**, a colorless alkaline fluid composed mostly of water along with proteins, globulins, salts, urea, neutral fats, and glucose. Lymph is carried in a network of very small, thin-walled vessels called **lymphatics** or lymphatic capillaries (Fig. 16–4). The cells present in lymph are called lymphocytes, which are WBCs; there are no erythrocytes.

Lymph is formed all over the body in tissues called **interstitial spaces** (Latin *interstitium*, space between, from *inter-*, and *-stituere*, stand). Lymph is gathered into the lymphatics, which carry it to two central points in the body where all of these vessels empty into either the right lymphatic duct or the left (thoracic) duct. These two ducts empty into the venous system, thus returning the tissue fluid to the circulating blood. The function of the lymphatic system is twofold: (1) to return to the circulating blood proteins that have leaked out of the capillaries and into the tissues, and (2) to filter foreign matter, especially bacteria, and destroy it through the phagocytic action of the lymphocytes.

All along the lymphatic vessels are accumulations of tissue called lymph **nodes** (Latin *nōdus*, knot) (Fig. 16–5). Within the nodes are spaces called lymph **sinuses** (Latin *sinus*, curve, hollow); lining the walls of these sinuses are phagocytes called **reticuloendothelial cells,*** which engulf and destroy foreign material and bacteria from the lymph as these substances pass through the nodes. It is this phagocytic activity in the nodes that causes the nodes to become swollen during severe infection. Lymph nodes are particularly abundant in the axillae (Latin *axilla*, armpit)

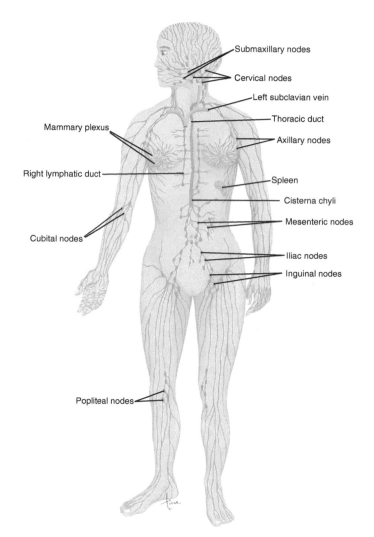

Figure 16–4. The lymphatic system. (From Scanlon, VC, and Sanders, T: Essentials of Anatomy and Physiology, ed 4. F.A. Davis, Philadelphia, 2003, p 309, with permission.)

---

*Latin *rēticulum*, diminutive of *rēte*, net, Greek *endon*, within, *thēlē*, nipple. Lymph sinuses are lined with endothelial tissue.

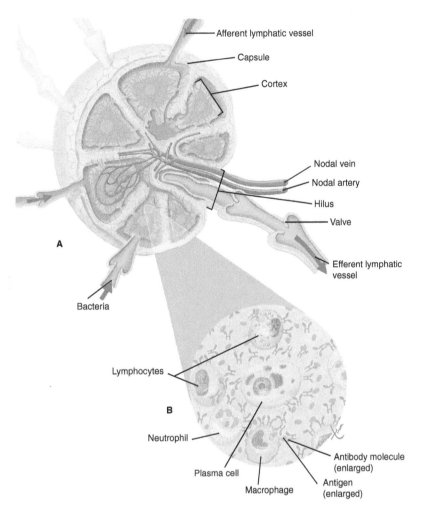

Figure 16–5. Lymph node. (From Scanlon, VC, and Sanders, T: Essentials of Anatomy and Physiology, ed 4. F. A. Davis, Philadelphia, 2003, p 310, with permission.)

and neck because the right and left lymphatic ducts empty into the right and left jugular veins (Latin *jugulum*, throat, neck) in the neck.

The phagocytes of the lymph nodes are able to destroy some cancer cells, but many of these malignant cells may be transferred to other parts of the body through the lymphatics, creating **metastases** (singular *metastasis*, from Greek *meta-*, change, and *stasis*, position), secondary growths of malignancies spread from the site of a primary growth.

Inflammation of the lymph nodes is called **lymphadenitis** and inflammation of the lymphatic vessels is called **lymphangitis**. Abnormal enlargement of the lymph nodes is one of the symptoms of **Hodgkin's disease**, named for British physician Thomas Hodgkin (1798–1866), a form of carcinoma characterized by inflammatory infiltration of lymphocytes into the bone marrow, which results in disturbed hematopoiesis and anemia. **Lymphoma** refers to any malignancy originating from lymphocytes.

VOCABULARY

Note: Latin combining forms appear in ***bold italics***.

Greek or Latin	Combining Form(s)	Meaning	Example
blastos	**BLAST-**	[bud, germ] primitive cell	myelo-**blast**
ēos	**EOS-**	red (stain)	**eos**-in
globus	***GLOB-***	round body, globe	**glob**-ulin

Greek or Latin	Combining Form(s)	Meaning	Example
grānulum	**GRANUL-**	granule	**granul**-ar
karyon	**KARY-**	[nut] nucleus	**kary**-ophage
lympha	**LYMPH-**	[clear water] lymph	**lymph**-atic
monos	**MON-**	single	**mon**-ochromatic
neuter	**NEUTR-***	neither	**neutr**-ophil
philein	**-PHIL-†**	having an affinity for	baso-**phil**

*In this terminology, words beginning with or containing NEUTR- refer to neutral dyes—those that are neither acid nor alkaline (basic).
†In this terminology, words containing the combining form PHIL- refer to the capacity of a cell to accept dye. A neutrophil is a cell that stains easily with neutral dyes.

ETYMOLOGICAL NOTES

The Greek and Latin languages are called cognate, which means literally "coming into being together," because both are derived from a parent language called Indo-European. Thus, just as there are many words in the Romance languages (which are all derived from Latin) with similar form and meaning, so there are words in Greek and in Latin with these similarities. The -penia in erythropenia, for example, is from the Greek *penia* (poverty, need), and is related in this way to the Latin noun *pēnūria* (want, need, scarcity). The words **penury**, poverty, and **penurious**, stingy, are from this Latin word. The same relationship exists between Greek *leukos* (white), and Latin *lux*, *lūcis* (light), as in the words **lucid** (clear) and **translucent** (transmitting light).

Another group of words with this same relationship is derived from the Greek verb *histanai* (stand) and the two Latin verbs *stāre*, *stātus* (stand), and *statuere*, *statūtus*, *-stituere*, *-stitūtus* (stand, set in place). These verbs have given rise to such words as **hemostat**, **stasis**, **metastasis**, **homeostasis**, **station**, **statue**, **interstitial**, **constitution**, and **consistent**.

Eosin, the red dye for which eosinophils have a special affinity, takes its name from the Greek word for the dawn, *ēōs*. In early Greek times, Eos (Dawn) was thought to be a goddess, a daughter of Hyperion and Theia, two of the Titans, primeval children of Sky and Earth. Dawn's sister was Selene, the moon, and her brother was Helios, the sun. In the Homeric poems, the new day was often heralded by the appearance of *rhododaktylos Eos*, rosy-fingered Dawn. On one occasion, Eos fell in love with a mortal, Tithonus, a brother of Priam, king of Troy at the time of the Trojan War. She carried the young man away to her home in Ethiopia, and secured immortality for him. But she neglected to obtain eternal youth for the unfortunate Tithonus, and although he was deathless, he continued to age. Some say that he was eventually changed into a grasshopper, a creature that renews its youth by casting off its old skin.

Tennyson recalls the sad story of this youth in his poem *Tithonus* (1860), in which the unhappy lover asks Dawn to release him from immortality:

Yet hold me not forever in thine East;
How can my nature longer mix with thine?
Coldly thy rosy shadows bathe me, cold
Are all thy lights, and cold my wrinkled feet
Upon thy glimmering thresholds, when the steam
Floats up from those dim fields about the homes
Of happy men that have the power to die,
And grassy barrows of the happier dead.
Release me, and restore me to the ground.
Thou seest all things, thou wilt see my grave;
Thou wilt renew thy beauty morn by morn,
I in earth forget these empty courts,
And thee returning on thy silver wheels.

Eos and Tithonus had two children, Emathion and Memnon. We know little about Emathion, but Memnon became king of the Ethiopians. In the closing phase of the Trojan War, Memnon came to the aid of the Trojans, leading his Ethiopian troops and wearing armor fashioned by the god Hephaestus himself. Shortly after his arrival, Memnon faced the great Greek hero Achilles in single combat and was mortally wounded in the battle. Ovid, in the *Metamorphoses*, tells us that Eos (Latin *Aurora*) appealed to Zeus to grant Memnon some special honor in death. Zeus agreed, and from the ashes that rose from Memnon's funeral pyre countless birds came into being and were named Memnonides, daughters of Memnon. The dew on the morning grass is said to be the tears shed daily by Eos for her unfortunate son.

Lymph, the clear, alkaline fluid found in the lymphatic vessels, is named from Latin *lympha* (clear water). This Latin word is adapted from the Greek *nymphē* (or *nymphā*), young girl, maiden, nymph. Nymphs were female spirits of nature and were usually represented as living in either the mountains, where they were called oreads; in the woods, where they were called dryads; or in the waters, where they were called naiads. Some nymphs were singled out in mythology for the unusual events surrounding them, and some do not appear to be oreads, dryads, or naiads. In Homer's *Odyssey*, the hero Odysseus spends 7 years on the island of Ogygia, detained by the beautiful nymph Calypso, who wants to make him immortal so that he can dwell with her forever. But his thoughts are on his home and on his wife Penelope and young son Telemachus.

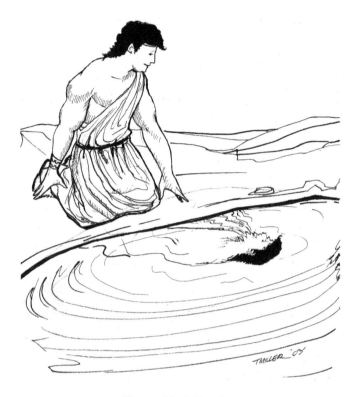

Figure 16–6. Narcissus.

Eventually, he is released from this unusual bondage by the order of Zeus and does, at long last, after almost 20 years, return to his home, wife, and son.

Another well-known nymph was the oread Echo. She fell in love with a handsome young man named Narcissus, the son of a naiad, Liriope, and a river god, Cephisus. Ovid tells us that when Narcissus was born, Liriope asked Tiresias, the blind prophet of Thebes, if her son would live to a ripe old age. Tiresias answered, "Only if he never knows himself."

Narcissus grew up to be a haughty young man and spurned all lovers. As the story goes, he, at last, fell in love with the image of a beautiful youth in a pool of clear water—himself (Fig. 16–6). In his frustration at this hopeless love, he pined away until only a flower remained, a flower with a yellow center surrounded by white petals. His last words to himself were, *Heu, frustra dilecte puer* (alas, dear boy, loved in vain). *Vale* (farewell). Echo repeated the same words back to him. Ovid tells us that even in the Underworld, his spirit gazes eternally at its image in the waters of the river Styx. Echo, desolate, mourning for her lost love, faded away until only her voice remained, echoing through the hills and valleys, repeating whatever she heard spoken.

Exercise 1: Analyze and Define

Analyze and define each of the following words. In this and in succeeding exercises, analysis should consist of separating the words into prefixes (if any), combining forms, and suffixes or suffix forms (if any) and giving the meaning of each. Be certain to differentiate between nouns and adjectives in your definitions. Consult a medical dictionary for the current meanings of these words.

1. agranulocyte _____

2. akaryocyte _____

3. blastocyst _____

4. ecchymoses _____

5. ecchymotic _____

6. eosin _____

7. erythroblastosis _____

8. erythropoiesis _____

9. erythropoietin _____

10. globin _____

11. granuloblast _____

12. granulocyte _____

13. granulocytopoiesis _____

14. hematin _____

15. hematophagia _____

16. hematopoiesis _____

17. hemoglobinocholia _____

18. hemoglobinolysis _____

19. hemoglobinuria _____

20. hemopathology _____

21. hypereosinophilic syndrome _____

22. karyochromatophil _____

23. karyochrome _____

24. karyophage _____

25. hemolysin _____

26. leukopoiesis _____

27. lymphadenectasis _____

28. lymphadenitis _____

29. lymphagogue _____

30. lymphangiectasis _____

31. lymphangioma _____

32. lymphangitis _____

33. lymphaticostomy* _____

34. lymphoblast _____

35. lymphocytopenia _____

36. lymphocytotoxin _____

37. lymphogranulomatosis _____

38. lymphoma _____

39. lymphopoiesis _____

40. monocyte _____

*From New Latin *lymphaticus* (lymphatic, a lymph vessel).

41. monocytopenia _____

42. monocytosis _____

43. myeloblast _____

44. polykaryocyte _____

45. thrombase _____

46. thrombin _____

47. thromboclasis _____

48. thrombocyte _____

49. thrombopenia _____

50. thrombophilia _____

MUSCULOSKELETAL

SYSTEM

The musculoskeletal system has several important functions in the body (Fig. 17–1). It serves to support the body, give it shape, and protect its vital organs. The musculoskeletal system makes movement possible. Muscle (Latin *musculus*, diminutive of *mūs*, mouse; used in Latin to mean both a little mouse and a muscle) is a type of tissue composed of contractile cells or fibers, the outstanding characteristic of which is their elasticity, their ability to

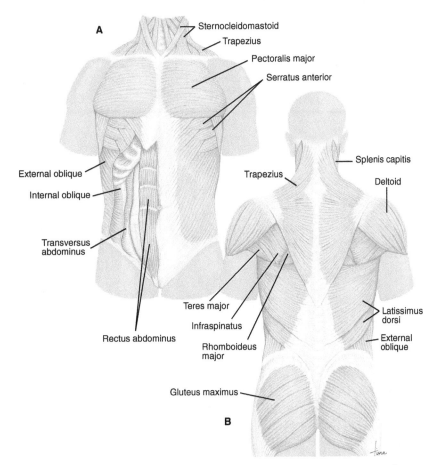

Figure 17–1. Muscles of the trunk. (*A*) Anterior, (*B*) posterior. (From Scanlon, VC, and Sanders, T: Essentials of Anatomy and Physiology, ed 4. F. A. Davis, Philadelphia, 2003, p 145, with permission.)

expand and contract. Muscle tissue possesses little inter-cellular material and, as a result, its cells or fibers lie close together.

Three types of muscle tissue are differentiated in the body: smooth, cardiac, and striated (also called skeletal) (Fig. 17–2). Smooth muscle tissue forms the involuntary muscles, so named because they are not under conscious control. These muscles are found mainly in the internal organs—for example, in the digestive tract, the respiratory passages, the urinary and genital ducts, and the walls of blood vessels. Spindle shaped in form, smooth muscle cells each contain a central nucleus and are arranged in sheets, or layers. They are sometimes found as isolated units in connective tissue.

Cardiac tissue is the tissue of the muscle of the heart. Cardiac muscle fibers branch and interconnect (**anasto-mose**), forming a continuous network, or **syncytium**. At intervals, the fibers are crossed by bands, or intercalated discs. Atypical muscle fibers beneath the endocardium, known as Purkinje fibers, form the impulse-conducting system of the heart.

Striated (or skeletal) muscle tissue composes the voluntary muscles, those that are under conscious control. It is these muscles that we are concerned with here (Fig. 17–3). Striated muscle fibers possess alternate light and dark bands, or striations, and are found in all skeletal muscles. These muscle fibers are grouped into bundles

called **fasciculi**, each of which is surrounded by a connec-tive tissue sheath called the **perimysium**. Delicate reticu-lar fibrils surround and hold together the fibers within a fasciculus forming the **endomysium**.

In anatomic terminology, body muscles are named for one of the following reasons:

1. After a physical characteristic of the muscle: **bipennate muscle** (Latin *bi-*, two, *penna*, feather), so named because the muscle fibers flow down either side of a central tendon like the barbs on the two sides of a feather.
2. After the organ or part to which the muscle is attached and which it controls: **nasalis muscle** (Latin *nāsus*, nose). The nasalis muscle keeps the nostrils of the nose open during inspiration.
3. A combination of the preceding two: **biceps brachii muscle** (Latin *biceps*, two-headed, from *caput*, head, *brāchium*, [upper] arm; genitive case, *brāchii*). The point of origin of a muscle is called the caput, or head. This muscle is bicipital (two headed), attached to both the scapula and the coracoid (Greek *korax, korakos*, crow) process, a process (outgrowth) on the upper surface of the scapula resembling a crow's beak. The biceps brachii muscle flexes the forearm and supinates the hand; that is, turns the hand so that the palm faces upward.

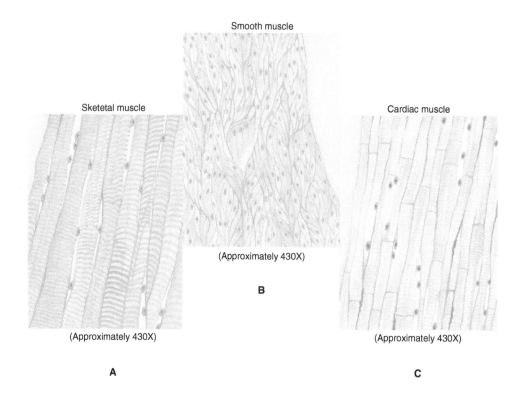

Smooth muscle

Sketetal muscle

Cardiac muscle

(Approximately 430X)

B

(Approximately 430X)

A

(Approximately 430X)

C

Figure 17–2. Comparison of properties of three types of muscle. (From Scanlon, VC, and Sanders, T: Essentials of Anatomy and Physiology, ed 4. F. A. Davis, Philadelphia, 2003, p 74, with permission.)

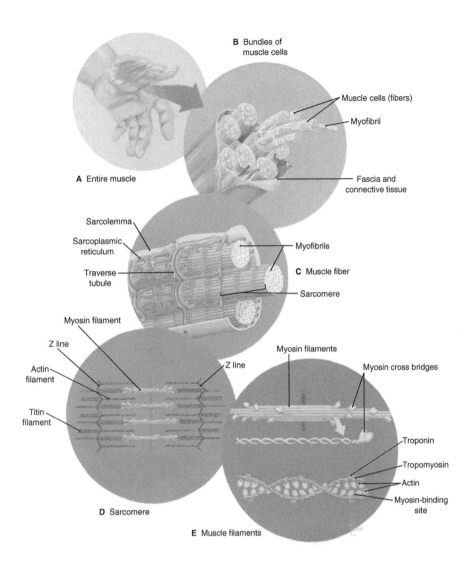

B Bundles of muscle cells

Muscle cells (fibers)

Myofibril

A Entire muscle

Fascia and connective tissue

Sarcolemma

Sarcoplasmic reticulum

Myofibrils

Traverse tubule

C Muscle fiber

Sarcomere

Myosin filament

Z line

Z line

Myosin filaments

Actin filament

Myosin cross bridges

Titin filament

Troponin

Tropomyosin

Actin

Myosin-binding site

D Sarcomere

E Muscle filaments

Figure 17–3. Skeletal muscle. (From Scanlon, VC, and Sanders, T: Essentials of Anatomy and Physiology, ed 4. F. A. Davis, Philadelphia, 2003, p 136, with permission.)

4. After the function that the muscle performs: a muscle that lifts a part is a **levator**; one that flexes a part is a **flexor**; one that moves a part away from the central plane of the body is an **abductor**; one that moves a part toward the central plane of the body is an **adductor**, and one that extends a part is an **extensor**. These terms are generally, but not always, used in combination with the part that the muscle moves. Sometimes the muscle is described as being long (Latin *longus*) or short (*brevis*). The **abductor pollicis brevis muscle** (*pollex, pollicis*, thumb) and **abductor* pollicis longus muscle** abduct and assist in extending the thumb. The **adductor**

longus muscle adducts the thigh. Note that it is not always possible to tell from the name of a muscle exactly which organ or part of the body it controls.

The names of muscles, as given in the preceding section, and other human anatomical structures are found in Terminologia Anatomica, usually abbreviated TA. TA is the official international terminology (nomenclature) of human anatomical structures, drafted by the Federative Committee on Anatomical Terminology (FCAT) in 1997 and accepted by the International Federation of Associations of Anatomists (IFAA) in 1999. TA replaced Nomina Anatomica (NA), the anatomic terminology adopted as official by the International Congress of Anatomists at various meetings after 1955. Latin was the standard in NA and remains the standard in TA, although

---

*The noun **abductor**, as well as other agent nouns ending in -or, is in apposition to the noun muscle; that is, it defines what kind of a muscle it is or what it does. It is easier to define these agent nouns as adjectives: the abductor muscle, that is, the muscle that abducts.

in TA Latin terms have English equivalents. For example, in TA, the Latin term **musculi intercostales interni** has an English equivalent, **internal intercostal muscles**.

NOUN DECLENSION

In the naming of muscles, Latin nouns and adjectives are found in the forms of different grammatical cases, and in both singular and plural. The cases most commonly used are the nominative (the form found in the vocabularies) and the genitive, or possessive, case, in both singular and plural.

As presented in Lesson 8, there are five categories, called declensions, of Latin nouns and two declensions of adjectives. First-declension Latin nouns end in *-a* and are feminine; second-declension nouns end in *-us* if masculine and *-um* if neuter gender. Third-declension nouns may be masculine, feminine, or neuter, and the nominative case (the vocabulary form) is not characterized by any particular ending. Nouns of the fourth and fifth declensions will not concern us here, with the exception of two fourth-declension nouns: *manus* (hand) is feminine, and the genitive singular is *manūs*; *genū* (knee) is neuter, and the genitive singular is *genūs*.

A Partial Declension of Typical Nouns

Singular		Plural	
Nominative	**Genitive**	**Nominative**	**Genitive**
auricula, f.,* ear	*auriculae*	*auriculae*	*auriculārum*
digitus, m., finger, toe	*digitī*	*digitī*	*digitōrum*
labium, n., lip	*labiī*	*labia*	*labiōrum*
mūs, m. and f., muscle	*mūris*	*mūrēs*	*mūrum*
manus, f., hand	*manūs*	*manūs*	*manuum*
genū, n., knee	*genūs*	*genua*	*genuum*

*The abbreviations m., f., and n. are for masculine, feminine, and neuter.

LATIN ADJECTIVES

There are two classes of Latin adjectives: they are either first and second declension, with endings like those of masculine, feminine, and neuter nouns of the first and second declensions; that is, they assume these endings depending on the gender of the nouns that they describe; or they are of the third declension and usually end in *-is*. The genitive singular of third-declension adjectives always ends in *-is*; thus, it is not always obvious whether a third-declension adjective, such as *brevis*, short (genitive, *brevis*), is in the nominative or genitive case. This must be determined from the way the adjective is used in the particular term in which it is found.

Adjectives that end in *-ior* are in the comparative degree: *superior* (higher); *inferior* (lower). This form is used for both masculine and feminine singular. The comparative degree of neuter nouns ends in *-ius* (*superius, inferius*). The genitive singular for both genders ends in *-is* (*superiōris, inferiōris*) and the nominative plural for both genders ends in *-ēs* (*superiōrēs, inferiōrēs*).

THE ORDER OF WORDS

In Latin, nouns in the genitive case, the possessive case, usually follow the noun on which they depend:

Nominative Singular	**Genitive Singular**	
rectus "the straight (muscle)	**femoris** of the thigh"	(that is, the thigh muscle)
extensor "the extensor (muscle)	**indicis** of the index finger"	(that is, the index finger's extensor muscle)

In Latin, adjectives follow the nouns they describe:

adductor longus "the long adductor (muscle)"	**adductor brevis** "the short adductor (muscle)"

In English, adjectives precede the nouns they describe:

flexor muscle	**adductor muscle**

SELECTED VOCABULARY FOR NAMES OF MUSCLES

Latin	Meaning
*abductor**	that which leads away, abductor
accelerātor	that which speeds up, accelerator
adductor	that which leads toward, adductor

* The word abductor is not found in Latin of the classical period, but has been formed on the model of other Latin words of similar construction. Such words (and terms), common in the terminology of anatomy and biology, are called New Latin. Several other words in this vocabulary are New Latin.

āla	wing; ala nasi (wing of the nose, the lateral wall of each nostril)
angulus	angle, corner
ānus	anus, opening of the rectum
arrector	that which raises, erector
articulāris	joint (adj.), pertaining to joints
auricula	ear, the external portion of the ear
biceps	two-headed
brevis	short
buccinātor	that which has to do with the cheek (*bucca*)
corrūgātor	that which wrinkles, "wrinkler"
cubitum	elbow
dēpressor	that which lowers or depresses, depressor
digitus	finger, toe
dīlātor	that which widens, dilator
extensor	that which extends, extensor
femur, femoris	thigh
flexor	that which flexes or bends, flexor
genū, genūs	knee
hallux, hallucis	big toe
index, indicis	index (first) finger
levātor	that which raises, levator
manus, manūs	hand
medius	middle
mentālis	of the chin (*mentum*)
minimus	smallest
nāris	nostril
nāsus	nose
oppōnēns	opposing
palpēbra	eyelid
pēs, pedis	foot
pilus	hair
pollex, pollicis	thumb
pūpilla	pupil (of the eye)
rotātor	that which turns, rotator
supercilium	eyebrow
superior, superiōris	upper, higher
sūra	calf (of the leg)
tensor	that which tenses, tensor
triceps	three-headed
tympanum†	ear drum, tympanic membrane

ETYMOLOGICAL NOTES

The abductor and adductor muscles take their name from the Latin verb *dūcere, ductus* (lead, draw). Related to this verb is the noun *dux, ducis* (leader, commander, chief). The Italian honorific title *Il Duce* (the Chief) was accorded to Benito Mussolini on his accession to the dictatorship of Italy in the years between World Wars I and II. Adherents of his party belonged to the political organization called *Fascista*, Fascists, named for the symbol of the party, the *Fasci*, from Latin *fascēs*, a bundle of rods bound around an axe and carried in procession in front of the high magistrates of Rome. A related Latin word is *fascia* (band, bandage), which has given the name to the anatomic term **fascia**, the fibrous membrane covering, supporting, and separating muscles.

The Latin word *cubitum* (elbow) is from the verb *cubāre, cubitus* (lie down). The sense was that, when reclining to dine, as the Romans did, the elbow was to lean upon. The verb meaning to recline at a dining table was *recumbere* (*re-*, back, and *-cumbere*, lie down), an alternate form of *cubāre*, which is used with prefixes. In Roman times, the term *cubitum* also meant the distance from the elbow to the tip of the extended middle finger, a term of measurement: a cubit. The distance is variously calculated as being from 18 to 21 inches.

There are a number of words in current use that are all related to the verb *cubāre* and its alternate form *–cumbere*: cubicle, from *cubiculum*, a diminutive noun meaning a (small) place for sleeping, bedroom. Procumbent means leaning forward and recumbent means leaning backward The incumbent is the one who is in office, and the expression "It is incumbent upon us" implies a burden "lying upon" us. The terms incubus and succubus refer to demons, or evil spirits, that visit one in the night for sexual intercourse. The incubus "lies upon" women and the succubus "lies under" men. Today, the term incubus is used to refer to anything that is oppressive, something that weighs one down. Chickens incubate their eggs. An incubator is an apparatus where eggs are artificially hatched, or a chamber used to provide a stable and healthful atmosphere for the development of premature or sick babies.

Latin *manus* (hand), has several interesting derivatives in English, among which are the words **maneuver** and **manure**, both with the same etymology, from *manus* and *opus, operis* (work), and both disguised as a result of their transition through French before entering the English language (Fig. 17–4). Maneuver is from French *manoeuvre*, from Medieval Latin *manuopera*, meaning something done by hand, from Latin *manuoperāre* (work by hand). Thus, a maneuver is literally "something done by hand." Today it means an evasive movement, a manipulation of affairs done for someone's advantage. (Note that the words manipulate and manipulation are from Latin *manipulus*, a handful.) Manure, barnyard refuse used as fertilizer, has the same ultimate etymology as maneuver but has undergone a secondary change in form during the Middle English period, the 12th through the 15th centuries. The Middle English form is *manouren*, a verb meaning to cultivate the land (by hand), with a secondary (and modern) meaning of using manure to enrich the soil. The second component of these words, *opus, operis*, has given us such words as **operate, opera, operation,** and **inoperable**.

The modern names for the bones of the body are those that were given by the ancient Roman anatomists and their successors in the Middle Ages and Renaissance. In some instances, the bones were named after some familiar object

BONES OF THE RIGHT HAND AND WRIST

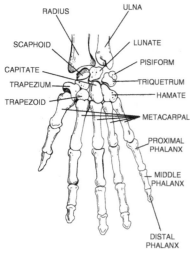

VIEW FROM PALMAR SIDE

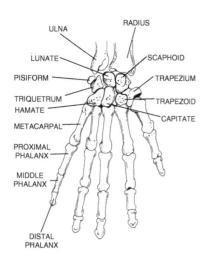

VIEW FROM BACK OF THE HAND

Figure 17–4. Bones of the right hand and wrist.

that they were thought to resemble, and, in others, there seems to be no etymology to the name or any reason for it. Most of the names of bones are Latin words, but an appreciable number were borrowed from the early Greek scientists such as Hippocrates, Aristotle, and Galen.

The Latin words *digitus* (finger, toe), *ulna* (elbow, arm),

femur, femoris (thigh), *humerus* (shoulder), *tibia* (shin), and *ilium* (flank) were originally used only to designate these parts of the body. Later, they were used to designate the bones underlying these parts. The following is a partial list of bones that includes some named after familiar objects:

clavicle, collar bone: "little key." Latin *clavis* (key)

patella, kneecap: "little dish." Latin *patena* (open dish), from *patere* (lie open)

mandible, jawbone: "capable of chewing." Latin *mandere* (chew)

fibula, outer bone of leg: "safety pin." Latin *fibula* (brooch)

scaphoid, bone of the ankle and wrist: "boat-shaped." Greek *skaphē* (boat)

zygoma, bone of the cheek: "arch." Greek *zygon* (yoke)

trapezium, bone of the wrist: "little table." Greek *trapeza* (table)

cuneiform, bone of the ankle: "wedge-shaped." Latin *cuneus* (wedge)

malleus, ossicle ("little bone") of the middle ear: "hammer." Latin *malleus* (hammer)

incus, ossicle ("little bone") of the middle ear: "anvil." Latin *incūs* (anvil)

sacrum, base of the vertebral column: "sacred thing." Latin *sacer* (sacred) (This part of the body of animals was burned in offerings to the gods.)

lunate, bone of the wrist: "moon shaped." Latin *lūna* (moon)

hamate, bone of the wrist: "hook shaped." Latin *hāmus* (hook)

pisiform, bone of the wrist: "pea shaped." Latin *pīsum* (pea)

tarsus, ankle: "framework." Greek *tarsos* (wicker frame)

phalanges, bones of the fingers or toes: "battle line." Greek *phalanges* (plural of *phalanx*, a military unit) (The Macedonian phalanx, a fighting group developed by Philip II, King of Macedonia and father of Alexander the Great, was made up of 256 men formed in a square 16 across and 16 deep and trained to maneuver with great dexterity on the field of battle.)

Exercise 1: Determine the Function

Using the vocabulary for this lesson, determine the function of each of the following muscles.

1. abductor* digiti minimi muscle _____

2. abductor digiti minimi pedis muscle _____

3. abductor hallucis muscle _____

4. abductor pollicis brevis muscle _____

5. abductor pollicis longus muscle _____

6. adductor brevis muscle _____

7. adductor hallucis muscle _____

8. adductor pollicis muscle _____

9. arrectores pilorum muscles _____

10. articularis cubiti muscle _____

11. articularis genus muscle _____

12. biceps brachii muscle _____

13. femoris muscle _____

14. buccinator muscle _____

15. corrugator supercilii muscle _____

16. depressor anguli oris muscle _____

17. depressor labii inferioris muscle _____

18. dilator naris muscle _____

---

* When the first word of the names of muscles ends in -or (singular, or -ores, plural), this word is usually a noun that explains what the muscle does. All of the first five muscles above, for example, are abductor muscles. The part of the body that is abducted is put in the genitive case. That is, each of these muscles is the abductor of something.

19. extensor digiti minimi muscle _____

20. extensor digitorum muscle _____

21. extensor hallucis brevis muscle _____

22. extensor indicis muscle _____

23. extensor pollicis brevis muscle _____

24. flexor digiti minimi brevis pedis muscle _____

25. flexor digiti minimi brevis manus muscle _____

26. flexor digitorum brevis pedis muscle _____

27. flexor hallucis brevis muscle _____

28. flexor pollicis brevis muscle _____

29. flexor pollicis longus muscle _____

30. levator anguli oris muscle _____

31. levator ani muscle _____

32. levator labii superioris muscle _____

33. levator labii superioris alaeque* nasi muscle _____

34. levator palpebrae superioris muscle _____

35. mentalis muscle _____

36. opponens digiti minimi muscle _____

37. opponens pollicis muscle _____

*Latin *alaeque* means "and of the wing." *-que* affixed to a noun means that this noun is to be connected with the noun that precedes it with "and." This *-que* (called an enclitic) can be affixed to any form of a noun or adjective. The initials S.P.Q.R., frequently seen on Roman inscriptions, stand for *Senatus Populusque Romanus* (the Senate and the Roman People).

38. rotatores cervicis muscles _____

39. sphincter ani externus muscle _____

40. sphincter ani internus muscle _____

41. sphincter pupillae muscle _____

42. sphincter urethrae muscle _____

43. tensor tympani muscle _____

44. triceps brachii muscle _____

45. triceps surae muscle _____

THE SKELETON

The **skeleton** (Greek *skeleton*, dried up [sc. *sōma*, body]; that is, "a dried up body") (Fig. 17–5) is the bony framework of the body consisting of 206 bones. The distribution of these 206 bones is as follows:

skull: 8 bones

face: 14 bones

hyoid bone: A single U-shaped bone lying at the base of the tongue

ear: 6 ossicles, "little bones"

vertebrae: 26 bones

ribs: 24 bones

sternum: the single breastbone

arms and shoulders: 10 bones

wrists: 16 bones

hands: 38 bones

legs and hips: 10 bones

ankles: 14 bones

feet: 38 bones

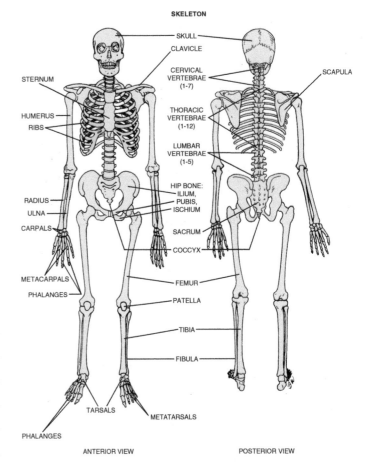

Figure 17–5. Skeleton. (From Taber's Cyclopedic Medical Dictionary, ed 19. F. A. Davis, Philadelphia, 2001, p 1903, with permission.)

Exercise 2: Identify Bones or Groups of Bones

Indicate, in ordinary, everyday terms, the location of each of the following bones or groups of bones.

1. clavicle _____

2. sternum _____

3. humerus _____

4. lumbar vertebrae _____

5. metacarpals _____

6. patella _____

7. fibula _____

8. phalanges (two different sets) _____

   a. _____

   b. _____

9. scapula _____

10. sacrum _____

11. radius _____

12. femur _____

13. tibia _____

14. ilium _____

15. metatarsals _____

NERVOUS SYSTEM

The human body is an infinitely complex and elegant organism composed of billions of cells that perform the many functions that keep it in the normal, healthy condition called **homeostasis**. The effective functioning of the body is regulated by two systems of communication: the **nervous system**, which is discussed here, and the **endocrine** system, which is discussed in Lesson 19.

The nervous system is divided into three parts: the **central nervous system** (CNS), the **peripheral nervous system** (PNS), and the **autonomic nervous system** (ANS) (Fig. 18–1). Each of these three systems is composed of cells called **neurons**, the structural and functional units of the nervous system. Some of these neurons are minute in length, measuring no more than a fraction of a millimeter, whereas others are up to 1 meter (39.37 inches) long. The longer neurons are usually called nerve fibers. The terms neuron, or nerve cell, and nerve fiber are not to be confused with the term **nerve**. A nerve consists of a bundle or a group of bundles of nerve fibers that connect the brain and the spinal cord with various parts of the body. A bundle of nerve fibers is called a **fasciculus** (diminutive of Latin *fascis*, bundle; see discussion in Lesson 17). Nerves transmit electrical and chemical signals between the CNS and body tissues. Signals carried from the brain to any part of the body are called **efferent impulses**, whereas signals carried to the brain from other parts of the body are called **afferent impulses**.

SUBDIVISIONS OF THE NERVOUS SYSTEM

The **CNS** consists of the spinal cord and the brain. The spinal cord conducts sensory impulses from the PNS to the brain, and motor impulses from the brain to the various effectors, such as the skeletal muscles. The brain receives sensory impulses from the spinal cord and its own nerves, and discharges motor impulses to the muscles and glands. The brain and the spinal cord are made up of two types of tissue called gray matter (**substantia grisea**) and white matter (**substantia alba**). **Gray matter** is nerve tissue

composed mainly of the cell bodies of neurons, whereas **white matter** is nerve tissue composed of myelinated nerve fibers. White matter in the brain and spinal cord transmits the afferent and efferent impulses.

The brain is enclosed within the skull for protection, and the spinal cord is enclosed within the spinal column, or spine, which is composed of bony vertebrae. The **meninges** are the three membranes that lie under the bony structures of the skull and the spinal column, and that cover and protect the spinal cord and the brain (Fig. 18–2). The outermost of the three meninges is a hard membrane called the **dura mater**. The term **epidural** refers to the space around the dura. The innermost of the three is a soft membrane called the **pia mater,**[*] and lying between these two is a weblike membrane called the **arachnoid** or the **arachnoidea**. A blow to the head, even one that seems to be trivial, can result in bleeding in the area under the dura mater called the subdural space. This bleeding, called **subdural hematoma**, may not be apparent for several days or even weeks after the initial injury.

Inflammation of any of the meninges is called **meningitis**. Inflammation of the membranes of the spine is **spinal meningitis**, and inflammation of the membranes of the brain is **cerebral meningitis**. Clinically, these two are not differentiated but are simply referred to as meningitis. Meningitis can be caused by infection from bacteria, a virus, or a fungus, and may also be caused by noninfectious inflammation, such as that which occurs with **systemic lupus erythematosus** (referred to as SLE or lupus).

Poliomyelitis (Greek *polios*, gray), inflammation of the gray matter of the spinal cord, is the disease usually called "polio." Development of the Salk vaccine by American microbiologist Dr. Jonas E. Salk (1914–1995) and later the Sabin vaccine, an oral vaccine developed by Russian-born American virologist Dr. Albert B. Sabin (1906–1993), significantly reduced the incidence of polio in the United States. Virtually all cases of polio that occurred in the United States after the introduction of the oral vaccine were associated with the vaccine itself, which was made

---

[*]See the Etymological Notes in this lesson for a discussion of the dura mater and pia mater

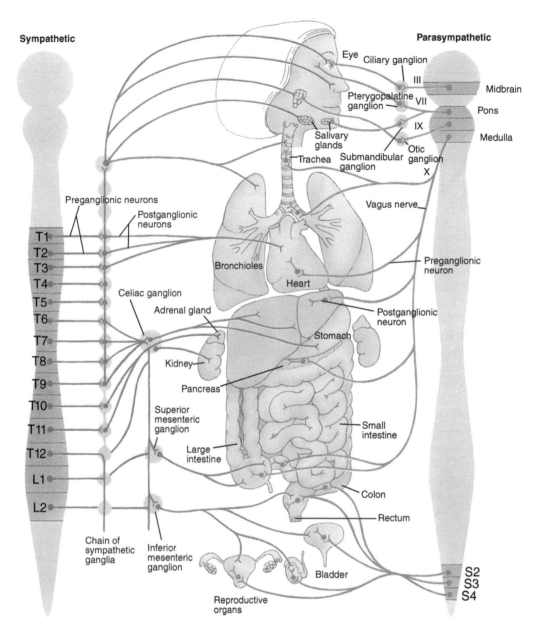

Sympathetic

Eye
Ciliary ganglion
III
Pterygopalatine ganglion
VII
Salivary glands
Submandibular ganglion
Trachea
Otic ganglion
IX
X

Parasympathetic

Midbrain
Pons
Medulla

Vagus nerve

Preganglionic neurons
Postganglionic neurons

T1
T2
T3
T4
T5
T6
T7
T8
T9
T10
T11
T12
L1
L2

Bronchioles
Heart

Preganglionic neuron

Celiac ganglion
Adrenal gland

Postganglionic neuron

Stomach

Kidney

Pancreas

Superior mesenteric ganglion

Large intestine

Small intestine

Colon

Rectum

Chain of sympathetic ganglia
Inferior mesenteric ganglion

Bladder

S2
S3
S4

Reproductive organs

Figure 18–1. Autonomic nervous system. (From Scanlon, VC, and Sanders, T: Essentials of Anatomy and Physiology, ed 4. F. A. Davis, Philadelphia, 2003, p 180, with permission.)

from live, attenuated virus. The current use of an inactivated, injectable poliovirus vaccine has eliminated polio caused by the live oral vaccine. In countries where the vaccine is not readily available, polio epidemics still happen and are usually seasonal, occurring in the summer and fall.

The peripheral nervous system or **PNS** consists of nerves and masses of nervous tissue called **ganglia** (plural of ganglion). The PNS, so called because its nerves extend to peripheral, or outlying, parts of the body, is the part of the nervous system that lies outside the CNS. Both the CNS and the PNS control the voluntary functions of the body.

The autonomic nervous system or **ANS** controls involuntary bodily functions. It regulates the action of

the salivary, gastric, and sweat glands, as well as the adrenal medulla, which produces epinephrine. The ANS is divided into two parts: the **sympathetic division** and the **parasympathetic division**, each with its own functions. Stimulation of the nerve fibers of the sympathetic division causes constriction of the vasomotor muscles, the muscles that surround the blood vessels of the body. **Vasoconstriction**, a decrease in the size of a blood vessel or vessels, causes a rise in blood pressure, erection of the hairs of the body ("gooseflesh" or "goosebumps"), dilation of the pupils of the eyes, depression of gastrointestinal activity, and acceleration of the action of the heart. These changes usually occur under the stimulation of fright.

Stimulation of the nerve fibers of the parasympathetic

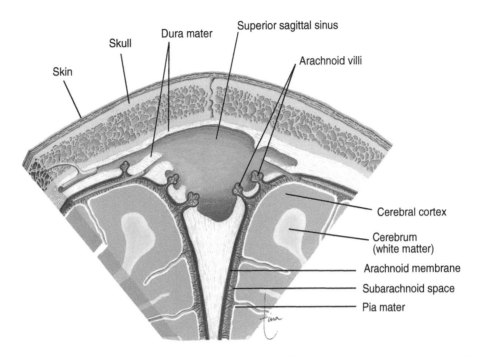

Figure 18–2. Meninges. (From Scanlon, VC, and Sanders, T: Essentials of Anatomy and Physiology, ed 4. F. A. Davis, Philadelphia, 2003, p 175, with permission.)

division produces **vasodilation**, an increase in the size of a blood vessel or vessels, which results in decreased blood pressure, contraction of the pupils of the eyes, increased gastrointestinal activity, and slowing of the heart action.

Stimulation of the nerve fibers of the sympathetic and the parasympathetic systems is effected through the action of two substances: **norepinephrine**, a hormone, and **acetylcholine**, an ester. The endings of the nerve fibers of the sympathetic nervous system secrete norepinephrine; thus these fibers are said to be **adrenergic** (named after adrenaline, the name given to synthetic epinephrine). Release of this hormone causes stimulation of the sympathetic system, and thus norepinephrine is said to be a **sympathetic mediator** or, sometimes, an **adrenergic mediator**.

The endings of nerve fibers of the parasympathetic nervous system secrete acetylcholine, and are thus said to be **cholinergic**. It is the action of these two substances, norepinephrine and acetylcholine, that stimulates these two divisions of the ANS to produce the effects on the body that they do; that is, vasoconstriction, caused by the sympathetic division, and vasodilation, caused by the parasympathetic division.

STRUCTURE OF THE NERVOUS SYSTEM

The nervous system is composed of nerve cells, called neurons (Fig. 18–3). If the neurons are of substantial length, they are called nerve fibers. Neurons form the gray matter of the nervous system, whereas nerve fibers form the white matter. The neurons make contact with each other at points called **synapses**. Through the synapses, the neurons form a network of infinite complexity.

In addition to the synapses, the neurons have structures called **dendrites** and **axons**. Dendrites, which under microscopy look like the branches of a tree, conduct impulses to the cell body and form synaptic connections with dendrites of other neurons. The axons are structures—"processes" is the term used for both dendrites and axons—that conduct impulses away from the cell body. The axons are usually long and straight, and most end in synapses through which these impulses are conducted to other neurons. In other words, dendrites conduct afferent impulses and axons conduct efferent impulses.

The brain contains approximately 50 billion neurons. Each neuron has contact with more than one synapse, and perhaps as many as 20 synaptic contacts. This brings the total number of synaptic contacts between neurons to the amazing figure of 1 trillion (1,000,000,000,000). In addition to the neurons, in the gray and white matter of the nervous system are cells known as accessory cells, called **glia cells**, or **neuroglia cells**. These glia cells bind the neurons in place and form supporting tissue for them. Tumors of the glia cells of the brain are not uncommon and are called **gliomas** or **neurogliomas**. These tumors can often be removed by modern surgical techniques.

The **spinal cord** is a cylindrical structure about the thickness of a pencil and about 18 inches in length. It runs through the spinal column from the base of the skull to just below the ribs. Thirty-one pairs of nerves issue from the spinal cord, and these spinal nerves conduct impulses between the brain and the trunk and limbs of the body (Fig. 18–4). If the spinal cord is severed or damaged

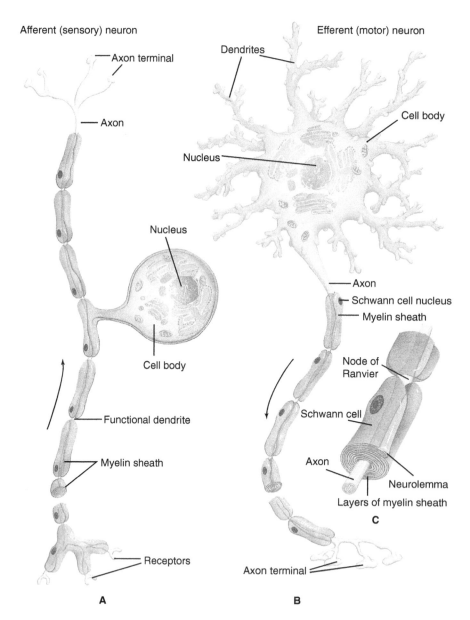

Afferent (sensory) neuron

— Axon terminal

— Axon

Nucleus

Cell body

Functional dendrite

Myelin sheath

Receptors

A

Efferent (motor) neuron

Dendrites

Cell body

Nucleus

— Axon
— Schwann cell nucleus
— Myelin sheath

Node of Ranvier

Schwann cell

Axon

Neurolemma

Layers of myelin sheath

C

Axon terminal

B

Figure 18–3. Neuron structure. (From Scanlon, VC, and Sanders, T: Essentials of Anatomy and Physiology, ed 4. F. A. Davis, Philadelphia, 2003, p 157, with permission.)

severely enough, sensation and control of all muscles below the point of the injury are lost. In the present state of medical knowledge, if the spinal cord is severed, the damage is irreparable, and permanent paralysis below the point of injury results.

The **brainstem** is the continuation of the spinal cord up into the skull (Fig. 18–5). Although it is only about 3 inches long, it contains several important structures, among which are the medulla oblongata, the pons, and the midbrain. The **medulla oblongata** (from Latin *medulla*, marrow, and *oblongata*, elongated), the lower part of the brainstem, is about 1 inch long and contains structures that regulate heart action, breathing, circulation, and control of body temperature. The **midbrain**, also called the **mesencephalon**, is the upper part of the brainstem and contains structures that regulate the senses of sight, touch,

and hearing as well as equilibrium and posture. The **pons** lies between the medulla and the cerebrum itself; that is, it bridges the area between these two structures. Functions of the pons include transmission of impulses from the 5th, 6th, 7th, and 8th cranial nerves, which control muscles of the face and the eyes. At the upper end of the brainstem are two masses of nerve cells called the **thalami**. All sensory stimuli except olfactory (the sense of smell) are received by the thalami, including the sensations of touch, pain, heat, cold, taste, sight, and hearing. These sensations are relayed by the thalami to the brain.

Just underneath the thalami is a structure called the **hypothalamus**. This structure controls certain metabolic activities, such as the maintenance of water balance, sugar and fat metabolism, and the regulation of body temperature.

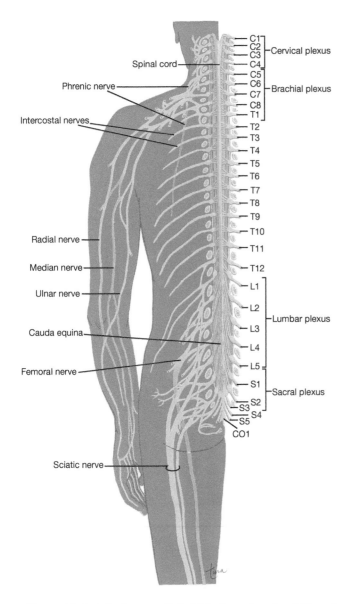

Figure 18–4. Spinal nerves (left side). (From Scanlon, VC, and Sanders, T: Essentials of Anatomy and Physiology, ed 4. F. A. Davis, Philadelphia, 2003, p 163, with permission.)

The actual brain, the **cerebrum**, is divided into two halves called the cerebral hemispheres. Each hemisphere is subdivided into four lobes: frontal, parietal, occipital, and temporal. Within these two hemispheres are four masses of gray matter called the **basal ganglia**. These ganglia control muscular movement, such as walking or lifting, and other voluntary movements. If these ganglia become damaged, the individual loses some control over these simple muscular movements, resulting in the disorders called cerebral palsy, Saint Vitus' dance (Sydenham's chorea), Bell's palsy, Parkinson's disease, and other abnormalities of voluntary muscular movement.

The **cerebral cortex** is the name given to the covering of the outer surface of each cerebral hemisphere (Fig. 18–6). The word *cortex* is from Latin and meant bark (of a

tree). Other organs of the body have outer coverings called **cortices** (singular, cortex), such as the adrenal gland. However, when the term cortex is used alone, it always refers to the cerebral cortex. The cortex is composed of gray matter; it controls the functions of sight, hearing, touch, smell, and taste—the five senses—and exerts motor control over certain muscles.

In addition to the functions just named, the cortex controls language, learning, and memory. The area of the cortex that controls language is called Broca's area (named after Pierre Paul Broca, a 19th-century French surgeon). Damage to Broca's area causes loss of control over the speech muscles, resulting in the abnormality called **motor aphasia**. Individuals with motor aphasia have difficulty in expressing themselves verbally or in writing, although there is no impairment of understanding or of intelligence. Another area of the cortex is called Wernicke's area (named after Karl Wernicke, a 19th-century German neurologist). Damage to Wernicke's area results in the loss of comprehension of spoken or written language, a condition called **Wernicke's aphasia**.

It was noted earlier that the cortex exercises control over memory, but this includes only immediate- or short-term memory. Apparently, long-term memory is associated with another part of the brain, an area called the **hippocampus**.* The hippocampus appears to be important in establishing new memories. Damage to the hippocampus results in the loss of ability to remember anything for more than a short time—a day, or even a few hours.

The **cerebellum** ("little brain") is an outgrowth of the brainstem and is located at the back of the skull (Fig. 18–7). Like the cerebrum, the cerebellum has two hemispheres and a cortex. This portion of the brain exercises control over the locomotor system of the body, the system that governs voluntary muscular movements other than those controlled by the cerebral hemispheres. Although the cerebellum does not initiate movements, it is involved in the execution of various movements, including walking and running.

EPILEPSY

Epilepsy, from the Greek *epilepsia*, was well known to the ancients and was vividly described by Hippocrates, the Greek physician of the 5th century BC, in a lengthy treatise on what he called "The Sacred Disease." This disease is the result of a disorder of neuronal activity in the brain causing abnormal sensations, emotions, and behavior, as well as convulsions, muscle spasms, and loss of consciousness. It is thought that epileptic seizures are mostly idiopathic; that is, they originate within the body and may be caused by abnormal brain development, or by an imbalance of chemicals, called neurotransmitters, in the brain. Illness, brain trauma, infection, and metabolic disturbances, as well as other factors that disturb the normal

*Greek *hippokampos*, a mythical sea horse, a creature with the head and nack of a horse and the body and tail of a fish.

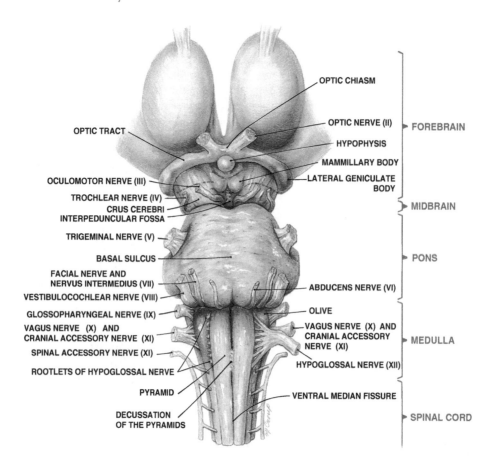

OPTIC CHIASM

OPTIC NERVE (II)

HYPOPHYSIS

MAMMILLARY BODY

LATERAL GENICULATE BODY

FOREBRAIN

OPTIC TRACT

OCULOMOTOR NERVE (III)

TROCHLEAR NERVE (IV)

CRUS CEREBRI

INTERPEDUNCULAR FOSSA

MIDBRAIN

TRIGEMINAL NERVE (V)

BASAL SULCUS

PONS

FACIAL NERVE AND NERVUS INTERMEDIUS (VII)

VESTIBULOCOCHLEAR NERVE (VIII)

ABDUCENS NERVE (VI)

GLOSSOPHARYNGEAL NERVE (IX)

VAGUS NERVE (X) AND CRANIAL ACCESSORY NERVE (XI)

SPINAL ACCESSORY NERVE (XI)

ROOTLETS OF HYPOGLOSSAL NERVE

OLIVE

VAGUS NERVE (X) AND CRANIAL ACCESSORY NERVE (XI)

HYPOGLOSSAL NERVE (XII)

MEDULLA

PYRAMID

DECUSSATION OF THE PYRAMIDS

VENTRAL MEDIAN FISSURE

SPINAL CORD

Figure 18–5. Brainstem. (From Gilman, S, and Newman, S: Manter and Gantz's Essentials of Clinical Neuroanatomy and Neurophysiology, ed 10. F. A. Davis, 2002, Philadelphia, p. 78, with permission.)

neuronal activity of the brain, can lead to seizures. A person is considered to have epilepsy once he or she has experienced two or more seizures unrelated to an underlying illness, such as meningitis.

Seizures are classified into two categories: partial and generalized. The two most common forms of generalized seizures are **absence seizures** (petit mal), which usually last between 2 and 10 seconds and are characterized by loss of consciousness without convulsions, and **tonic-clonic seizures** (grand mal), which are characterized by falling and loss of consciousness along with stiffening and twitching or jerking of the extremities. In most cases, seizure disorder can be prevented and/or controlled with antiepileptic medications. In some cases, surgical therapy can be used to manage seizures that cannot be well controlled with other therapies.

NERVE PLEXUSES

In certain areas of the body, nerves from the spine and the brain, of both the voluntary and the autonomic systems, join each other (anastomose) to form an interlacing network of nerves called a **plexus** (plural plexus or plexuses).

Some characteristic plexuses and their location include the following:

- **Brachial plexus**: lower part of the neck to the axilla (armpit)
- **Celiac plexus**: behind the stomach and in front of the aorta
- **Cervical plexus**: opposite the first four cervical vertebrae; that is, the top four of the seven vertebrae of the spinal column
- **Lumbar plexus**: psoas muscle (one of two muscles of the loins, the area known as the lumbar region)
- **Myenteric plexus**: the muscles that surround the walls of the intestine
- **Solar plexus**: celiac plexus

CRANIAL NERVES

The **cranial nerves** are 12 pairs of nerves that originate on either side of the brain; that is, one of each pair arises in the left hemisphere, and one in the right (Fig. 18–8). The name, function, and distribution of these 12 pairs of nerves are listed in Table 18–1.

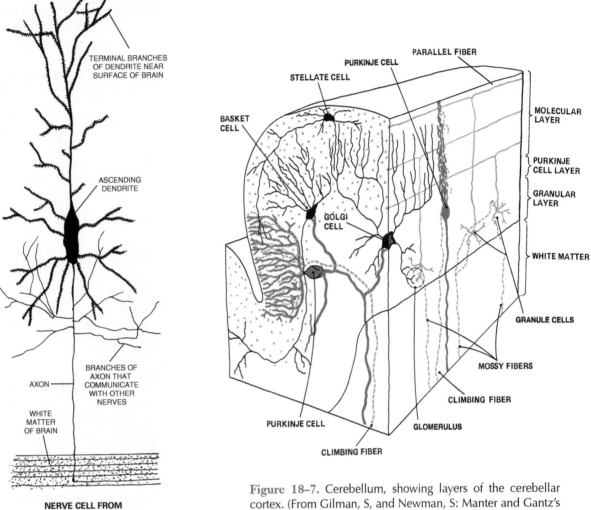

Figure 18–6. Nerve cell from cerebral cortex.

Figure 18–7. Cerebellum, showing layers of the cerebellar cortex. (From Gilman, S, and Newman, S: Manter and Gantz's Essentials of Clinical Neuroanatomy and Neurophysiology, ed 10. F. A. Davis, 2002, Philadelphia, p. 138, with permission.)

Table 18–1. Cranial Nerves

Number	Name	Function	Distribution
1st	Olfactory	Smell	Nasal mucous membrane
2nd	Optic	Sight	Retina
3rd	Oculomotor	Motor	Most muscles of the eyes
4th	Trochlear	Motor	Superior oblique muscles of the eye
5th	Trigeminal	Motor and chief sensory nerve of the face	Skin of the face, tongue, teeth, muscles of mastication
6th	Abducens	Motor	Lateral rectus muscle of the eye
7th	Facial	Motor	Muscles of facial expression
8th	Vestibulocochlear	Hearing and equilibrium	Internal auditory meatus[*]
9th	Glossopharyngeal	Motor and sensory	Pharynx and posterior third of the tongue, parotid gland, ear, meninges

[*]Latin *meatus*, opening

Number	Name	Function	Distribution
10th	Vagus	Motor and sensory	Pharynx, larynx, heart, lungs, esophagus, stomach, abdominal viscera
11th	Accessory	Motor	Sternomastoid and trapezius muscles
12th	Hypoglossal	Motor	Muscles of the tongue

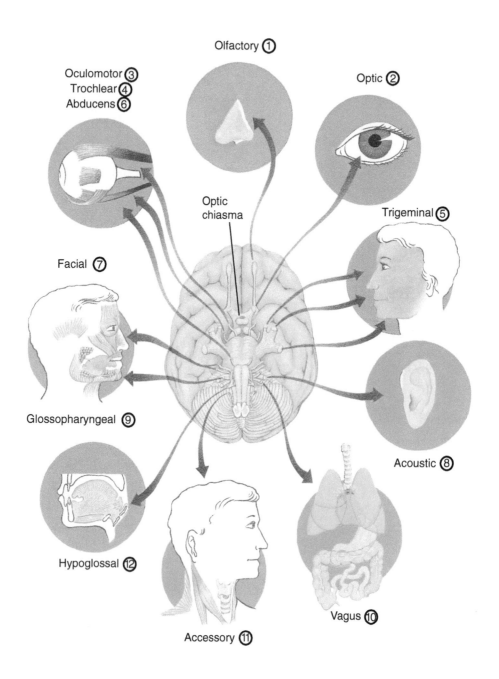

Figure 18–8. Cranial nerves and their distributions. (From Scanlon, VC, and Sanders, T: Essentials of Anatomy and Physiology, ed 4. F. A. Davis, Philadelphia, 2003, p 178, with permission.)

VOCABULARY

Note: Latin forms are given in ***bold italics***.

Greek or Latin	Combining Form	Meaning	Example
arachnē	**ARACHN-**	spider, web; arachnoid membrane	**arachn**-oidea
axōn	**AX-, AXON-**	axis, axon	**ax**-olemma
cerebrum	***CEREBR-***	brain	**cerebr**-oid
cholē	**CHOL(E)-**	bile, gall	**chol**-inergic
cortex, corticis	***CORTIC-, CORTEX***	[bark, rind] outer layer (of an organ)	cerebral **cortex**
dendron	**DENDR-**	[tree] dendrite, dendron	**dendr**-ic
dendritēs	**DENDRIT-**	[pertaining to a tree] dendrite, dendron	**dendrit**-es
fasciculus[*]	***FASCICL-, FASCICUL-***	[little bundle] fasciculus	**fascicul**-ation
ganglion	**GANGLI-**	[knot] ganglion	**gangli**-oma
glia	**GLI-, -GLIA-**	[glue] glia, neuroglia	neuro-**glia**
medulla	***MEDULL-***	marrow, medulla oblongata	**medull**-ary
mēninx, mēningos (plural *mēninges*)	**MENING-, -MENINX**	meningeal membrane, meninges	**mening**-es
myelos	**MYEL-**	myelin, spinal cord, bone marrow	**myel**-in
neuron	**NEUR-**	[tendon] neuron, nerve, nervous system	**neur**-obiology
plexus	***PLEX-***	[braid] plexus	**plex**-opathy
pons, pontis	***PONT-, PONS***	[bridge] pons	**pont**-ile nuclei
synapsis[†]	**SYNAP-, SYNAPS-**	[point of contact] synapse	**synap**-tic
thalamos	**THALAM-**	[inner chamber] thalamus	**thalam**-ic

[*]Diminutive of Latin, *fascis*, bundle

[†]From Greek, *haptein*, touch

ETYMOLOGICAL NOTES

The spinal cord and the brain are covered with three layers of protective membrane called the meninges (singular, meninx). Before the 1st century AD, the Greek word *mēninx* was applied to any membrane of the body; Hippocrates used it to refer to the membrane of the eye, and Aristotle used it to refer to the eardrum. After the 1st century, the term came to be used exclusively to refer to the meninges in their modern anatomic sense. The three meninges are named the **pia mater**, the delicate inner covering; the **dura mater**, the tough outer coat; and the **arachnoid**, the membrane between these two. The arachnoid (resembling a web) takes its name from Greek *arachnē* (spider, web), because of its delicate structure. However, the names pia mater, meaning "devout mother" in Latin, and dura mater, "hard mother," make little sense until it is realized that they are translations from the Arabic.

By the 4th century AD, the Roman Empire was split into two halves, with Rome the capital of the West and Byzantium (later named Constantinople by the emperor Constantine, and today called Istanbul) the capital of the East. The two halves were separated linguistically as well as geographically, with Latin used as the language of the West and Greek used in the East. The writings that survived in the West in the period after this were preserved, for the most part, by the Roman church and were principally the works of Latin authors. Greek ceased to be taught in the schools, and the knowledge of this language gradually was lost, along with the works of Hippocrates, Aristotle, and others. Nevertheless, these works were very much alive in the East, not only in Byzantium/Constantinople, but also in other lands of the Eastern Empire.

With the rise and spread of Islam during and after the 7th century, Arabic became the common language of almost the entire East. Works of the ancient Greek writers were translated into Arabic and read in the great centers of learning all over the Islamic empire, including Spain. These Arabic translations, and Arabic literature in general, escaped the notice of most of western Europe for the simple reason that there were few who could read Arabic. Thus, by the early Middle Ages, practically all knowledge of ancient Greek literature, including the medical works, was lost in the West.

In the 11th and 12th centuries, monks of the Roman church began translating some of the Arabic versions of the Greek writers into Latin. In Syria, a churchman known as Stephen of Antioch produced a Latin translation of Galen from the Arabic version. At this time, only two of the three meninges were known: the dura and the pia. Galen, writing in Greek, had named the outer (the dura) the *mēninx sklēra pacheia* (the hard, thick, membrane), and the inner (the pia), the *mēninx leptē* (the thin membrane). In the Arabic translation of Galen, the Greek terms were translated as "hard mother" and "thin mother." The Arabic use of the word for mother to translate the Greek *mēninx* may have implied that the protection afforded the spinal cord by the meninges could be compared with the protection that a mother gives to her young. Stephen translated these two terms into the Latin *dura mater* and *pia mater*, "hard mother" and "devout mother." The pia (feminine of *pius*, devout, pious) should have been *tenuis* (thin), but Stephen, a monk, apparently decided that pia was a more appropriate term, and it has remained. The arachnoid membrane was not identified until the 17th century, when the Dutch anatomist Frederick Ruysch realized its existence and named it.

Exercise 1

Answer each of the following questions.

1. To what part of the nervous system does each of the following refer?

   a. CNS _____

   b. PNS _____

   c. ANS _____

2. The _____ are the structural and functional units of the nervous system.

3. What is the name given to a bundle of nerve fibers? _____

4. What is the difference between an afferent and an efferent impulse? _____

   _____

5. Name the three membranes that cover and protect the spinal cord and the brain and lie under the bony structure of the skull and the spinal column.

   a. _____

   b. _____

   c. _____

6. What is a common cause of subdural hematoma? _____

7. Immunity against the disease polio was achieved with which two vaccines? _____

8. What is the difference between a nerve fiber that is adrenergic and one that is cholinergic? _____

_____

9. A/An _____ is the process that conducts impulses away from the cell body.

A/An _____ is the process that conducts impulses to the cell body.

10. Glia cells, often called neuroglia cells, have what function? _____

11. What are gliomas and neurogliomas? _____

12. The brainstem, the continuation of the spinal cord up into the skull, contains several important structures. What are they, and where are they found? _____

_____

13. Beneath the thalami is a structure called the _____

14. The four lobes that subdivide each cerebral hemisphere are the:

a. _____

b. _____

c. _____

d. _____

15. Disorders such as Sydenham's chorea, Parkinson's disease, and Bell's palsy are caused by damage to the _____

_____

16. A person who has motor aphasia as a result of damage to Broca's area, has difficulty doing what? _____

_____

17. What does the term "idiopathic" mean when it is used in reference to seizures? _____

_____

18. What is a plexus? _____

19. Give five plexuses (plexus) and their location.

    a. _____   _____

    b. _____   _____

    c. _____   _____

    d. _____   _____

    e. _____   _____

20. What is another name for a tonic-clonic seizure? _____

ENDOCRINE SYSTEM

The state of equilibrium within the body, when all organs are functioning perfectly, is called **homeostasis**. The body is kept in homeostasis by two systems: the **nervous system**, discussed in Lesson 18, and the **endocrine system** (Greek *endo-*, within, and *krinein*, separate, secrete), the subject of this chapter (Fig. 19–1). The endocrine system is made up of glands that produce **hormones** (Greek *horman*, set in motion), internal secretions that are discharged into the blood and then circulated throughout the body. The **endocrine glands** (Table 19–1), known as ductless glands, do not transmit their secretions by way of ducts as do the sweat glands and the tear glands. Glands that send their secretions by way of ducts are called **exocrine glands**, or sometimes **eccrine glands** (in particular, the eccrine sweat glands). Hormones, which can originate in a gland, an organ, or a body part, are carried to other parts of the body by the bloodstream and, through chemical action, increase or decrease the functional activity of those parts. The hormones secreted by the ductless glands may have a specific effect, as in the case of estrogens, which are secreted by the ovaries and stimulate the development and maintenance of female sexual characteristics. Alternately, they may have a general effect on the entire body, as in the case of thyroid hormone, which regulates the rate of metabolism of the whole body. The principal endocrine glands and their functions follow.

THE PITUITARY GLAND

The pituitary gland, also called the **hypophysis cerebri**, is a small, round gland (about the size of a bean) situated at the base of the brain (Fig. 19–2). It is sometimes referred to as the master gland of the body because its secretions stimulate other endocrine glands into increased (or decreased) activity. It consists of three sections: the anterior lobe, the posterior lobe, and the intermediate lobe. The **intermediate lobe** seems to have no function in warm-blooded animals. In cold-blooded animals, this lobe produces intermedin, which influences the activity of pigment cells in some reptiles, fish, and amphibians. The **anterior lobe** of the pituitary secretes six principal hormones:

1. **Growth hormone (GH)**, or **somatotropic hormone (STH)**, regulates growth. Increased production of this hormone can cause giantism (abnormal growth) and/or **acromegaly**, abnormal enlargement of the hands, feet, jaw, and other extremities. Decreased production of GH can cause dwarfism and/or **acromicria**, abnormal smallness of the extremities.

2. **Adrenocorticotropic hormone (ACTH)**, also called **corticotropin**, regulates the activity of the adrenal cortex, the outer layer of the adrenal gland. Secretions of the **adrenal cortex** include two groups of hormones that belong to the family of chemicals called **steroids**. The first of these is a group called **mineralocorticoids**, which regulate the metabolism of sodium. The second of these hormones is a group of chemicals called **glucocorticoids**, which act mainly on the metabolis of glucose. This group of steroids is also effective in protecting the body against stress and in promoting the healing process. In addition to these steroids, the

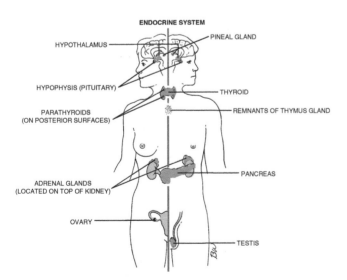

Figure 19–1. Endocrine system. (From Scanlon, VC, and Sanders, T: Essentials of Anatomy and Physiology, ed 4. F. A. Davis, Philadelphia, 2003, p 839, with permission.)

237

Table 19–1. Principal Endocrine Glands

Name	Position	Function	Endocrine Disorders
Adrenal cortex	Outer portion of gland on top of each kidney	Cortisol regulates carbohydrate and fat metabolism; aldosterone regulates salt and water balance	Hypofunction: Addison's disease Hyperfunction: Adrenogenital syndrome; Cushing's syndrome
Adrenal medulla	Inner portion of adrenal gland; surrounded by adrenal cortex	Effects of epinephrine and norepinephrine mimic those of sympathetic nervous system; increases carbohydrate use for energy	Hypofunction: Almost unknown Hyperfunction: Pheochromocytoma
Pancreas (endocrine portion)	Abdominal cavity; head adjacent to duodenum; tail close to spleen and kidney	Secretes insulin and glucagon, which regulate carbohydrate metabolism	Hypofunction: Diabetes mellitus Hyperfunction: If a tumor produces excess insulin, hypoglycemia
Parathyroid	Four or more small glands on back of thyroid	Parathyroid hormone regulates calcium and phosphorus metabolism; indirectly affects muscular irritability	Hypofunction: Hypocalcemia; tetany Hyperfunction: Hypercalcemia; resorption of bone; kidney stones; nausea; vomiting; altered mental status
Pituitary, anterior	Front portion of small gland below hypothalamus	Influences growth, sexual development, skin pigmentation, thyroid function, and adrenocortical function through effects on other endocrine glands (except for growth hormone, which acts directly on cells)	Hypofunction: Dwarfism in child; decrease in all other endocrine gland functions except parathyroid's Hyperfunction: Acromegaly in adult; giantism in child
Pituitary, posterior	Back portion of small gland below hypothalamus	Oxytocin increases uterine contractions	Unknown
		Antidiuretic hormone increases absorption of water by kidney tubules	Hypofunction: Diabetes insipidus
Testes and ovaries	Testes—in the scrotum Ovaries—in the pelvic cavity	Testosterone and estrogen regulate sexual maturation and development of secondary sex characteristics; some effects on growth	Hypofunction: Lack of sex development or regression in adult Hyperfunction: Abnormal sex development
Thyroid	Two lobes in anterior portion of neck	Thyroxine and T_3 increase metabolic rate and influence growth and maturation; calcitonin regulates calcium and phosphorus metabolism	Hypofunction: Cretinism in young; myxedema in adult; goiter Hyperfunction: Goiter; thyrotoxicosis

Source: *Taber's Cyclopedic Medical Dictionary*, ed 19. F. A. Davis, Philadelphia, 2001, p 840, with permission.

adrenal cortex secretes sex hormones: androgens in men and estrogens and progesterone in women.

3. **Thyroid-stimulating hormone (TSH)** regulates the activity of the thyroid gland.

4. (Ovarian) **follicle-stimulating hormone (FSH)** stimulates development of follicles (Latin *folliculus*, a little sac, diminutive of *follis*, sac) in the ovaries, and sper-

matogenesis in the testes. The ovarian follicles are spherical structures that produce an ovum every month in women of childbearing age.

5. **Luteinizing hormone (LH),** in conjunction with FSH, induces secretion of estrogens and progesterone, stimulates ovulation each month, and regulates the development of the *corpus luteum* (Latin, yellow body), a small

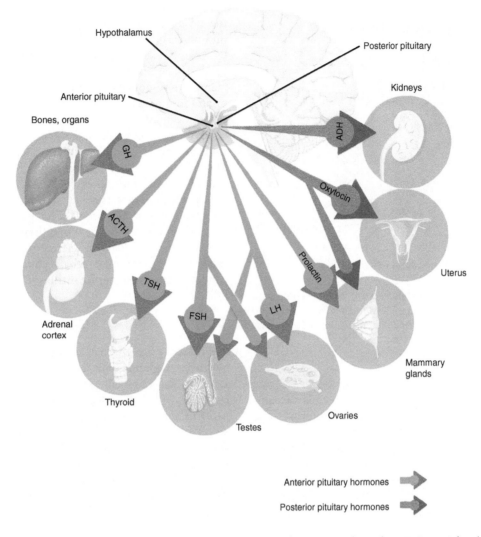

Figure 19–2. Pituitary gland. (Reproduced from Scanlon, VC, and Sanders, T: Essentials of Anatomy and Physiology, ed 4. F. A. Davis, Philadelphia, 2003, p 218, with permission.)

yellow structure that develops within a ruptured ovarian follicle when the ovum is released each month.

6. **Prolactin** or **lactogenic hormone**, in conjunction with progesterone and estrogens, stimulates breast development and induces the secretion of milk during pregnancy.

The **posterior lobe** of the pituitary gland secretes a hormone called **oxytocin** (Greek *oxys*, rapid, and *tokos*, childbirth), which increases uterine contractions during labor. Another hormone secreted within the posterior lobe is **antidiuretic hormone** (**ADH**), also called vasopressin, which contracts the muscles of blood vessels and elevates blood pressure. ADH also acts as an antidiuretic, preventing excessive loss of fluids through the kidneys.

THE THYROID GLAND

The **thyroid gland** is situated at the base of the neck on both sides of the lower part of the larynx and upper part of

the trachea (Fig. 19–3). The name comes from Greek *thyreos* (shield), thyroid, "shield shaped." As noted previously, the thyroid gland is stimulated by TSH (also called **thyrotropin**), which is secreted within the anterior lobe of the pituitary gland. One of the principal hormones secreted by the thyroid gland is **thyroxine**. Oversecretion of thyroxine produces the condition called **hyperthyroidism**. This increases the rate of basal metabolism and leads to excessive stimulation of the sympathetic nervous system. Symptoms of hyperthyroidism can include increased nervousness, tremors, heat intolerance, increased heart rate, and weight loss. If the overproduction of this hormone is excessive, the condition called **thyrotoxicosis** may occur. This can be clinically associated with protruding eyes (**exophthalmos**) and, often, goiter, or enlargement of the thyroid.

Deficient production of thyroxin produces the condition called **hypothyroidism**, which results in a lowered basal metabolic rate. Symptoms of hypothyroidism are the opposite of those of hyperthyroidism and include

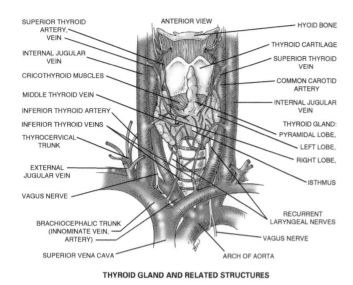

THYROID GLAND AND RELATED STRUCTURES

Figure 19–3. Thyroid gland and related structures. (Reproduced from Scanlon, VC, and Sanders, T: Essentials of Anatomy and Physiology, ed 4. F. A. Davis, Philadelphia, 2003, p 2099, with permission.)

sluggishness, low blood pressure, slow pulse, and decreased muscular activity. However, goiter may accompany hypothyroidism as well as hyperthyroidism. The underlying cause of hyperthyroidism and hypothyroidism is associated with the maintenance of proper levels of iodine in the diet. In certain regions of the world where the water is deficient in iodine salts, hypothyroidism is endemic. In recent years, however, the use of iodized salt has reduced the incidence of hypothyroidism in areas where iodine salts are at low levels in the drinking water.

Severe lack of iodine in childhood produces the condition known as **cretinism**, characterized by lack of growth and mental development. The term cretin comes from Swiss French *creitin*, from Latin *Christiānus* (Christian). Use of this term originated in Switzerland where, because the land has long been separated geologically from the sea, the water lacks iodine salts. The Swiss are said to have used this term to indicate their realization that these cretins were, after all, children of God.

When hypothyroidism becomes severe, a condition known as **myxedema** (Greek *myxa*, mucus, and *edema*, swelling) can occur. Myxedema occurs when thick, gelatinous materials called mucopolysaccharides infiltrate the skin, giving it a waxy or coarsened appearance. Symptoms include sluggishness, cold intolerance, apathy, fatigue, and constipation. Thyroid hormone replacement reverses the symptoms and re-establishes normal metabolic function.

THE PARATHYROID GLANDS

There are four parathyroid glands, which are located close to the thyroid gland. These glands secrete **parathyroid hormone (PTH)**, which regulates the metabolism of cal-

cium and phosphorus. **Hypoparathyroidism** results when the level of blood calcium falls, and the level of blood phosphorus rises. This condition is characterized mainly by loss of calcium in the teeth and bones, with resultant tooth defects and bone lesions. In general, the parathyroid glands are responsible for the proper maintenance of vitamin D in the body. Without normal levels of this vitamin, calcium cannot be properly utilized.

Hyperparathyroidism is the opposite of hypoparathyroidism, and results when blood calcium rises and blood phosphorus falls. Symptoms of hyperparathyroidism include muscular weakness and increased fragility of the bones, which occurs when calcium escapes from the bones into the circulating blood. The presence of abnormal amounts of calcium in the blood (**hypercalcemia**) and the inability of the kidneys to excrete this excess calcium can cause the formation of renal calculi—kidney stones—a condition known as **nephrolithiasis**.

THE ADRENAL GLANDS

There are two adrenal glands, sometimes called the **suprarenal glands**, one above each kidney (Fig. 19–4). Each adrenal gland consists of two distinct parts: the outer covering, called the **adrenal cortex**, and the inner structure, called the **adrenal medulla**. The adrenal cortex secretes chemical substances called **steroids**, principally those called **mineralocorticoids**, which help regulate the mineral content of the blood, and **glucocorticoids**, which help maintain proper levels of glucose in the blood. Another important hormone secreted by the adrenal cortex is **cortisone**, which regulates the metabolism of fats, carbohydrates, sodium, potassium, and proteins.

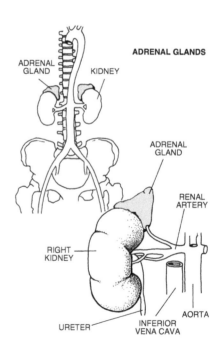

Figure 19–4. Adrenal glands.

Cortisone is also manufactured synthetically and used as an anti-inflammatory agent.

Also secreted in small amounts in the renal cortex are **androgens**, the male hormones, and **estrogens** and **progesterone**, the female hormones. Irregularities in the production of these hormones can result in increased or decreased sexual development in both males and females.

The **adrenal medulla** secretes three groups of chemical substances called **catecholamines: dopamine, norepinephrine**, and **epinephrine**. The principal effects of **dopamine** on the body are dilation of the arteries and increased cardiac output, with resultant increased flow of blood to the kidneys.

The principal effect of **norepinephrine** is constriction of the arterioles and venules, the ends of the arteries and veins, where they anastomose, or join, with the capillaries. This results in increased resistance to the flow of blood through the systemic circulation, which in turn causes elevated blood pressure and slowing of the heart action (**bradycardia**).

Epinephrine increases heart activity and dilates the bronchi. Adrenalin (synthetic epinephrine) is useful in treating people with asthma, increases the level of glucose in the blood, and diminishes the activity of the gastrointestinal system.

The adrenal medulla is under the control of the sympathetic nervous system, and thus is part of the autonomic nervous system. The secretion of epinephrine and norepinephrine is closely related to emotional states. Fear, stress, and emergency situations can cause the sympathetic nervous system to "send a message" to the adrenal medulla, which can result in the immediate secretion of norepinephrine or epinephrine, giving a quick boost to the energy level of the body, the "fight-or-flight" response.

THE ISLETS OF LANGERHANS

The **islets of Langerhans**, named for Paul Langerhans, a 19th-century German pathologist, are clusters of cells in the pancreas. There are three types of cell clusters in the islets of Langerhans: alpha, beta, and delta cells. The beta cells, which produce insulin, are found in the greatest number.

Insulin (Latin *insula*, island) is essential for the proper metabolism of blood sugar (glucose), and for the proper maintenance of glucose levels in the blood. Insufficient secretion of insulin results in deficient metabolism of carbohydrates and fats, and brings on the conditions called **hyperglycemia**, excessive amounts of blood sugar, and **glycosuria**, the presence of glucose in the urine. These two conditions characterize the disease called **diabetes**.

Excessive secretion of insulin brings about the condition called **hypoglycemia**, characterized by acute fatigue, irritability, and general weakness. In extreme cases, insulin shock, usually associated with excessive exogenous insulin, can bring about mental disturbances, coma, and even death.

Diabetes mellitus, or sugar diabetes, is a chronic disease characterized by the inability, in varying degrees, to metabolize carbohydrates. (See Lesson 15 for a further explanation of diabetes mellitus.) Manifestations of the disease are hyperglycemia and glycosuria. Symptoms include **polydipsia, polyuria**, loss of weight (despite **polyphagia**), and fatigue. There are two types of diabetes mellitus. Type 1 diabetes mellitus, also called insulin-dependent diabetes mellitus (IDDM), is caused by insufficient insulin production and usually begins early in life. The isolation and eventual synthesization of insulin by the Canadian physicians Sir Frederick Banting and Charles H. Best (for which Banting won the Nobel prize in 1923) made it possible for type 1 diabetics to live with their disease by the administration of insulin via injection.

Type 2 diabetes mellitus, called non–insulin-dependent diabetes mellitus (NIDDM), usually begins later in life, and is characterized by resistance to the effects of insulin at the cellular level. Often type 2 diabetes can be controlled with changes in diet and exercise. Tests for blood sugar (glucose) should be made frequently, however, and if glucose concentration remains high in the blood, it may be necessary to administer medications, such as the sulfonylureas, which stimulate the pancreas to release insulin. Newer medications that work on a cellular level to increase sensitivity to insulin may also be used.

GONADS: THE TESTES AND OVARIES

The gonads are the male and female sex glands. The male gonads, the testes, secrete spermatozoa; the female gonads, the ovaries, produce an ovum each month during parturient (childbearing) years.

The testes (or testicles) produce the male hormone testosterone, an androgen that stimulates and maintains secondary male sexual characteristics, including muscle strength, facial hair, and deepening of the voice.

The ovaries produce the female hormones estrogen and progesterone, which stimulate and maintain secondary female sexual characteristics, including body fat distribution, growth of the mammary glands, and voice quality. (For a complete discussion of ovulation, see Lesson 14.)

ETYMOLOGICAL NOTES

The Greek verb *krinein* (separate), which supplies the element **-crine** in the words endocrine and exocrine, has also provided other, nontechnical, words. In ancient times, the verb had the additional meanings of to pick out or choose, and then to judge. There was a noun, *krisis*, related to this verb that meant a separating, picking out, or choosing. Extended meanings of this noun included trial, judgment, and decision. From these varied but related meanings comes the word **crisis**. Also related to the verb *krinein* was the noun *kritēs* (judge or arbiter); the adjectival form of this noun was *kritikos* (able to decide or judge, critical). This word was found in Latin as the noun *criticus* (judge or critic). Another related word was *kritērion* (a means of judging, a standard, criterion).

Estrogen, the female hormone, takes its name from Greek *oistros* (gadfly), an insect that infected cattle, plus the form **-gen**. This unusual etymology has at its root a secondary meaning of this noun: a sting, anything that excites, madness, frenzy, or vehement passion. The term estrus (or oestrus) designates the cyclic period of sexual activity in females; thus, estrogen is the name of the hormone that causes or promotes the period of estrus. The ancients were unaware of the reasons for the cyclic periods of women between menarche and menopause, and the word *oistros* (Latin *oestrus*) was used by the writers in its original sense: that which excites (something or somebody) to action; a stinging insect. Virgil writes:

est lucos Silari circa ilicibusque virentem
plurimus Alburnum volitans, cui nomen asilo
Romanum est, oestrum Grai vertere vocantes…

Around the groves of Silarus and around
Alburnus green with oak trees
there flies a creature which the Romans call *asilus*,
but called *oestrus* by the Greeks… (*Georgics*, 3.146–148).

Greek legend tells us of a young girl named Io, daughter of the river Inachus, who had the misfortune to be desired by Zeus (Fig. 19–5). Just as he was about to consummate his desires, his wife, Hera, came upon the scene; in the instant before her appearance, Zeus changed Io into a heifer, a young cow. Hera, rightfully suspicious, asked that the creature be given to her. Zeus had no choice but to comply. Hera then stationed a hundred-eyed watchman, Argus, to stand guard over the luckless Io. Zeus, unable to tolerate this state of affairs, sent his messenger, Hermes, with orders: "Kill Argus!" Hermes did as ordered, and Io was free, but still in bovine form. Hera took the hundred eyes of Argus and placed them in the tail of her favorite bird, the peacock. She then sent a stinging insect, the gad-

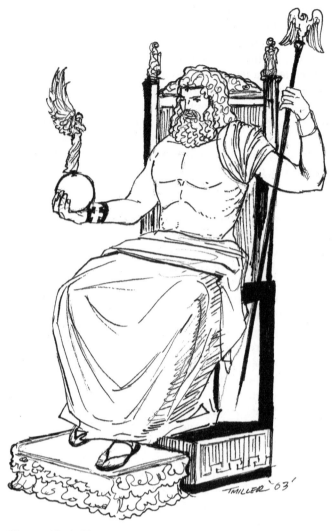

Figure 19–5. Zeus.

fly (*oistros*), to drive poor Io into flight all over the face of the earth. Eventually Zeus restored her to human form, and she settled down in the land of Egypt, where she became the mother of a son, Epaphus, sired by Zeus.

Exercise 1

Answer each of the following questions.

1. What name is given to glands that transmit their secretions through ducts? _____

2. What is the difference between the endocrine and the exocrine glands? _____

   What glands are commonly called eccrine? _____

3. What is the more common term for the gland called the hypophysis cerebri? _____

4. Which endocrine gland is often called the master gland of the body? _____

   What is the reason for this? _____

5. What are the functions of each of the following hormones, secreted in the anterior lobe of the pituitary gland?

   (a) growth hormone (GH) _____

   (b) adrenocorticotropic hormone (ACTH) _____

   (c) lactogenic hormone _____

6. Deficient secretion of the hormone STH can cause acromicria. What is the meaning of this term? _____

7. What is the main function of the hormone oxytocin, secreted in the posterior lobe of the pituitary gland? _____

   _____

8. What effect does vasopressin have on the body? _____

9. If there is excessive secretion of the hormone thyroxine by the thyroid gland, the result may be thyrotoxicosis. What is the meaning of each of the following two salient features of thyrotoxicosis? _____

   _____

   (a) exophthalmos _____

   (b) goiter _____

10. What is the cause of the condition known as cretinism? _____

11. Myxedema is a condition characterized by the accumulation of mucus in the tissues of the face and hands. What is the cause of myxedema, as far as glandular function is concerned?

   _____

12. Hypoparathyroidism can result in the condition known as hypercalcemia. What does this term mean? _____

    _____

13. Hypercalcemia can result in nephrolithiasis. What does this term mean? _____

14. What name is given to the outside covering of the adrenal gland? _____

15. What name is given to the inside portion of the adrenal gland? _____

16. Epinephrine, secreted in the adrenal glands, can be produced synthetically. When it is produced in this way, what is it called?

    _____

17. What hormone is secreted in the islets of Langerhans? _____

18. What is the meaning of each of the following five principal symptoms of diabetes mellitus?

    (a) hyperglycemia _____

    (b) glycosuria _____

    (c) polyuria _____

    (d) polydipsia _____

    (e) polyphagia _____

19. The hormone testosterone is an androgen. What does this term mean? _____

20. What hormones provide sudden energy to the body in emergency situations? _____

BIOLOGICAL NOMENCLATURE

UNIT

5

20

BIOLOGICAL
NOMENCLATURE

With the advance of human knowledge concerning the living organisms that inhabit the world around us—plants, birds, insects, fish, and all other living things from the smallest, the virus, a minute organism not visible under ordinary light microscopy, to the largest, the whale—it became desirable to classify these living organisms into convenient groupings. Following this classification, the next and immediate step was to name the members of each group. The term used for this classification is **taxonomy** (Greek *taxis*, arrangement, *nomos*, law), and the term used for the naming of these groups is **nomenclature** (Latin *nōmenclātūra*, a calling by name: *nōmen*, name, *c[a]lātus*, called, and -ura, a noun-forming suffix). The Latin noun *nōmenclātūra* was first used by Pliny, the Roman scientist, in his encyclopedic *Naturalis Historia* (Natural History), completed in 77 AD. The groups that are distinguishable from each other, and thus classified, are called taxa (singular, taxon), and the allocation of names to these taxa is called nomenclature.

Nomenclature follows classification and is independent of it. However, the objectives of both are the same: first, to provide a system whereby each and every living thing can be grouped according to shared characteristics and, second, to give names to these groups so that they may be referred to and discussed intelligently by all members of the scientific community in all countries, regardless of the different languages of these members. Traditionally, the language of biological and scientific nomenclature has been Latin. Included in the term "Latin" are words borrowed from other languages, mainly ancient Greek, and given the **form** of Latin words, so that they look like Latin.

The reasons for the use of Latin as the language of scientific nomenclature are compelling. Latin ceased to be a spoken language centuries ago and thus is not subject to the changes that constantly influence living, spoken languages. Latin remains forever static. Perhaps the most

cogent reason for selecting Latin as a means of communication among scientists of all nations is the fact that, in the Western world, Latin was the language of learned communities, whether the object of this learning was medicine, law, religion, philosophy, or science. The monumental work of British physician William Harvey on the circulation of the blood, published in 1628, was written in Latin: *Exercitatio Anatomica de Motu Cordis et Sanguinis* (An Anatomical Treatise concerning the Movement of the Heart and Blood). The Polish astronomer Copernicus wrote his great work, a treatise entitled *De Revolutionibus Orbium Coelestium* (Concerning the Revolutions of the Heavenly Bodies) in Latin in 1543, and the works of the Dutch theologian Erasmus (1466–1536) were written in Latin.

The Swedish botanist Carl von Linné, better known as Linnaeus (1707–1778), first formulated the principles that are still used for botanical taxonomy and nomenclature. His *Genera Plantarum* and *Classes Plantarum* (Genera of Plants and Classes of Plants), published in 1737 and 1738, are considered the beginning of systematic classification and terminology for modern botany. Following other important publications, his *Philosophia Botanica* (1751) explained fully his system for botanical nomenclature, and the 10th edition of his *Systema Naturae* (1758) established the rules for zoological nomenclature. All of these works were written in Latin and, for the first time, laid down the rules for the formulation of all subsequent biological terminology.

The system, based on Linnaeus' rules for botanical and zoological nomenclature, applies a binomial (Medieval Latin *binōmius*, having two names: Latin *bi-*, two, and *nōmen*, name) nomenclature to all living organisms. Every living organism is given two Latin names: the first identifies the **genus** (Latin *genus*, *generis*, race, stock, kind) to which it belongs, and the second is a name peculiar to each member of the genus, in order to differentiate it from other members of the same genus. For example, there are many members of the cat family—the lion, the leopard, the tiger, and so forth—obviously related to one another and, just as obviously, not related to members of the dog family—the household dog, the coyote, and so forth. The genus (plural genera) of cats to which many of the great cats belong, including the lion, leopard, and tiger, is named *Panthera*. In the binomial system, the lion is *Panthera leo*; the leopard, *Panthera pardus*; and the tiger, *Panthera tigris*. The second name—the specific or **species** name–distinguishes these great cats from each other, and the first, the genus or generic name, distinguishes them from the best-known member of the cat family, a member of the genus *Felis*, the domesticated feline, *Felis catus* (or *domesticus*), the common household cat. (Fig. 20–1).

SPECIES AND GENERA

The binomial terms mentioned above are names of **species**. As mentioned above, the first word of the name, *Panthera* or *Felis*, is the genus or **generic** name. The second word, *leo*, *pardus*, or *tigris*, is the species or **specific** name that, following the generic name, indicates the species. Note that in the names of species, the generic name is capitalized, whereas the specific name is not. Both names are customarily italicized, and it takes at least two words to name a species.

A species can be defined as a group that shares similar characteristics and is usually capable of interbreeding, although not all members of each species are identical in appearance. That is, all household cats look more or less alike, although they are not identical; all leopards look more or less alike, but household cats do not look much like leopards and cannot interbreed with this species. All species of cat belong to the family Felidae, which has 18 genera, one of which is the genus *Felis*, and another, the genus *Panthera*. All species of bears belong to the family Ursidae, which has six genera, the most diverse of which is the genus *Ursus*. The polar bear (*Ursus maritimus*), the American black bear (*Ursus americanus*), and the brown or grizzly bear (*Ursus arctos*) are species that resemble each other, but none of them resembles any of the species of the genus *Felis*. The household dog (*Canis familiaris*) and the coyote (*Canis latrans*) are two species of the same genus. They resemble each other, but neither resembles any members of the genus *Felis* or *Ursus*.

It should be noted that the specific name in binomial nomenclature is not used by itself. The specific names *catus*, *maritimus*, and *latrans* have no validity standing alone in this terminology.

FAMILIES

The **family** is the name for a group of closely related genera. The name for the cat family is Felidae and includes all its genera. The name for the bear family is Ursidae, and that for the dog family is Canidae. Names for families consist of one name only and therefore are uninomial (Latin *ūnus*, one). Family names are capitalized. Under the codes of nomenclature now in existence, the names of families of animals and protista are formed by adding -**idae** to the stem of the generic name, and names of families of plants, fungi, and prokaryotae (monera) are formed by adding -**aceae** to the stem of the generic name, with some exceptions: Compositae, Palmae, Gramineae, Leguminosae, Guttiferae, Umbelliferae, Labiatae, and Cruciferae.

These codes are drawn up in meetings of the appropriate international organizations. The naming of animals is governed by the *International Code of Zoological Nomenclature* (ICZN); of plants, by the *International Code of Botanical Nomenclature* (ICBN) and the *International Code of Nomenclature for Cultivated Plants* (ICNCP); of bacteria, by the *International Code of Nomenclature of Bacteria* (ICNB), and of viruses and subviral agents, by the *International Code of Virus Classification and Nomenclature* (ICVCN). In 1995, the International Committee on Bionomenclature (ICB) was established to expedite work toward a unified system of bionomenclature among the five codes.

TAXONOMIC HIERARCHY

The grouping of taxa into ranks or levels follows what is called the **taxonomic hierarchy** (Greek *hieros*, sacred, *archein*, rule). The smallest of the main groups within the principal ranks is the species. Secondary ranks are general-

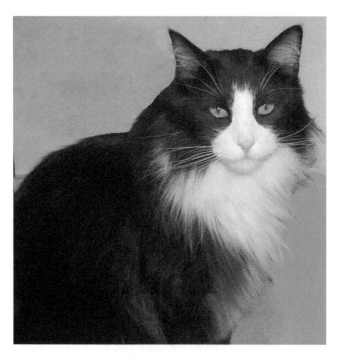

Figure 20–1. Genus *Felis* (cat). (Photograph by Laine McCarthy, 2000.)

ly used to subdivide large groups. Within a major group, a subgroup and supergroup may exist.

Species are grouped into genera, genera into families, families into orders, orders into classes, classes into phyla,* and phyla into kingdoms.

RANK†
Kingdom
Phylum
Class
Order
Suborder
Infraorder
Superfamily
Family
Subfamily
Genus
Subgenus
Species
Subspecies

The kingdom is the largest taxon. Controversy exists concerning the actual number of kingdoms. Most taxonomies identify five kingdoms: Animalia, Plantae, Fungi, Protista, and Prokaryotae (Monera). Some taxonomists believe that the five-kingdom paradigm is inadequate because it does not recognize the diversity of Protista and Prokaryotae. Molecular taxonomic studies, however, identify only three kingdoms, placing Animalia, Plantae, Fungi (Fig. 20–2), and Protista into one kingdom called Eukarya,

and splitting the Prokaryotae (Monera) into two kingdoms: Eubacteria and Archaea.‡

The phylum (singular of phyla, from Greek *phylon*, clan, tribe) of invertebrate animals called Arthropoda is the largest animal phylum, containing over 900,000 species. It includes the crustaceans, insects, myriapods (centipedes and millipedes), arachnids (spiders and scorpions), and other, similar forms. This phylum was well named because the term Arthropoda means "jointed feet," from Greek *arthron* (joint) and *pous, podos* (foot). All members of this group have jointed exoskeletons, segmented bodies, and jointed appendages (Fig. 20–3).

THE FORM AND ETYMOLOGICAL SIGNIFICANCE OF NAMES

All of the codes of nomenclature require that scientific names be in the form of Latin words, even if, as noted above, the terms used are originally from a language other than Latin (e.g., Greek, Arabic, or English). Whatever their ultimate linguistic source, these names must follow the rules of Latin grammar; that is, the names must be in the proper Latin grammatical form. An adjective that modifies a noun, for example, must agree with the noun in gender and number—feminine singular, masculine plural, neuter singular, and so forth. In the binomial nomenclature for species, the specific name—the second of the two terms—may be an adjective; thus, it must agree in gender

*In botanical nomenclature, "division" is used instead of "phylum."
†Source: *www.ecosystemworld.com/taxa003.htm*

‡Source: Universal Phylogenic Tree (*http://www.brunel.ac.uk/depts/blproject/microbio/bactax/classif/phylogen.htm*)

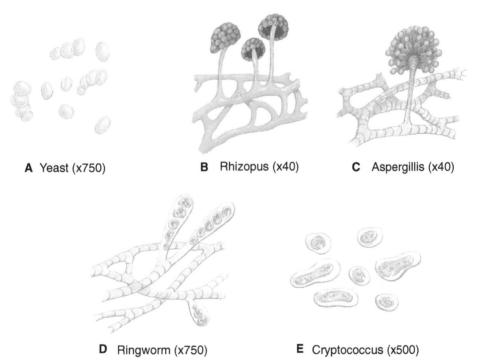

A Yeast (x750) **B** Rhizopus (x40) **C** Aspergillis (x40)

D Ringworm (x750) **E** Cryptococcus (x500)

Figure 20–2. Fungi. (From Scanlon, VC, and Sanders, T: Essentials of Anatomy and Physiology, ed 4. F. A. Davis, Philadelphia, 2003, p 490, with permission.)

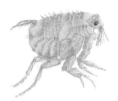

Flea (x15)

Figure 20–3. Genus *Xenopsylla* (flea). (From Scanlon, VC, and Sanders, T: Essentials of Anatomy and Physiology, ed 4. F. A. Davis, Philadelphia, 2003, p 493, with permission.)

and number with the first, or generic, name, which is always a noun.

Spirochaeta pallida (the causative organism of syphilis) is a spiral, hairlike microorganism. Its generic name is from Greek *speira* (spiral), and *chaitē* (hair). It should be noted that the Greek form for this word would be *speirochaitē* (if it ever existed in the ancient Greek language). However, the rules of the Codes say that all of the names must be in the form of Latin. In the latinization of Greek words, the Greek diphthong *ei* usually becomes *i*, the diphthong *ai* usually becomes *ae* (often *e*), and a final *-ē* becomes *-a*. The reason for these changes is that Greek words, when borrowed by the Latin language in antiquity, were spelled in this way. The word *Spirochaeta* is a feminine noun (because the Greek noun *chaitē* was feminine) and is singular in number. The specific name, *pallida*, which identifies this particular spirochete from others of the same genus, is a Latin adjective in the form of the feminine singular, agreeing with the feminine singular noun *Spirochaeta*. The Latin adjective *pallida* means pale, pallid. Thus, *Spirochaeta pallida* means a pale, spiral, hairlike microorganism. It belongs to the family Spirochaetaceae.

Another common name for *Spirochaeta pallida* is *Treponema pallidum*. The generic name, *Treponema*, means the same etymologically as *Spirochaeta*. It is formed from the stem trep- from the Greek verb *trepein* (turn, twist),

and the noun *nēma* (thread). The noun *nēma* is neuter in gender and singular in number; thus, the Latin adjective *pallidum*, the specific name, is in the form of the Latin neuter singular: *Treponema pallidum*, pale, twisted thread, is another name for *Spirochaeta pallida*, pale, spiral hair. The family name for the genus *Treponema* is Treponemata-ceae.

The second term, the specific name of the species, does not have to be an adjective modifying the generic name. It may be a noun in the genitive (possessive) case, or it may be a noun in the nominative singular. Examples of specific names in the form of the Latin nominative singular include *Panthera leo*, *Panthera tigris*, and *Panthera pardus*, in which the Latin nouns *leo*, *tigris*, and *pardus* meant lion, tiger, and leopard, respectively. Examples of specific names in the form of the Latin genitive singular include *Bacillus anthracis* (*anthrax, anthracis*, carbuncle), the causative agent of anthrax, a disease of animals, and *Entamoeba colī* (*colon, colī*, colon), a species of nonpathogenic, parasitic amoeba normally found in the human intestinal tract.

It should be noted that uninomial names for genera, orders, classes, and phyla give no indication by themselves as to taxon. Thus, for example, Lepidoptera is an order of the class Insecta that includes the moths and butterflies. Annelida is the name of the phylum to which the earthworms belong. Acanthocephala is the name of a class of wormlike enterozoa related to the Platyhelminthes, a phylum of flatworms that includes the tapeworms. Anoplura is the name of the order of insects that includes the sucking lice, and *Rhinosporidium* is a genus of fungi.

A number of genera have been named after the individual who first realized their existence. These names have been put into the form of a Latin word, usually by the addition of either the suffix -ia or the diminutive -ella: *Salmonella* (Daniel E. Salmon, American pathologist, 1850–1914); *Brucella* (Sir David Bruce, British bacteriologist, 1855–1931); *Shigella* (Kiyoshi Shiga, Japanese physician, 1870–1957); *Yersinia* (Alexandre Yersin, Swiss bacteriologist, 1863–1943); *Giardia* (Alfred Giard, French biologist, 1846–1908); and *Wuchereria* (Otto Wucherer, German physician, 1820–1873).

VOCABULARY

Note: Latin combining forms are in ***bold italics***.

Greek or Latin	Combining Form	Meaning	Example
akari	**ACAR-**	mite	**Acar**-ina
amoibē	**AMOEBA**	[change] amoeba	*Ent-**amoeba***
anōphelēs[*]	**ANOPHELES**	useless, harmful	***Anopheles***
askos	**ASC-**	sac, bag	**Asc**-omycetes
aspergere[†]	***ASPERG-***	sprinkle	***Asperg-illus***
aureus	***AURE-***	golden yellow	*Staphylococcus **aure**-us*

[*]Greek *an-* + *ōpheleia*, help
[†]Latin *ad-* + *spargere*, scatter

Greek or Latin	Combining Form	Meaning	Example
blatta	**BLATTA**	cockroach	**Blatta** orientalis
botulus	**BOTUL-**	sausage	Clostridium **botul**-inum
bōs, bovis	**BOV-**	ox, bull, cow	Actinomyces **bov**-is
chaitē	**CHAET-**	hair	Spiro-**chaet**-a pallida
cīmex	**CIMEX**	bug	**Cimex** lectularius
klōstēr	**CLOSTR-**	spindle	**Clostr**-idium
culex	**CULEX**	gnat	**Culex** pipiens
duodēnalis	**DUODENAL-**	of the duodenum	Ancylostoma **duodenal**-e
fēlineus‡	**FELINEUS**	of or belonging to a cat	Opisthorchis **felineus**
flāvus	**FLAVUS**	golden yellow	Aspergillus **flavus**
fluere	**FLU-**	flow	in-**flu**-enza
Germānicus	**GERMANIC-**	of Germany, German	Blatta **germanic**-a
glaukos	**GLAUCUS**	bluish gray	Aspergillus **glaucus**
Helvetius	**HELVET-**	Helvetian, Swiss	Lactobacillus **helvet**-icus
hex	**HEX-**	six	**Hex**-apoda
lectulus	**LECTUL-**	couch, bed	Cimex **lectul**-arius
lepis, lepidos	**LEPID-**	scale (of an animal)	**Lepid**-optera
nēma, nēmatos	**NEMA, NEMAT-**	thread	Trepo-**nema**
opisthen	**OPISTH-**	located in the back	**Opisth**-orchis
orchis	**ORCHIS**	testicle	Opisth-**orchis**
orientalis	**ORIENTAL-**	of the east, oriental	Blatta **oriental**-is
pallidus	**PALLID-**	pale, lacking color	**pallid**-um
phtheir	**PHTHIR-**	louse	**Phthir**-us (Fig. 20–4)
pīpīre	**PIP-**	peep, chirp	Culex **pip**-iens
platys	**PLATY-**	flat	**Platy**-helminthes
prōtos	**PROT-**	first	**Prot**-ozoa
pteron	**PTER-**	wing	Hemi-**pter**-a
pūbes, pūbis	**PUB-**	pubic region	Phthirus **pub**-is
speira	**SPIR-**	coil, spiral	**Spir**-ochaeta
staphylē	**STAPHYL-**	bunch of grapes	**Staphyl**-ococcus
streptos	**STREPT-**	twisted	**Strept**-ococcus
tabānus	**TABAN-**	horsefly	**Taban**-idae
trepein	**TREP-**	turn, twist	**Trep**-onema

‡Latin *fēlēs*, cat

ETYMOLOGICAL NOTES

The language that was used by Linnaeus and other scientists and scholars of the Renaissance and the period following (after 1500 AD) is called New Latin. The Latin found in the writings of Cicero, Julius Caesar, and other literary figures of their time is called Classical Latin. Although the language of the Classical Period (1st century BC to 2nd century AD) was kept alive by scholars, churchmen, and literary figures in the centuries preceding the Renaissance, the spoken tongue had changed so dramatically that it resembled Classical Latin in only the vaguest outlines. This phenomenon precipitated the development of the Romance languages—Italian, Spanish, French—from the Latin spoken in the various parts of the great Roman Empire. At any age and in any place, the spoken language differs from the literary language, just as today our everyday, informal speech tends to be more idiomatic than the language that we use in writing. The spoken language of the ancient Romans is called Vulgar Latin, from

LOUSE

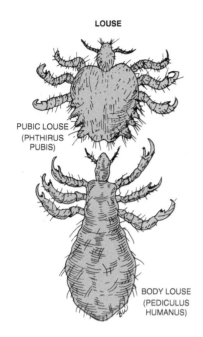

PUBIC LOUSE
(PHTHIRUS
PUBIS)

BODY LOUSE
(PEDICULUS
HUMANUS)

Figure 20–4. *Phthirus pubis* (pubic louse) and *Pediculus humanus* (body louse). (From Taber's Cyclopedic Medical Dictionary, ed 19. F. A. Davis, Philadelphia, 2001, p 1205, with permission.)

the adjective *vulgāris* (of the people, commonplace), from the noun *vulgus* (the people, the multitude). The first great document in Vulgar Latin was the Vulgate (from *vulgata editio*, the vulgar edition), the translation of the Scriptures from Greek by Jerome (later Saint Jerome) in the early 5th century AD.

Scientists and writers of the Renaissance and the period following, schooled in Classical Latin, tried to emulate the classical writers and to revive the style of Cicero and others. They were successful to varying degrees. Although their Latin often lacks the polish of a writer like Cicero, it is clear and straightforward, and can be read with relative ease by anyone with a background in Classical Latin. Linnaeus's *Genera Plantarum*, *Classes Plantarum*, *Philosophia Botanica*, and *Systema Naturae* are good examples of this style. The language is called New Latin. Some of these New Latin writers went so far as to change their given names to the form of Latin. As noted above, Linnaeus's given name was Carl von Linné. Other well-known personages who Latinized their names include the composer Wolfgang Mozart, who changed his middle name, Gottlieb (God-loving) to Amadeus (Latin *amāre*, love, *deus*, god). The 15th/16th century Polish astronomer, Nicolaus Koppernigk, changed his name to the familiar Copernicus, and the Swiss/German physician of the same period, Aureolus Theophrastus Bombastus von Hohenheim, already given a Latin name in part, preferred to be called Paracelsus, perhaps suggesting that he was the equal of, or even superior to, the early Roman physician Celsus.

Exercise 1

Using the vocabulary of this lesson, determine the etymological meaning of each of the following uninomial and binomial terms. Find the modern biological meaning of each of these terms in a medical dictionary.

1. Acarina _____

2. *Actinomyces bovis* _____

3. *Ancylostoma duodenale* _____

4. *Anopheles* _____

5. Arthropoda _____

6. Ascomycetes _____

7. *Aspergillus flavus* _____

8. *Aspergillus glaucus* _____

9. *Blatta germanica* _____

10. *Blatta orientalis* _____

11. *Bordetella*[*] pertussis _____

12. *Cimex lectularius* _____

13. *Clostridium*[†] botulinum _____

14. *Clostridium septicum* _____

15. *Culex pipiens* _____

16. *Diplococcus pneumoniae* _____

17. Diptera _____

18. *Entamoeba coli* _____

19. *Entamoeba gingivalis* _____

20. Hemiptera _____

21. Hexapoda _____

22. *Lactobacillus helveticus* _____

23. Lepidoptera _____

24. *Opisthorchis felineus* _____

25. *Phthirus pubis* _____

[*]Named for Jules Bordet, Belgian physician (1870-1961)
[†]Here the Greek-derived suffix *-ium* (*-ion*) is a diminutive ending: clostridium, a little thing resembling a spindle.

26. Platyhelminthes _____

27. Protozoa _____

28. *Salmonella typhi* _____

29. Sarcophagidae _____

30. *Spirochaeta pallida* _____

31. *Staphylococcus aureus* _____

32. *Streptococcus pyogenes* _____

33. Tabanidae _____

34. *Treponema pallidum* _____

35. *Trichinella spiralis* _____

APPENDICES

INDEX OF COMBINING FORMS

This index includes all of the combining forms found in this text, along with their basic meanings and the Greek or Latin term from which each is formed (in italics). The combining forms are in capital letters and **bold** type; Latin combining forms are in ***bold italic*** type. The number of the lesson in which each is found is included in parentheses.

A

ABDOMIN-, *abdōmen, abdōminis*, belly, abdomen (8)

ACANTH-, *akantha*, thorn, spine (1)

ACAR-, *akari*, mite (20)

ACOU-, *akouein*, hear (5)

ACOUS-, *akouein*, hear (5)

ACR-, *akron*, [highest point] extremities (particularly the hands and feet) (2)

ACTIN-, *aktis, aktinos*, [ray] radiation (15)

ACU-, *akouein*, hear (5)

ACUS-, *akouein*, hear (5)

ADEN-, *adēn*, gland (7)

ADIP-, *adeps, adipis*, fat (8)

AER-, *aēr*, air, gas (7)

AGOG-, *agōgos*, leading, drawing forth (14)

-AGRA, *agra*, [hunting] (sudden) pain, gout (15)

ALG-, *algos*, pain (1)

ALGES-, *algēsis*, sensitivity to pain (1)

ALL-, *allos*, other, divergence, difference from (1)

ALVE-, *alveus*, hollow, cavity (11)

AMBLY-, *amblys*, dull, faint (2)

AMNI-, *amnion*, fetal membrane, amniotic sac, amnion (5)

AMOEBA, *amoibē*, [change] amoeba (20)

AMYGDAL-, *amygdalē*, [almond] tonsil (11)

AMYL-, *amylon*, starch (10)

ANCYL-, *ankylos*, fused, stiffened; hooked, crooked (6)

ANDR-, *anēr, andros*, man, male (6)

ANGI-, *angeion*, (blood) vessel, duct (1)

ANGIN-, *angina*, choking pain, angina pectoris (10)

ANKYL-, *ankylos*, fused, stiffened; hooked, crooked (6)

ANOPHELES, *anōphelēs*, useless, harmful (20)

ANTER-, *anterior*, front, in front (9)

ANTHRAC-, *anthrax, anthrakos*, coal; anthrax (11)

ANTHRAX, *anthrax, anthrakos*, coal; anthrax (11)

AORT-, *aortē*, aorta (10)

APHRODIS-, *Aphrodisios*, sexual desire (6)

APHRODISI-, *Aphrodisios*, sexual desire (6)

ARACHN-, *arachnē*, spider, web; arachnoid membrane (3, 18)

ARCH-, *archē*, beginning, origin (14)

-ARCHE, *archē*, beginning, origin (14)

ARCT-, *arctāre*, *arctātus*, compress (10)

ARCTAT-, *arctāre*, *arctātus*, compress (10)

ARTERI-, *arteria*, [air passage] artery (1)

ARTHR-, *arthron*, joint (1)

ASC-, *askos*, [leather bag] sac, bag, bladder (5, 20)

ASCIT-, *askos*, [leather bag] sac, bag, bladder (5)

ASPERG-, *aspergere*, sprinkle (20)

ATHER-, *athērē*, [soup] fatty deposit (10)

ATRI-, *ātrium* [entrance hall] atrium (10)

AUR-, *auris*, ear (8)

AURE-, *aureus*, golden-yellow (20)

AUT-, *autos*, self (4)

AUX-, *auxein*, grow, increase (11)

-AUXE, *auxein*, grow, increase (11)

-AUXIS, *auxein*, grow, increase (11)

AX-, *axōn*, axis, axon (18)

AXON-, *axōn*, axis, axon (18)

B

BACILL-, *bacillus*, [rod, staff] bacillus (8)

BACTER-, *baktērion*, [small staff] bacterium (11)

BACTERI-, *baktērion*, [small staff] bacterium (11)

BARY-, *barys*, heavy, dull, hard (5)

BI-, *bios*, life (1)

BILI-, *bīlis*, bile (12)

BLAST-, *blastos*, [bud, germ] primitive cell (16)

BLATTA, *blatta*, cockroach (20)

BLENN-, *blennos*, mucus (7)

BLEPHAR-, *blepharon*, eyelid (13)

BOL-, *bolē*, a throwing (10)

BOTUL-, *botulus*, sausage (20)

BOV-, *bōs*, *bovis*, ox, bull, cow (20)

BRACHI-, *bracchium*, (upper) arm (9)

BRACHY-, *brachys*, short (6)

BRADY-, *bradys*, slow (1)

BRONCH-, *bronchos*, [windpipe] bronchus (11)

BRONCHI-, *bronchos*, [windpipe] bronchus (11)

BURS-, *bursa*, [leather sack] bursa (8)

C

CALC-, *calx*, *calcis*, stone, calcium, lime (salts) (8)

CALOR-, *calor*, heat, energy (8)

CAPILL-, *capillus*, [hair] capillary (10)

CAPIT-, *caput*, *capitis*, head (8)

CAPN-, *kapnos*, [smoke] carbon dioxide (11)

CARCIN-, *karkinos*, [crab] carcinoma, cancer (2)

CARDI-, *kardia*, heart (1)

CARDI-, *kardia*, cardia (12)

CEC-, *caecus*, [blind] cecum (12)

CEL-, *koilia*, abdomen (7)

-CEL-, *kēlē*, hernia, tumor, swelling (2)

CELI-, *koilia*, abdomen (7)

CENTE-, *kentein*, pierce (5)

CEPHAL-, *kephalē*, head (1)

-CEPT-, *capere*, *captus*, take (9)

CEREBR-, *cerebrum*, brain (8, 18)

CERVIC-, *cervix*, *cervīcis*, neck (of the uterus), cervix uteri (14)

CERVIX, *cervix*, *cervīcis*, neck (of the uterus), cervix uteri (14)

CHAET-, *chaitē*, hair (20)

CHEIL-, *cheilos*, lip (7)

CHEIR-, *cheir*, hand (2)

CHIL-, *cheilos*, lip (7)

CHIR-, *cheir*, hand (2)

CHLOR-, *chlōros*, green (3)

CHOL-, *cholē*, bile, gall (2, 18)

CHOLE-, *cholē*, bile, gall (2, 18)

CHONDR-, *chondros*, cartilage (3)

CHOROID-, *chorioeidēs*, [skinlike] choroid (13)

CHROM-, *chrōma*, *chrōmatos*, color, pigment (5)

CHROMA-, *chrōma, chrōmatos*, color, pigment (5)

CHROMAT-, *chrōma, chrōmatos*, color, pigment (5)

CHRON-, *chronos*, time, timing (7)

-CID-, *caedere, caesus*, cut, kill (9)

CIMEX, *cīmex*, bug (20)

-CIP-, *capere, captus*, take (9)

CIRS-, *kirsos*, dilated and twisted vein, varix (10)

-CIS-, *caedere, caesus*, cut, kill (9)

CLA-, *klān*, break (up), destroy (7)

CLAS-, *klān*, break (up), destroy (7)

-CLAST, *klān*, something that breaks or destroys (7)

CLOSTR-, *klōstēr*, spindle (20)

-CLUD-, *claudere, clausus*, close (10)

-CLUS-, *claudere, clausus*, close (10)

CLY-, *klyzein*, rinse out, inject fluid (12)

CLYS-, *klyzein*, rinse out, inject fluid (12)

COCC-, *kokkos*, [berry] coccus (11)

-COCCUS, *kokkos*, [berry] coccus (11)

COL-, *kolon*, colon (2)

COLI-, *kolon*, *Escherichia coli* (2)

COLON-, *kolon*, colon (2)

COLP-, *kolpos*, vagina (14)

CONI-, *konis*, dust (11)

COPR-, *kopros*, excrement, fecal matter (12)

COR, *cor, cordis*, heart (10)

COR-, *korē*, [girl] pupil (of the eye) (13)

CORD-, *cor, cordis*, heart (10)

CORE-, *korē*, [girl] pupil (of the eye) (13)

CORON-, *corōna*, crown (10)

CORTEX, *cortex, corticis*, [bark, rind] outer layer (of an organ) (15, 18)

CORTIC-, *cortex, corticis*, [bark, rind] outer layer (of an organ) (15, 18)

COST-, *costa*, rib (8)

CRANI-, *kranion*, skull (1)

CREAT-, *kreas, kreatos*, flesh (12)

CRESC-, *crescere, crētus*, (begin to) grow (9)

-CRET-, *crescere, crētus*, (begin to) grow (9)

CRIN-, *krinein*, [separate] secrete, secretion (4)

CRY-, *kry(m)os*, icy cold (15)

CRYM-, *kry(m)os*, icy cold (15)

CRYPT-, *kryptos*, hidden, latent (6)

CULEX, *culex*, gnat (20)

CUSP-, *cuspis, cuspidis*, point (10)

-CUSPID, *cuspis, cuspidis*, point (10)

CYAN-, *kyanos*, blue (2)

CYCL-, *kyklos*, circle; the ciliary body (13)

CYE-, *kyein*, be pregnant (14)

CYST-, *kystis*, bladder, cyst (2)

CYSTI-, *kystis*, bladder, cyst (2)

-CYSTIS, *kystis*, bladder, cyst (2)

CYT-, *kytos*, [hollow container] cell (1)

D

DACRY-, *dakryon*, tear; lacrimal sac or duct (13)

DACTYL-, *daktylos*, finger, toe (3)

DEM-, *dēmos*, people, population (6)

DENDR-, *dendron*, [tree] dendrite, dendron (18)

DENDRIT-, *dendritēs*, [pertaining to a tree] dendrite (18)

DENT-, *dens, dentis*, tooth (8)

DERM-, *derma, dermatos*, skin (3)

-DERMA, *derma, dermatos*, skin (3)

DERMAT-, *derma, dermatos*, skin (3)

-DESIS, *desis*, binding (7)

DESM-, *desmos*, [binding] ligament, connective tissue (7)

DEXTR-, *dexter*, right (side) (10)

DIGIT-, *digitus*, finger, toe (9)

DIPLO-, *diploos*, double, twin (2)

DIPS-, *dipsa*, thirst (5)

-DOCH-, *dochos*, duct (12)

DOLICH-, *dolichos*, long, narrow, slender (6)

DORS-, *dorsum*, back (of the body) (8)

DROM-, *dromos*, a running (6)

DUC-, *dūcere*, *ductus*, lead, bring, conduct (9)

DUCT-, *dūcere*, *ductus*, lead, bring, conduct (9)

DUODEN-, *duodēnī*, [twelve] duodenum (12)

DUODENAL-, *duodēnalis*, of the duodenum (20)

DYNAM-, *dynamis*, force, power, energy (7)

E

ECHO-, *ēkhō*, reverberating sound, echo (5)

EDEMA, *oidēma*, *oidēmatos*, swelling (5)

EDEMAT-, *oidēma*, *oidēmatos*, swelling (5)

ELC-, *helkos*, ulcer (3)

-EM-, *haima*, *haimatos*, blood (2)

EME-, *emein*, vomit (5)

ENCEPHAL-, *enkephalon*, brain (1)

ENTER-, *enteron*, (small) intestine (2)

EOS-, *ēōs*, red (stain) (16)

ER-, *Erōs*, *Erōtos*, sexual desire (6)

ERG-, *ergon*, action, work (2)

EROT-, *Erōs*, *Erōtos*, sexual desire (6)

ERYTHR-, *erythros*, red, red blood cell (1)

ESOPHAG-, *oisophagos*, esophagus (12)

ESTHE-, *aisthēsis*, sensation, sensitivity, sense (4)

ESTHES-, *aisthēsis*, sensation, sensitivity, sense (4)

EURY-, *eurynein*, widen, dilate (14)

EURYN-, *eurynein*, widen, dilate (14)

EXTERN-, *externus*, *-a*, *-um*, outer (8)

F

FAC-, *facere*, *factus*, make (9)

FACI-, *faciēs*, face, appearance, surface (9)

FACIES, *faciēs*, face, appearance, surface (9)

FASCICL-, *fasciculus*, [little bundle] fasciculus (18)

FASCICUL-, *fasciculus*, [little bundle] fasciculus (18)

FEBR-, *febris*, fever (9)

FEBRIS, *febris*, fever (9)

FEC-, *faex*, *faecis*, [sediment] excrement, fecal matter (12)

-FECT, *facere*, *factus*, make (9)

FELINEUS, *felineus*, of or belonging to a cat (20)

FER-, *ferre*, *lātus*, carry, bear (9)

FIBR-, *fibra*, fiber, filament (8)

-FIC-, *facere*, *factus*, make (9)

-FICI-, *faciēs*, face, appearance, surface (9)

FISTUL-, *fistula*, (tube, pipe) fistula, an abnormal tube-like passage in the body (8)

FLAVUS, *flāvus*, golden-yellow (20)

FLECT-, *flectere*, *flexus*, bend (9)

FLEX-, *flectere*, *flexus*, bend (9)

FLU-, *fluere*, flow (20)

-FORM, *forma*, shape (10)

FRIG-, *frīgus*, *frīgoris*, cold (8)

FRIGOR-, *frīgus*, *frīgoris*, cold (8)

FUNG-, *fungus*, [mushroom] fungus (9)

FUS-, *fundere*, *fūsus*, pour (9)

G

GAL-, *gala*, *galaktos*, milk (14)

GALACT-, *gala*, *galaktos*, milk (14)

GANGLI-, *ganglion*, [knot] ganglion (18)

GASTR-, *gastēr*, *gastros*, stomach (2)

GEN-, *gignesthai*, come into being; produce (4)

GENE-, *gignesthai*, come into being; produce (4)

GENIT-, *gignere*, *genitus*, bring forth, give birth (9)

GER-, *gēras*, old age (7)

GER-, *gerere*, *gestus*, carry, bear (9)

GERMANIC-, *Germānicus*, of Germany, German (20)

GEST-, *gerere*, *gestus*, carry, bear (9)

GEUS-, *geuein*, taste (12)

GEUST-, *geuein*, taste (12)

GINGIV-, *gingīva*, gum (of the mouth) (12)

GLAUCUS, *glaukos*, bluish-gray (20)

GLI-, *glia*, [glue] glia, neuroglia (18)

-GLIA-, *glia*, [glue] glia, neuroglia (18)

GLOB-, *globus*, round body, globe (16)

GLOSS-, *glōssa*, tongue (12)

GLYC-, *glykys*, sugar (15)

-GN-, *(g)nascī, nātus*, be born (14)

GNATH-, *gnathos*, (lower) jaw (7)

GNO-, *gignōskein*, know (5)

GNOS-, *gignōskein*, know (5)

GONAD-, *gonad*, sex glands, sex organs (14)

GRAM-, *gramma*, [something written] a record (4)

GRANUL-, *grānulum*, granule (16)

GRAPH-, *graphein*, write, record (4)

GRAVID-, *gravidus*, pregnant (14)

GURGIT-, *gurgitāre, gurgitātus*, flood, flow (10)

GURGITAT-, *gurgitāre, gurgitātus*, flood, flow (10)

GYN-, *gynē, gynaikos*, woman, female (6)

GYNEC-, *gynē, gynaikos*, woman, female (6)

H

HELC-, *helkos*, ulcer (3)

HELMINT-, *helmins, helminthos*, (intestinal) worm (6)

HELMINTH-, *helmins, helminthos*, (intestinal) worm (6)

HELVET-, *Helvetius*, Helvetian, Swiss (20)

HEM-, *haima, haimatos*, blood (2)

HEMAT-, *haima, haimatos*, blood (2)

HEPAR-, *hēpar, hēpatos*, liver (2)

HEPAT-, *hēpar, hēpatos*, liver (2)

HERPES, *herpēs, herpētos*, [shingles] herpes, a creeping skin disease (13)

HERPET-, *herpēs, herpētos*, [shingles] herpes, a creeping skin disease (13)

HEX-, *hex*, six (20)

HIDR-, *hidrōs, hidrōtos*, sweat (3)

HIDROT-, *hidrōs, hidrōtos*, sweat (3)

HIST-, *histos*, [web] tissue (3)

HISTI-, *histos*, [web] tissue (3)

HYDR-, *hydōr, hydatos*, water, fluid (3)

HYMEN-, *hymēn*, membrane; hymen (14)

HYPN-, *hypnos*, sleep (3)

HYSTER-, *hystera*, uterus (14)

I

IATR-, *iatros*, healer, physician; treatment (4)

ICTER-, *ikteros*, jaundice (3)

IDI-, *idios*, of one's self (4)

-IDR-, *hidrōs, hidrōtos*, sweat (3)

ILE-, *ileum*, ileum (12)

IMMUN-, *immūnis*, [exempt] safe, protected (9)

IN-, *is, inos*, fiber, muscle (3)

INFERIOR-, *inferior*, below (9)

INGUIN-, *inguen, inguinis*, groin (15)

INOS-, *is, inos*, fiber, muscle (3)

INSUL-, *insula*, island (8)

INTERN-, *internus, -a, -um*, inner (8)

IR-, *iris, iridos*, [rainbow] iris (13)

IRID-, *iris, iridos* [rainbow] iris (13)

IS-, *isos*, equal, same, similar, alike (3)

ISCH-, *ischein*, suppress, check (7)

J

JEJUN-, *jējūnus*, [empty] jejunum (12)

JUNCT-, *jungere, junctus*, join (13)

K

KARY-, *karyon*, [nut] nucleus (16)

KERAT-, *keras, keratos*, [horn] cornea (13)

KINE-, *kinein*, move (4)

KINES-, *kinēsis*, movement, motion (4)

KINESI-, *kinēsis*, movement, motion (4)

KLEPT-, *kleptein*, steal, theft (7)

KONI-, *konis*, dust (11)

L

LAB-, *lābī, lapsus*, slide, slip (9)

LABI-, *labium*, lip (11)

LACRIM-, *lacrima*, tear (13)

LACT-, *lac, lactis*, milk (14)

-**LAGNIA**, *lagneia*, abnormal sexual excitation or gratification (15)

LAL-, *lalein*, talk (5)

LAPAR-, *lapara*, abdomen, abdominal wall (5)

LAPS-, *lābī*, *lapsus*, slide, slip (9)

LARYNG-, *larynx*, *laryngos*, larynx (11)

LARYNX, *larynx*, *laryngos*, larynx (11)

LAT-, *ferre*, *lātus*, carry, bear (9)

LATER-, *latus*, *lateris*, side (9)

LECTUL-, *lectulus*, couch, bed (20)

LEI-, *leios*, smooth (7)

LEP-, *lēpsis*, attach, seizure (7)

LEPID-, *lepis*, *lepidos*, scale (of an animal) (20)

LEPT-, *leptos*, thin, fine, slight (1)

LEUK-, *leukos*, white, white blood cell (1)

LEX-, *legein*, read (5)

LIEN-, *liēn*, spleen (12)

LINGU-, *lingua*, tongue (12)

LIP-, *lipos*, fat (2)

LITH-, *lithos*, stone, calculus (1)

LOG-, *logos*, word, study (1)

LY-, *lyein*, destroy, break down (4)

LYMPH-, *lympha*, [clear water] lymph (16)

LYS-, *lyein*, destroy, break down (4)

M

MACR-, *makros*, (abnormally) large or long (2)

MALAC-, *malakos*, soft (1)

MAMM-, *mamma*, breast (14)

MAN-, *mainesthai*, be mad (7)

MAST-, *mastos*, breast (14)

MAZ-, *mastos*, breast (14)

MEAT-, *meātus*, passage, opening, meatus (8)

MEDULL-, *medulla*, marrow, medulla oblongata (18)

MEGA-, *megas*, *megalou* (abnormally) large or long (2)

MEGAL-, *megas*, *megalou* (abnormally) large or long (2)

MEL-, *melos*, limb (7)

MELAN-, *melas*, *melanos*, dark, black (2)

MEN-, *mēn*, [month] menstruation (14)

MENING-, *mēninx*, *mēningos*, meningeal membrane, meninges (3)

-**MENINX**, *mēninx*, *mēningos*, meningeal membrane, meninges (3)

MES-, *mesos*, middle, secondary, partial, mesentery (1)

-**METER**, *metron*, instrument for measuring (1)

METR-, *metron*, measure (1)

METR-, *mētra*, uterus (14)

-**METRA**, *mētra*, uterus (14)

MICR-, *mikros*, (abnormally) small (2)

MNE-, *mimnēskein*, remember (5)

MON-, *monos*, single (16)

MORPH-, *morphē*, form, shape (7)

MY-, *mys*, *myos*, [mouse] muscle (3)

MY-, *myein*, close, shut (13)

MYC-, *mykēs*, *mykētos*, [mushroom] fungus (3)

MYCET-, *mykēs*, *mykētos*, [mushroom] fungus (3)

MYEL-, *myelos*, bone marrow, spinal cord, myelin (3, 18)

MYS-, *mys*, *myos*, [mouse] muscle (3)

MYX-, *myxa*, mucus (4)

N

NARC-, *narkē*, stupor, numbness (3)

NAS-, *nāsus*, nose (8)

NAT-, *(g)nascī*, *nātus*, be born (14)

NE-, *neos*, new (5)

NECR-, *nekros*, corpse; dead (3)

NEMA, *nēma*, *nēmatos*, thread (worm) (6, 20)

NEMAT-, *nēma*, *nēmatos*, thread (worm) (6, 20)

NEPHR-, *nephros*, kidney (1)

NEUR-, *neuron*, [tendon] nerve, nervous system, neuron (1, 18)

NEUTR-, *neuter*, neither (16)

NO-, *nous*, mind, mental activity, comprehension (5)

NOM-, *nomos*, law (7)

NOS-, *nosos*, disease, illness (6)

NYCT-, *nyx*, *nyctos*, night (2)

O

OCUL-, *oculus*, eye (13)

ODONT-, *odous*, *odontos*, tooth (6)

ODYN-, *odynē*, pain (2)

OLIG-, *oligos*, few, deficient (3)

OMPHAL-, *omphalos*, navel, umbilicus (7)

ONC-, *onkos*, tumor (2)

ONYCH-, *onyx*, *onychos*, fingernail, toenail (3)

OOPHOR-, *oophoron*, ovary (14)

OP-, *ōps*, vision (13)

OPHTHALM-, *ophthalmos*, eye (13)

OPISTH-, *opisthen*, located in the back (20)

OPS-, *ōps*, vision (13)

OPT-, *optos*, [seen] vision; eye (13)

OR-, *ōs*, *ōris*, mouth, opening (9)

ORCH-, *orchis*, *orchios*, testicle (15)

ORCHE-, *orchis*, *orchios*, testicle (15)

ORCHI-, *orchis*, *orchios*, testicle (15)

ORCHID-, *orchis*, *orchios*, testicle (15)

ORCHIS, *orchis*, *orchios*, testicle (20)

OREC-, *oregein*, have an appetite (5)

OREX-, *oregein*, have an appetite (5)

ORIENTAL-, *orientalis*, of the east, oriental (20)

ORTH-, *orthos*, straight, erect; normal (4)

OS, *ōs*, *ōris*, mouth, opening (9)

OSM-, *osmē*, sense of smell; odor (12)

OSPHR-, *osphrēsis*, sense of smell (12)

OSS-, *ossa*, bone (9)

OSTE-, *osteon*, bone (1)

OT-, *ous*, *ōtos*, ear (4)

OV-, *ōvum*, egg (14)

OVARI-, *ōvārium*, ovary (14)

OX-, *oxys*, acute, pointed; rapid; oxygen (5)

OXY-, *oxys*, acute, pointed; rapid; oxygen (5)

P

PACHY-, *pachys*, thick (2)

PALI-, *palin*, back, again (6)

PALIN-, *palin*, back, again (6)

PALLID-, *pallidus*, pale, lacking color (20)

PAN-, *pas*, *pantos*, all, entire, every (6)

PANT-, *pas*, *pantos*, all, entire, every (6)

-*PARA*, *parere*, *partus*, give birth (14)

PARESIS, *paresis*, slackening of strength, paralysis (11)

PART-, *parere*, *partus*, give birth (14)

PATH-, *pathos*, [suffering] disease (4)

PECTOR-, *pectus*, *pectoris*, breast, chest (10)

PED-, *pais*, *paidos*, child (7)

PEDICUL-, *pediculus*, louse (9)

PELV-, *pelvis*, [basin] pelvis (14)

PEN-, *penia*, decrease, deficiency (7)

PEN-, *pēnis*, [tail] penis (15)

PEPS-, *peptein*, digest (12)

PEPT-, *peptein*, digest (12)

-**PEX**-, *pexis*, fixing, (surgical) attachment (7)

PHA-, *phēnai*, speak, communicate (5)

PHAC-, *phakos*, [lentil] lens (13)

PHAG-, *phagein*, swallow, eat (5)

PHAK-, *phakos*, [lentil] lens (13)

PHALL-, *phallos*, penis (15)

PHARMAC-, *pharmakon*, medicine, drug (5)

PHARMACEU-, *pharmakon*, medicine, drug (5)

PHARYNG-, *pharynx*, *pharyngos*, [throat] pharynx (11)

PHARYNX, *pharynx*, *pharyngos*, [throat] pharynx (11)

PHEM-, *phēmē*, speech (5)

-**PHIL**-, *philein*, love; have an affinity for (4, 16)

PHLEB-, *phleps*, *phlebos*, vein (10)

PHOB-, *phobos*, (abnormal) fear (5)

PHON-, *phonē*, voice, sound (5)

PHOR-, *phoros*, bearing, carrying (6)

PHOS-, *phōs, phōtos*, light, daylight (6)

PHOT-, *phōs, phōtos*, light, daylight (6)

PHRAC-, *phrassein*, enclose, obstruct (5)

PHRAG-, *phrassein*, enclose, obstruct (5)

PHRAS-, *phrazein*, speak (5)

PHREN-, *phrēn*, mind; diaphragm (5)

PHTHIR-, *phtheir*, louse (20)

PHYLAC-, *phylattein*, protection (against disease) (5)

PHYS-, *physis*, nature, appearance (5)

PHYS-, *physa*, air, gas (11)

PHYSI-, *physis*, nature, appearance (5)

PHYT-, *phyton*, plant (organism), growth (5)

PIP-, *pīpire*, peep, chirp (20)

PLAS-, *plassein*, form, develop (7)

PLAST-, *plassein*, form, develop (7)

PLATY-, *platys*, flat (20)

PLEC-, *plēssein*, strike, paralyze (6)

PLEG-, *plēssein*, strike, paralyze (6)

PLEUR-, *pleura*, [side] pleura (11)

PLEX-, *plēssein*, strike, paralyze (6)

PLEX-, *plexus*, [braid] plexus (18)

PNE-, *pnein*, breathe (11)

PNEUM-, *pneuma, pneumatos*, [breath] air, gas (11)

PNEUM-, *pneumōn*, lung (11)

PNEUMAT-, *pneuma, pneumatos*, [breath] air, gas (11)

PNEUMON-, *pneumōn*, lung (11)

POD-, *pous, podos*, foot (3)

POIE-, *poiein*, produce, make (5)

POLI-, *polios*, [gray] gray matter of the brain and spinal cord (3)

POLY-, *polys*, many, excessive (3)

PONS, *pons, pontis*, [bridge] pons (18)

PONT-, *pons, pontis*, [bridge] pons (18)

POR-, *poros*, passage, opening, duct, pore, cavity (3)

POSTER-, *posterior*, behind, in back (9)

-POSTERIOR, *posterior*, behind, in back (9)

PRESBY-, *presbys*, old, old age (7)

PROCT-, *proktos*, anus (12)

PROSOP-, *prosōpon*, face (1)

PROSTAT-, *prostatēs*, [one who stands before] prostate gland (7)

PROT-, *prōtos*, first, primitive, early (1, 20)

PSEUD-, *pseudēs*, false (2)

PSYCH-, *psychē*, [soul] mind (3)

PT-, *piptein*, fall, sag, drop, prolapse (4)

PTER-, *pteron*, wing (20)

PTY-, *ptyein*, spit (7)

PTYAL-, *ptyalon*, saliva (7)

PUB-, *pūbēs*, pubic hair, pubic bone, pubic region, pubis (14, 20)

PUBER-, *pūbertās*, [manhood] puberty (14)

PUBERT-, *pūbertās*, [manhood] puberty (14)

PULM-, *pulmō, pulmōnis*, lung, pulmonary artery (10)

PULMON-, *pulmō, pulmōnis*, lung, pulmonary artery (10)

PUR-, *pus, puris*, pus (8)

PY-, *pyon*, pus (2)

PYEL-, *pyelos*, renal pelvis (15)

PYLE-, *pylē*, [gate] portal vein (12)

PYLOR-, *pylōrus*, [gatekeeper] pylorus (12)

PYR-, *pyr, pyros*, [fire] fever, burning (4)

PYRET-, *pyretos*, fever (4)

PYREX-, *pyressein*, be feverish (4)

R

RACHI-, *rhachis*, spine (6)

RAD-, *rādix, rādīcis*, root (8)

RADIC-, *rādix, rādīcis*, root (8)

RADIX, *rādix, rādīcis*, root (8)

RECT-, *rectus*, [straight] rectum (12)

REN-, *rēn, rēnis*, kidney (8)

RET-, *rēte, rētis*, [net] retina; network, plexus (13)

RETIN-, *rēte, rētis*, [net] retina; network, plexus (13)

RHABD-, *rhabdos*, rod (15)

RHACHI-, *rhachis*, spine (6)

RHAG-, *rhēgnynai*, [burst forth] flow profusely, hemorrhage (4)

RHE-, *rhein*, [run] flow, secrete (4)

RHEX-, *rhēxis*, rupture (4)

RHIN-, *rhis, rhīnos*, nose (4)

RHYTHM-, *rhythmos*, [steady motion] heartbeat (10)

-RRHAPH-, *rhaptein*, suture (7)

S

SALPING-, *salpinx, salpingos*, [war trumpet] fallopian tube (14)

-SALPINX, *salpinx, salpingos*, [war trumpet] fallopian tube (14)

SANGUI-, *sanguis, sanguinis*, blood (8)

SANGUIN-, *sanguis, sanguinis*, blood (8)

SAPR-, *sapros*, rotten, putrid, decaying (5)

SARC-, *sarx, sarcos*, flesh, soft tissue (2)

SCAT-, *skōr, skatos*, excrement, fecal matter (12)

-SCHE-, *ischein*, suppress, check (7)

-SCHISIS, *schizein*, split, cleft, fissure (6)

SCHIST-, *schizein*, split, cleft, fissure (6)

SCHIZ-, *schizein*, split, cleft, fissure (6)

SCLER-, *skleros*, hard (1)

SCOP-, *skopein*, look at, examine (4)

SCROT-, *scrōtum*, [bag] scrotum (15)

SECT-, *secāre, sectus*, cut (9)

SEM-, *sēmen, sēminis*, [seed] semen (15)

SEMIN-, *sēmen, sēminis*, [seed] semen (15)

SEP-, *sēpein*, [be putrid] be infected (4)

SEPT-, *saeptum*, wall, partition (10)

SIAL-, *sialon*, saliva, salivary duct (12)

SIDER-, *sidēros*, iron (11)

SIGM-, *sigma*, sigmoid colon (12)

SIN-, *sinus*, [curve, hollow] sinus (10)

SINISTR-, *sinister*, left (side) (10)

SINUS-, *sinus*, [curve, hollow] sinus (10)

SIT-, *sitos*, food (7)

SOM-, *sōma, sōmatos*, body (3)

-SOMA, *sōma, sōmatos*, body (3)

SOMAT-, *sōma, sōmatos*, body (3)

SOMN-, *somnus*, sleep (9)

SON-, *sonus*, sound (8)

SPASM-, *spasmos*, spasm, involuntary muscular contraction (2)

SPERM-, *sperma, spermatos*, seed, sperm, semen (15)

SPERMAT-, *sperma, spermatos*, seed, sperm, semen (15)

SPHINCTER-, *sphincter*, sphincter muscle (12)

SPHYGM-, *sphygmos*, pulse (10)

SPIR-, *spīrāre, spīrātus*, breathe (11)

SPIR-, *speira*, coil, spiral (20)

SPIRAT-, *spīrāre, spīrātus*, breathe (11)

SPLANCHN-, *splanchnon*, internal organ, viscus (12)

SPLEN-, *splēn*, spleen (2)

SPONDYL-, *spondylos*, vertebra (6)

STA-, *histanai*, stand, stop (7)

STABIL-, *stabilis*, stable, fixed (9)

STABL-, *stabilis*, stable, fixed (9)

STAL-, *stellein*, send, contraction (10)

STAPHYL-, *staphylē*, [bunch of grapes] uvula, palate; staphylococci (11, 20)

STAT-, *histanai*, stand, stop (7)

-STAT, *histanai*, device or agent for stopping the flow (of something) (7)

-STAXIA, *staxis*, dripping, oozing (of blood) (6)

-STAXIS, *staxis*, dripping, oozing (of blood) (6)

STEAR-, *stear, steatos*, fat, sebum, sebaceous glands (5)

STEAT-, *stear, steatos*, fat, sebum, sebaceous glands (5)

STEN-, *stenos*, narrow (1)

STERE-, *stereos*, solid, having three dimensions (1)

STERN-, *sternon*, chest, breast, breastbone (11)

STETH-, *stēthos*, chest, breast (11)

STHEN-, *sthenos*, strength (3)

STIGM-, *stigma, stigmatos*, point, mark, spot (13)

STIGMAT-, *stigma, stigmatos*, point, mark, spot (13)

STOL-, *stellein*, send, contraction (10)

STOM-, *stoma, stomatos*, mouth, opening (2)

STOMAT-, *stoma, stomatos*, mouth, opening (2)

STREPT-, *streptos*, [twisted] streptococci (11, 20)

SUD-, *sūdor*, sweat, fluid (11)

SUDOR-, *sūdor*, sweat, fluid (11)

SUPERIOR-, *superior*, above (9)

SYNAP-, *synapsis*, [point of contact] synapse (18)

SYNAPS-, *synapsis*, [point of contact] synapse (18)

SYNOV-, *synovia*, synovial fluid, synovial membrane or sac (8)

SYRING-, *syrinx, syringos*, [pipe] fistula, cavity, oviduct, sweat glands, syringe (14)

-SYRINX, *syrinx, syringos*, [pipe] fistula, cavity, oviduct, sweat glands, syringe (14)

T

TA-, *tasis*, stretching (4)

TABAN-, *tabānus*, horsefly (20)

TACHY-, *tachys*, rapid (1)

TAX-, *taxis*, (muscular) coordination (7)

TEL-, *telos*, end, completion (4)

TEN-, *tenōn, tenontos*, tendon (4)

TENON-, *tenōn, tenontos*, tendon (4)

TENONT-, *tenōn, tenontos*, tendon (4)

TENS-, *tendere, tensus*, stretch (10)

TENSI-, *tendere, tensus*, stretch (10)

THALAM-, *thalamos*, [inner chamber] thalamus (18)

THAN-, *thanatos*, death (6)

THANAT-, *thanatos*, death (6)

THE-, *tithenai*, place, put (6)

THEL-, *thēlē*, nipple (14)

THELE-, *thēlē*, nipple (14)

THERAP-, *therapeuein*, treat medically, heal (4)

THERAPEU-, *therapeuein*, treat medically, heal (4)

THERM-, *thermē*, heat, (body) temperature (7)

THORAC-, *thōrax, thōrakos*, chest cavity, pleural cavity, thorax (11)

THORAX, *thōrax, thōrakos*, chest cavity, pleural cavity, thorax (11)

THROMB-, *thrombos*, blood clot (10)

THYR-, *thyreos*, [shield] thyroid gland (7)

TOC-, *tokos*, childbirth, labor (14)

TOM-, *tomē*, a cutting, slice, incision (4)

TON-, *tonos*, [a stretching] (muscular) tone, tension (4)

TOP-, *topos*, place (10)

TOX-, *toxon*, poison (1)

TOXI-, *toxon*, poison (1)

TRACH-, *trachys*, [rough] trachea (11)

TRACHE-, *trachys*, [rough] trachea (11)

TRACHEL-, *trachēlos*, neck, cervix (3)

TRACHY-, *trachys*, [rough] trachea (11)

TREP-, *trepein*, turn, twist (20)

TRICH-, *thrix, trichos*, hair (6)

TROP-, *tropē*, turning (7)

TROPH-, *trophē*, nourishment (6)

TUB-, *tuba*, [trumpet] tube (8)

TUM-, *tumēre*, be swollen (9)

TUME-, *tumēre*, be swollen (9)

TUSS-, *tussis*, cough (8)

TYPHL-, *typhlos*, [blind] cecum (12)

U

UR-, *ouron*, urine, urinary tract, uric acid (15)

URETER-, *ourētēr*, ureter (15)

URETHR-, *ourēthra*, urethra (15)

UTER-, *uterus*, womb, belly, uterus (14)

V

VACC-, *vacca*, cow (8)

VAG-, *vagus*, [wandering] the vagus nerve (10)

VAGIN-, *vāgina* [sheath] vagina (14)

VARIC-, *varix, varicis*, dilated and twisted vein, varix (10)

VARIX, *varix, varicis*, dilated and twisted vein, varix (10)

VAS-, *vās*, (blood) vessel; vas deferens (10)

VEN-, *vēna*, vein (10)

VENTR-, *venter*, *ventris*, belly, abdomen, abdominal cavity (10)

VESIC-, *vēsīca*, (urinary) bladder (15)

VIR-, *vīrus*, [poison, venom] virus (8)

VIRUS-, *vīrus*, [poison, venom] virus (8)

VISCER-, *viscus*, *visceris*, internal organ(s) (8)

VISCUS-, *viscus*, *visceris*, internal organ (8)

X

XANTH-, *xanthos*, yellow (3)

XER-, *xēros*, dry (13)

Z

ZO-, *zōon*, animal, organism (15)

ZYM-, *zymē*, [leaven] ferment, enzyme, fermentation (12)

INDEX OF PREFIXES

Prefixes modify or qualify in some way the meaning of the word to which they are affixed. It is often difficult to assign a single specific meaning to each prefix, and often it is necessary to adapt a meaning that fits the particular use of a word. Words can have more than one prefix and a prefix can follow a combining form.

Entries for Latin prefixes are in *italics*.

---

a- (an- before a vowel or *h*): not, without, lacking, deficient

---

ab- (*a-* rarely before certain consonants; *abs-* before *c* and *t*): away from

---

ad- (*ac-* before *c*; *af-* before *f*; *ag-* before *g*; *al-* before *l*; *an-* before *n*; *ap-* before *p*; *as-* before *s*; *a-* before *sp*; *at-* before *t*): to, toward

---

ambi-: both

---

amphi-, ampho-: on both sides, around, both

---

ana-: up, back, against

---

ante-: before, forward

---

anti- (ant- often before a vowel or *h*; hyphenated before *i*): against, opposed to, preventing, relieving

---

apo-: away from

---

bi- (*bin-*, *bis-*): two, twice, double, both

---

cata- (cat- before a vowel or *h*): downward; disordered

---

circum-: around

---

con- (*co-* before *h*; *col-* before *l*; *com-* before *e*, *m*, and *p*; *cor-* before *r*): together, with; thoroughly, very

---

contra-: against, opposite

---

de-: down, away from, absent

---

di- (rarely dis-): two, twice, double

---

dia- (di- before a vowel): through, across, apart

---

dis- (*di-* before *g*, *v*, and usually before *l*; *dif-* before *f*): apart, away

---

dys-: difficult, painful, defective, abnormal

---

ec- (ex- before a vowel): out of, away from

---

ecto- (ect- often before a vowel): outside of

---

en- (em- before *b*, *m*, and *p*): in, into, within

---

endo-, ento- (end-, ent- before a vowel): within

---

epi- (ep- before a vowel or *h*): upon, over, above

---

eso-: within, inner, inward

---

eu-: good, normal, healthy

---

ex- (*e-* before certain consonants; *ef-* before *f*): out of, away from

---

exo-: outside, from the outside, toward the outside

---

extra- (rarely *extro-*): on the outside, beyond

---

hemi-: half, partial; (often) one side of the body

---

heter-, hetero-: different, other, relationship to another

---

homo-, homeo-: same, likeness

---

hyper-: over, above, excessive, beyond normal

---

hypo- (hyp- before a vowel or *h*): under, deficient, below normal

---

in- (*il-* before *l*; *im-* before *b*, *m*, and *p*; *ir-* before *r*): in, into

---

in- (*il-* before *l*; *im-* before *b*, *m*, and *p*; *ir-* before *r*): not

in- (*il-* before *l*; *im-* before *b*, *m*, and *p*; *ir-* before *r*): very, thoroughly

infra-: beneath, below

inter-: between

intra- (rarely *intro-*): within

meta- (met- before a vowel or *h*): change, transformation, after, behind

mono- (mon-before a vowel or *h*): one, single

mult- (often *multi-*): many, much, affecting many parts

non-: not

ob- (*oc-* before *c*; *op-* before *p*): against, toward; very, thoroughly

para- (often par- before a vowel): alongside, around, abnormal, beyond

per- (*pel-* before *l*): through; very, thoroughly

peri-: around, surrounding

post-: after, following, behind

pre-: before, in front of

pro-: before

pro-: forward, in front

pros-, prosth-: in place of

re-: back, again

retro-: backward, in back, behind

se-: apart, away from

semi-: half

sub- (*suf-* before *f*; *sup-* before *p*): under

super- (often *supra-*): over, above; excess

trans-: across, through

syn- (sym- before *b*, *p*, and *m*; *n* assimilates or is dropped before *l* and *s*): together, with, joined

ultra-: beyond, excess

APPENDIX C

INDEX OF SUFFIXES

Suffixes form either nouns or adjectives (or, in some instances, verbs or adverbs). Most of the nouns in medical terminology are abstract, indicating a state, quality, condition, procedure, or process. Noun-forming suffixes that have special meanings, such as -itis, inflammation, will be so indicated. Adjectival suffixes usually have the general meaning of pertaining to, referring to, having to do with, in a condition or state of, caused by, causing, or located in. Only those meanings most commonly found are indicated here. Entries for Latin suffixes are in *italics*.

-a: forms abstract nouns: state, condition

-able: forms adjectives: capable of (being), able to

-ac (rare): forms adjectives: pertaining to, located in

-ad: forms adverbs: indicates direction toward a part of the body: toward

-al: forms adjectives: pertaining to, located in

-an: forms adjectives: pertaining to, located in

-ant: forms adjectives translated with -ing added to the meaning of a verb; forms nouns meaning a person who or thing that does something

-ar: forms adjectives: pertaining to, located in

-arium: forms nouns: denotes a place for something: place for

-ary: forms adjectives: pertaining to

-ary: forms nouns: denotes a place for something: place for

-ase: forms names of enzymes

-asia, -asis (rare): form abstract nouns: state, condition

-ate: forms names of chemical substances

-ate: forms adjectives: having the form of, possessing

-ation: forms nouns indicating an action or process: the act of (being), the result of (being), something that is

-ce: forms nouns: the act of (being), **the state of (being)**

-cle: forms diminutives: small

-culus, -cula, -culum: form diminutives: **small**

-cy: forms nouns: the act of (being), **the state of (being)**

-eal: forms adjectives: pertaining to, **located in**

-ean: forms adjectives: pertaining to, **located in**

-ellus, -ella, -ellum: form names of **biological genera**

-ellus, -ella, -ellum: form diminutives: **small**

-ema: forms abstract nouns: state, **condition**

-ent: forms adjectives translated with **-ing** added to the meaning of a verb; forms nouns that mean a person who or thing that does something

-esis: forms abstract nouns: state, condition, procedure

-etic: forms adjectives, often from nouns ending in -esis: pertaining to

-ia: forms abstract nouns. In many instances -ia appears in English as -y: state, condition

-ia: forms abstract nouns: state, condition

-iac (rare): forms nouns: person afflicted with

-ian: forms nouns: indicates an expert in a certain field

-iasis: forms abstract nouns: disease, abnormal condition, abnormal presence of

-ible: forms adjectives: capable of (being)

-ic: forms adjectives: pertaining to, located in; many words ending in -ic have come to be used as nouns: drug, agent

-ic: forms adjectives: pertaining to

-ics, -tics: form nouns indicating a particular science or study: science or study of

-id: see -oid

-id: forms adjectives: pertaining to; in a state or condition of

-ide: forms names of chemical substances

-ient: forms adjectives translated with -ing added to the meaning of a verb; forms nouns that mean a person who or thing that does something

-il: forms diminutives: small

-ile: forms adjectives: pertaining to, capable of (being), like

-illus, -illa, -illum: form diminutives: small

-in, -ine: form names of substances

-ine: forms adjectives: pertaining to, located in

-ion: forms nouns: the act of

-ism: forms abstract nouns: state, condition, quality

-ismus: forms abstract nouns: state, condition; muscular spasm

-ist: forms nouns: a person interested in

-ite: forms names of chemical substances

-itic: forms adjectives: pertaining to; pertaining to inflammation; many words ending in -itic have come to be used an nouns: drug, agent

-itides: plural of -itis: forms plural nouns: inflammation

-itis: forms nouns indicating an inflamed condition: inflammation

-ium (rarely -eum): forms nouns: sometimes names a body region; membrane, connective tissue

-ive: forms adjectives: pertaining to

-ize: forms verbs: make, become, cause to be, subject to, engage in

-lent: forms adjectives: full of

-ma: forms nouns: (often) abnormal or diseased condition; sometimes forms names of substances

-ment: forms nouns: agent or instrument

-oid, (rarely) -ode, -id: form both nouns and adjectives indicating a particular shape, form, or resemblance: resembling

-ole: forms diminutives: small

-olus, -ola, -olum: form diminutives: *small*

-oma: forms abstract nouns: usually tumor; occasionally disease

-one: forms names of chemical substances

-or: forms nouns: agent or instrument

-orium: forms nouns: place for (something)

-ory: forms adjectives: pertaining to

-ory: forms nouns: place for (something)

-ose: forms adjectives: full of, resembling; also used to form names of chemical substances

-osis: forms abstract nouns: abnormal or diseased condition

-otic: forms adjectives from nouns in -osis: pertaining to

-ous: forms adjectives: pertaining to, characterized by, full of

-sia: forms abstract nouns: state, condition

-sis: forms abstract nouns: state, condition

-ter: forms nouns: instrument, device

-tic: forms adjectives from nouns in -sis: pertaining to; many words ending in -tic have come to be used as nouns: drug, agent; person suffering from a certain disability

-tics: see -ics

-ty: forms abstract nouns: state, condition

-ule: forms diminutives: small

-ulus, -ula, -ulum: form diminutives: small

-ure, -ura: form nouns: result of (an action)

-us: forms nouns: condition, person (sometimes a malformed fetus)

-y: forms abstract nouns: state, condition

-y: forms abstract nouns: state, condition

INDEX OF SUFFIX FORMS* AND COMPOUND SUFFIX FORMS

-ectasia, **-ectasis**: dilation, enlargement

-ectomy: surgical excision; removal of all (total excision) or part (partial excision) of an organ

-gen: substance that produces (something)

-genesis: formation, origin

-genic, **-genous**: causing, producing, caused by, produced by or in

-gram: a record of the activity of an organ (often an x-ray)

-graph: an instrument for recording the activity of an organ

-graphy: (1) the recording of the activity of an organ (usually by x-ray examination), (2) a descriptive treatise (on a subject)

-logy: study, science, the study or science of

-logist: one who specializes in a certain study or science

-lysis: dissolution, reduction, decomposition, disintegration

-lytic: pertaining to dissolution or decomposition, disintegration (forms adjectives from words ending in or containing -lysis)

-malacia: the softening (of tissues) of

-pathy: disease

-ptosis: dropping, sagging (of an organ or part)

-rrhagia: profuse discharge, hemorrhage

-rrhea: profuse discharge, excessive secretion

-rrhexis: bursting (of tissues), rupture

-sclerosis: the hardening (of tissues) of

-scope: an instrument for examining

-scopy: examination

-stenosis: the narrowing (of a part of the body)

-tome: a surgical instrument for cutting

-tomy: surgical incision

-toxic: poisonous (to an organ)

-toxin: a substance poisonous to (a part of the body)

*-logy, -logist, -malacia, -sclerosis, -stenosis, -toxic, and –toxin are suffix forms; the remaining terms are compound suffix forms.

GLOSSARY OF ENGLISH-TO-GREEK/LATIN

This glossary contains the English meaning of the Greek and Latin combining forms, prefixes, suffixes, suffix forms, and compound suffix forms found in Lessons 1 to 15 of this text. It is included as an aid for your completion of Exercise 2 in each of these lessons. Verbs are given in the present infinitive form and nouns, and adjectives are given in dictionary form.

A

abdomen: abdomin-, cel(i)-, gastr-, lapar-, ventr-,

abdominal cavity: ventr-

abdominal wall: lapar-

abnormal: dys-, para-, par-

above: epi, super-, superior-

absent: de-

across: dia-, trans-

action: erg-

acute: ox(y)-

after: meta-, post-

again: pali(n)-, re-

against: ana-, anti-, contra-, ob-

agent: -e, -ment, -or

agent that induces secretion: -agogue

air: aer-, pneum(at)-, phys-

alike: is-

all, entire, every: pan(t)-

alongside: para-, par-

amnion: amni-

amniotic sac: amni-

angina pectoris: angin-

animal: zo-

anthrax: anthrax, anthrac-

anus: proct-

aorta: aort-

apart: dia-, dis-, se-

appearance: phys(i)-, faci-, -fici-, facies

(have an) appetite: orec-, orex-

arachnoid membrane: arachn-

(upper) arm: brachi-

around: amphi-, ampho-, circum-, para-, par-, peri-

atrium: atri-

(surgical) attachment: -pex-

attack: lep-

away: dis-

away from: ab-, apo, de-, ec-, ex-, se-

B

bacillus: bacill-

back: ana-, re-, retro-; pali(n)-

back of the body: dors-

backward: retro-

bacterium: bacter(i)-

bear: fer-, lat-, ger-, gest-

bearing, carrying: phor-

before: ante-, pre-, pro-

beginning: arch-, -arche

behind: meta-, post-, retro-; poster-, -posterior

belly: abdomin-, ventr-, uter-

below: infra-; inferior-

below normal: hypo-

bend: flect-, flex-

beneath: infra-

between: inter-

beyond: extra-, para-, par-, ultra-

bile: chol(e)-, bili-

binding: -desis, desm-

(give) birth: genit-, part-, -para

black: melan-

bladder: cyst(i)-, -cystis, vesic-

blood: hem-, hemat-, -em-, sangui(n)-

blood clot: thromb-

blood vessel: vas-

blue: cyan-

body: som(at)-, -soma

bone: oss-

bone marrow: myel-

born: -gn-, nat-

(be) born: -gn-, nat-

both: ambi-, amphi-, ampho-, bi-

brain: cerebr-

break (up): cla(s)-

breast: pector-, mamm-, mast-, maz-, stern-, steth-

breastbone: stern-

breathe: pne-, spir(at)-

bring: duc-, duct-

bring forth: genit-

bronchus: bronch(i)-

bunch of grapes: staphyl-

burning: pyr-

bursa: burs-

bursting (of tissues): -rrhexis

C

calcium: calc-

cancer: carcin-

capillary: capill-

carbon dioxide: capn-

carcinoma: carcin-

cardia: cardi-

carry: fer-, lat-, ger-, gest-

cartilage: chondr-

caused by: -genic, -genous

causing: -genic, -genous

cavity: alve-, por-, syring-, -syrinx

cecum: cec-, typhl-

cervix uteri: cervic-, cervix, trachel-

change: meta-

check: isch-, -sche-

chemical substance: -ide, -ite, -one, -ate

chest: pector-, stern-, steth-

chest cavity: thorax, thorac-

child: ped-

childbirth: toc-

choking pain: angin-

choroid: choroid-

ciliary body: cycl-

circle: cycl-

cleft: schiz-, schist-, -schisis

close: -clud-, -clus-, my-

coal: anthrax, anthrac-

coccus: cocc-, -coccus

cold: frig-, frigor-

(icy) cold: cry(m)-

colon: col-, colon-

color: chrom-, chroma-, chromat-come into being: gen(e)-, -gen

communicate: pha-

completion: tel-

comprehension: no-

compress: arct(at)-

conduct: duc-, duct-

connective tissue: -ium (rarely-eum); desm-

contraction: stal-, stol-

(muscular) coordination: tax-

cornea: kerat-

corpse: necr-

cough: tuss-

cow: vacc-

crown: coron-

cut: -cid-, -cis, sect-

cyst: cyst(i)-, -cystis

D

dark: melan-

daylight: phos-, phot-

dead: necr-

death: than(at)-

decaying: sapr-

decomposition: -lysis

decrease: pen-

defective: dys-

deficiency: pen-

deficient: a-, an-, hypo-; olig-

destroy: cla(s)-, -clast, ly(s)-

develop: plas(t)-

device: -ter

device or agent for stopping the flow (of something): -stat

diaphragm: phren-

different: heter-, hetero-

difficult: dys-

digest: peps-, pept-

dilate: eury(n)-

dilation: -ectasia, -ectasis

discharge: -rrhea

disease: nos-, path-, -pathy

disintegration: -lysis

disordered: cata-

double: bi-, di-, dis-, diplo-

down: de-

downward: cata-

drawing forth: agog-

dripping (of blood): -staxis, -staxia

drop: pt-

drug: -ic, -tic, -itic; pharmac(eu)-

dry: xer-

duct: -doch-, por-

dull: ambly-, bary-

duodenum: duoden-

dust: coni-, koni-

E

Escherichia coli: coli-

ear: aur-, ot-

eat: phag-

echo: echo-

egg: ov-

enclose: phrac-, phrag-

end: tel-

energy: calor-, dynam-

enlargement: -ectasia, -ectasis

entire: pan(t)-

enzyme: -ase; zym-

equal: is-

erect: orth-

esophagus: esophag-

every: pan(t)-

examination: -scopy

examine: scop-

excess: super-, ultra-

excessive: hyper-, poly-

(surgical) excision: -ectomy

excrement: copr-, fec-, scat-

expert (in a certain field): -ian, -ist

extremities: acr-

eye: ocul-, ophthalm-, opt-

eyelid: blephar-

F

face: faci-, -fici-, facies

faint: ambly-

fall: pt-

falling: -ptosis

fallopian tube: salping-, -salpinx

false: pseud-

fat: adip-, lip-, stear-, steat-

fatty deposit: ather-

(abnormal) fear: phob-

fecal matter: copr-, fec-, scat-

female: gyn(ec)-

ferment: zym-

fermentation: zym-

fetal membrane: amni-

fever: febr-, febris, pyr-, pyret-

feverish: pyrex-

few: olig-

fiber: fibr-, is-, inos-

filament: fibr-

finger: dactyl-, digit-

fingernail: onych-

first: prot-

fissure: schiz-, schist-, -schisis

fistula: fistul-, syring-, -syrinx

fixed: stabil-, stabl-

fixing: -pex-

flesh: creat-, sarc-

flood: gurgit-, gurgitat-

flow: gurgit-, gurgitat-, rhe-

fluid: hydr-, sud(or)-

following: post-

food: sit-

foot: pod-

force: dynam-

form: morph-, plas(t)-

formation: -genesis

formation (of a passage): -stomy

forward: ante-, pro-

front: pro-; anter-

(in) front (of): pre-, pro-; anter-

fungus: fung-, myc(et)-

fused: ankyl-, ancyl-

G

gall: chol(e)-

gas: aer-, phys-, pneum(at)-

gland: aden-

good: eu-

gout: -agra

gray matter (of the brain and spinal cord): poli-

green: chlor-

groin: inguin-

grow: aux-, -auxe, -auxis

(begin to) grow: cresc-, -cret-

growth: phyt-

gum (of the mouth): gingiv-

H

hair: trich-

half: hemi-, semi-

hand: cheir-, chir-

hard: bary-

hardening (of tissues) of: -sclerosis

head: capit-

heal: therap(eu)-

healer: iatr-

healthy: eu-

hear: acou(s)-, acu(s)-

heart: cor, cord-

heartbeat: rhythm-

heat: calor-, therm-

heavy: bary-

hemorrhage: rhag-, -rrhagia

hernia: -cel-

herpes: herpes, herpet-

hidden: crypt-

hollow: alve-

hooked, crooked: ankyl-, ancyl-

hymen: hymen-

I

ileum: ile-

illness: nos-

in, into: in-, en-

in place of: pros-, prosth-

incision: tom-, -tomy

increase: aux-, -auxe, -auxis

increased: hyper-

infected: sep-

inflammation: -itis (pl. -itides)

inject fluid: cly(s)-

inner: eso-; intern-

instrument: -ment, -or, -ter

instrument (for breaking or crushing): -clast

instrument (for cutting): -tome

instrument (for examining): -scope

instrument (for recording the activity of an organ): -graph

internal organ: splanchn-, viscer-, viscus-

intestine: enter-

into: en-

inward: eso-

iris: ir(id)-

iron: sider-

island: insul-

J

jaundice: icter-

(lower) jaw: gnath-

jejunum: jejun-

join: junct-

joined: syn-

K

kidney: ren-

kill: -cid-, -cis-

know: gno(s)-

L

labor: toc-

lack: a-, an-

lacrimal sac or duct: dacry-

large: macr-, mega-, megal-

larynx: larynx, laryng-

latent: crypt-

law: nom-

lead: duc-, duct-

leading: agog-

left side: sinistr-

lens: phac-, phak-

ligament: desm-

light: phos-, phot-

limb: mel-

lip: ch(e)il-, labi-

little: use diminutive suffix

liver: hepar-, hepat-

located in the back: opisth-, dolich-

long: macr-, mega-, megal-

louse: pedicul-

love: phil-

lung: pneum(on)-, pulm(on)-

lymph: lymph-

M

(be) mad: man-

make: fac-, -fic-, -fect, poie-

male: andr-

man: andr-

many: mult-, multi-, poly-

mark: stigm-, stigmat-

marrow: medull-

measure: metr-

meatus: meat-

medicine: pharmac(eu)-

membrane: -ium (rarely-eum); hymen-

meningeal membrane: mening-, -meninx

meninges: mening-, -meninx

menstruation: men-

mental activity: no-

mesentery: mes-

milk: gal-, galact-, lact-

mind: no-, phren-, psych-

motion: kines(i)-

mouth: or-, os, stom-, stomat-

move: kine-

movement: kines(i)-

much: mult-, multi-

mucus: blenn-, myx-

muscle: is-, inos-, my(s)-

muscular spasm: -ismus

N

narrow: dolich-

narrowing (of a part of the body): stenosis

nature: phys(i)-

navel: omphal-

neck (of the uterus): cervic-, cervix

neck: trachel-

neither: neutr-

nerve: neur-

nervous system: neur-

network: ret-, retin-

new: ne-

night: nyct-

nipple: thel(e)-

normal: eu-; orth-

nose: nas-, rhin-

not: a-, an-, in-, non-

nourishment: troph-

numbness: narc-

O

obstruct: phrac-, phrag-

odor: osm-

of one's self: idi-

old age: ger-, presby-

on both sides: amphi-, ampho-

on the outside: extra-

one: mono-

oozing (of blood): -staxis, -staxia

opening: meat-, or-, os, por-, stom-, stomat-

opposed to: anti-

opposite: contra-

organism: zo-

origin: arch-, -arche; -genesis

out of: ec-, ex-

outer layer (of an organ): cortic-, cortex

outer: extern-

outside: exo-

outside of: ecto-

ovary: oophor-, ovari-

over: epi-, super-

oviduct: syring-, -syrinx

oxygen: ox(y)-

P

pain: odyn-

(sudden) pain: -agra

painful: dys-

palate: staphyl-

paralysis: paresis

paralyze: plec-, pleg-

partition: sept-

passage: meat-, por-

pelvis: pelv-

penis: pen-, phall-

people: dem-

pharynx: pharynx, pharyng-

physician: iatr-

pierce: cente-

pigment: chrom-, chroma-, chromat-

place for: -arium, -ary, -orium, -ory

place: the-, top-

plant organism: phyt-

plastic surgery: -plasty

pleura: pleur-

pleural cavity: thorax, thorac-

point: cusp, -cuspid

pointed: ox(y)-

poisonous (to an organ): -toxic

poisonous substance: -toxin

population: dem-

pore: por-

portal vein: pyle-

pour: fus-

power: dynam-

pregnant: gravid-, cye-

preventing: anti-

produce: gen(e)-, -gen, poie-

produced by or in: -genic, -genous

producing: -genic, -genous

prolapse: pt-

prostate gland: prostat-

protected: immun-

protection (against disease): phylac-

puberty: puber(t)-

pubic bone: pub-

pubic region: pub-

pubis: pub-

pulmonary artery: pulm(on)-

pulse: sphygm-

pupil (of the eye): cor(e)-

pus: pur-, py-

put: the-

putrid: sapr-

pylorus: pylor-

R

radiation: actin-

rapid: ox(y)-

read: lex-

record: graph-

(written) record: gram-

record of the activity of an organ (often an x-ray): -gram

rectum: rect-

reduction: -lysis

relieving: anti-

remember: mne-

renal pelvis: pyel-

resembling: -ile, -oid, -ose

retina: ret-, retin-

reverberating sound: echo-

rib: cost-

right side: dextr-

rinse out: cly(s)-

rod: rhabd-

root: radic-, rad-, radix

rotten: sapr-

rupture: rhex-, -rrhexis

S

safe: immun-

sag: pt-

sagging (of an organ or part): -ptosis

saliva: ptyal-, sial-

salivary duct: sial-

same: homo-, homeo-; is-

science, study of: -ics, -tics; -logy

scrotum: scrot-

sebaceous glands: stear-, steat-

sebum: stear-, steat-

secrete: crin-, rhe-

secretion: crin-

seed: sem-, semin-, sperm(at)-

seizure: lep-

self: aut-

semen: sem-, semin-, sperm(at)-

send: stal-, stol-

sensation: esthe(s)-

sense: esthe(s)-

sense of smell: osm-, osphr-

sensitivity: esthe(s)-

sex glands: gonad-

sex organs: gonad-

sexual desire: aphrodis(i)-, er-, erot-

(abnormal) sexual excitation or gratification: -lagnia

shape: -form, morph-

short: brachy-

shut: my-

side: later-

sigmoid colon: sigm-

similar: is-

single: mon-, mono-

sinus: sin-, sinus-

skin: derm(at)-, -derma

slackening (of strength): paresis

sleep: hypn-, somn-

slender: dolich-

slide: lab-, laps-

slip: lab-, laps-

small: micr-; use diminutive suffix

smooth: lei-

soft tissue: sarc-

softening (of tissues) of: -malacia

sound: phon-, son-

spasm: spasm-

speak: pha-, phras-

specialist: -logist

specialty: -logy

speech: phem-

sperm: sperm(at)-

sphincter muscle: sphincter-

spider: arachn-

spinal cord: myel-

spine: r(h)achi-

spit: pty-

spleen: lien-, splen-

split: schiz-, schist-, -schisis

spot: stigm-, stigmat-

stable: stabil-, stabl-

stand: sta(t)-

staphylococci: staphyl-

starch: amyl-

steal: klept-

stomach: gastr-

stone: calc-

stop: sta(t)-

straight: orth-

strength: sthen-

streptococci: strept-

stretch: tens(i)-

stretching: ta-

strike: plec-, pleg-

study: -logy

stupor: narc-

substance: -in, -ine

substance that produces (something): -gen

sugar: glyc-

suppress: isch-, -sche-

surface: faci-, -fici-, facies

surrounding: peri-

suture: -rrhaph-

swallow: phag-

sweat: hidr(ot)-, -idr-, sud(or)-

sweat glands: syring-, -syrinx

swelling: -cel-, edema, edemat-

swollen: tum(e)-

synovial fluid, synovial membrane or sac: synov(i)-

syringe: syring-, -syrinx

T

take: -cip-, -cept-

talk: lal-

taste: geus(t)-

tear: dacry-, lacrim-

(body) temperature: therm-

tendon: ten-, tenon(t)-

tension: ton-, tens(i)-

testicle: orchi(d)-, orch(e)-

theft: klept-

thick: pachy-

thirst: dips-

thorax: thorax, thorac-

thoroughly: con-, in-, ob-, per-

thread (worm): nemat-

through: dia-, per-, trans-

(a) throwing: bol-

thyroid gland: thyr-

time: chron-

timing: chron-

tissue: hist(i)-

to: ad-

toe: dactyl-, digit-

toenail: onych-

together: con-, syn-

tone: ton-

tongue: gloss-, lingu-

tonsil: amygdal-

tooth: dent-, odont-

toward: ad-, ob-

trachea: trach(e)-, trachy-

transformation: meta-

treatise (on a subject): -graphy

treat medically: therap(eu)-

treatment: iatr-

tube: tub-

tumor: -oma; -cel-, onc-

turning: trop-

twice: bi-, di-, dis-

twin: diplo-

twisted: strept-

two: bi-, di-, dis-

U

ulcer: (h)elc-

umbilicus: omphal-

under: sub-

up: ana-

upon: epi-

ureter: ureter-

urethra: urethr-

uric acid: ur-

urinary tract: ur-

urine: ur-

uterus: hyster-, metr-, -metra, uter-

uvula: staphyl-

V

vagina: colp-, vagin-

vagus nerve: vag-

varix: cirs-, varic-, varix

vas deferens: vas-

(dilated and twisted) vein: cirs-, varic-, varix

vein: phleb-, ven-

vertebra: spondyl-

very: con-, in-, ob-, per-

virus: vir(u)-, virus-

viscus: splanchn-

vision: op(s)-, opt-

voice: phon-

vomit: eme-

W

wall: sept-

water: hydr-

web: arachn-

widen: eury(n)-

with: con-

within: en-, endo-, ento-, eso-, intra-

without: a-, an-

woman: gyn(ec)-

womb: uter-

work: erg-

(intestinal) worm: helmint(h)-

write: graph-

Y

yellow: xanth-

MEDICAL TERMINOLOGY USED IN LESSONS 1 TO 15

The following is a complete list of terms used in the exercises in Lessons 1 to 15, the main body of this text. Terms from the supplemental lessons (Lessons 16 to 19) and the biological nomenclature lesson (Lesson 20) are not included. This list is provided as a reference source and spelling guide.

A

abdominalgia
abdominocystic
abdominoplasty
abdominoscrotal
abduct
abenteric
abiosis
ablation
aborad
aboral
abrachia
acanthocyte
acanthocytosis
acanthoid

acanthoma
acanthopelvis
acanthosis
acapnia
acardia
achlorhydria
achromatopsia
achromatosis
acroanesthesia
acrocyanosis
acrohyperhidrosis
acromegaly
acromicria
actinodermatitis
actinogenic
actinoneuritis

actinotherapy
adduct
adenectopia
adenoidectomy
adenoids
adenotome
adipectomy
adipocyte
adipose
adiposuria
adoral
adrenal cortex
adrenalin
aerobe
aerothermotherapy
aerotitis

aerotropism
afebrile
afferent
ageusia
aglycemia
agnathia
agnosia
akinesia
algolagnia
algophobia
allochiria
allodynia
allolalia
allophasis
alloplasia
allostery

alveolar

alveolitis

amblyacousia

amblychromasia

amblychromatic

amblyopia

amenorrhea

amnesia

amniocentesis

amniography

amniorrhexis

amphibious

amphocyte

amygdalolith

amygdalopathy

amylase

amylogenesis

amylolysis

amylophagia

amyosthenia

amyotrophia

amyxia

analgesic

analgia

anamniotic

anaphrodisiac

anaphylaxis

anastomosis

androgynoid

androgynous

android

anemic

anergia

anerythroplasia

anerythropsia

anesthesia

anesthesiology

angiitis

anginoid

anginophobia

angiocarditis

angiogram

angiolith

angiorrhaphy

angiorrhexis

angiosclerosis

angiosclerotic myasthenia

angiosis

angiostenosis

anhydrous

aniridia

anisochromatic

anisocytosis

anisomastia

anisomelia

anisometropia

anisopia

ankyloblepharon

ankylochilia

ankylodactylia

ankyloproctia

ankylosis

anodyne

anonychia

anorchidism

anorexia

anoxia

antaphrodisiac

antasthenic

antatrophic

antebrachium

antenatal

antepartum

antepyretic

anterolateral

anteroposterior

anthelmintic

anthracosis

anthrax

antianemic

antiarthritic

antibiotic

anticytotoxin

antifungal

antigalactic

antigen

antihemorrhagic

antihypnotic

anti-icteric

antilithic

antinarcotic

antistaphylococcic

antisudorific

antitoxin

antitussive

anuresis

aortarctia

aortoclasia

aphagia

aphemia

aphrodisiac

aplasia

apnea

apoplexy

aptyalia

apyrexia

apyrogenic

arachnodactyly

arachnolysin

archenteron

archigaster

arctation

areflexia

arrhythmia

arteriolith

arteriomyomatosis

arteriosclerosis

arteriostenosis

arteriostosis

arteritis

arthritides

arthritis

arthrocentesis

arthroclasia

arthrodynia

arthroneuralgia

arthropyosis

arthrosclerosis

arthrosteitis

ascus

aspiration

asthenia

astigmatism

astigmometer

asynergy

asystolia

ataxophobia

atelocardia

atelocheiria

ateloglossia

atelognathia

atelopodia

atheroma

atheromatosis

atheronecrosis

atoxic

atrichia

atriotome

atrophy

auricula

auris externa

auris interna

autism

autoantitoxin

autoerotism

autohemolysis

autosepticemia

auxin

avirulent

azoospermia

azymia

B

bacillar

bacillophobia

bacteriolysin

bacteriophage

bacteriostatic

bacteroid

barylalia

baryophobia

baryphonia

biceps

biliary

biligenesis

bilious

binaural

binocular

binotic

biotoxin

bisection

blennadenitis

blennemesis

blennoid

blennorrhagia

blepharism

blepharodiastasis

blepharorrhea

blepharostat

brachia

brachial

brachialgia

brachycephalous

brachycheilia

brachydactylia

brachygnathia

bradyarrhythmia

bradycardia

bradykinesia

bradylexia

bradypnea

bradytachycardia

bronchiolectasis

bronchomycosis

bronchorrhagia

bursae

bursolith

bursopathy

C

calcemia

calciferous

calcification

calcipenia

calcium

calculogenesis

calorie

calorifacient

calorific

calorimeter

capillarectasia

capillaropathy

capillaroscopy

capitulum

capnography

capnophilic

captate

carcinogenic

cardia

cardiac

cardioangiology

cardiomalacia

cardioptosis

cardiopyloric

cardiospasm

cardiotomy

cecopexy

cecoptosis

cecostomy

celiac

celiocentesis

celiohysterectomy

celioma

centesis

cephalalgia

cephalodynia

cerebellar ataxia

cerebellar cortex

cerebellum

cerebropathy

cervicitis

cervicovaginitis

cervicovesical

cheilophagia

cheiloschisis

cheilotomy

cheirognostic

cheirology

cheirospasm

chloroleukemia

chloropia

chlorosis

cholangioma

cholecystenterostomy

cholecystic

choledochal

choledochorraphy

cholelithiasis

cholemesis

cholestasia

chondralgia

chondrectomy

chondritis

chondroangioma

chondrocostal

chondrocyte

chondrodystrophy

chondroplasty

choroid

choroidoretinitis

chromatogenous

chromatophore

chromidrosis

chromophobia

chromophore

chromotherapy

chronobiology

chronognosis

chronograph

circumrenal

cirsectomy

cirsomphalos

cirsotome

cirsotomy

clysis

coccobacilli

coccoid

colicolitis

colicystitis

coliform

colinephritis

colitis

coloenteritis

colonalgia

colonitis

colorectostomy

colostomy

colpocystocele

colpomicroscope

concrescence

coniofibrosis

coniology

coniosis

conjunctivitis

conjunctivoplasty

contralateral

copremesis

coprolalia

coprolith

coprozoa

cordate

cordiform

corectopia

coremorphosis

coreometry

corestenoma

corona dentis

coronavirus

coroner

coronoid

cortical

corticoadrenal

costalgia

costochondral

costotome

craniology

craniomalacia

craniorhachischisis

craniosclerosis

creatorrhea

crinogenic

cryalgesia

crymodynia

crymophilic

cryobiology

cryotherapy

cryptanamnesia

cryptesthesia

cryptocephalus

cryptogenic

cryptolith

cryptorchidism

cusp

cyanhidrosis

cyanoderma

cyanomycosis

cyanopia

cyanosis

cyanotic

cyclectomy

cyclokeratitis

cycloplegia

cyesis

cystigerous

cystocele

cystoid

cystolith

cystoma

cystopexy

cystorrhexis

cystoscopy

cytobiology

cytocidal

cytoclastic

cytometer

cytotoxin

D

dacryadenalgia

dacryagogue

dacryelcosis

dacryocyst

dacryohemorrhea

dacryopyorrhea

dactyledema

dearterialization

decalcification

decalcify

decimeter

defecation

demography

denticle

dentigerous

dentilabial

dentin

dentoalveolitis

dentofacial

dentoid

deossification

dermalgia

dermatoconiosis

dermatocyst

dermatomycosis

dermatomyoma

dermatophyte

dermatosclerosis

dermatotherapy

dermonosology

desmocyte

desmoneoplasm

desmopathy

desmorrhexis

detoxify

dextrad

dextral

dextrocardia

dextrogastria

diaphoresis

diaphoretic

diaphragmitis

diencephalon

digestion

digitate

digiti

digitiform

digitus

diplegia

diplobacillus

diploccoccemia

diplocephaly

diplocoria

dipsophobia

dipsosis

dolichocephalic

dolichocolon

dolichofacial

dolichomorphic

dolichosigmoid

dorsad

dorsiduction

dorsiflect

dorsocephalad

dorsodynia

dromomania

dromotropic

ductile

ductule

duodenoenterostomy

duodenohepatic

duodenojejunostomy

dynamic

dynamogenic

dysacousia

dysarthrosis

dyscephaly

dysentery

dysgraphia

dyshidrosis

dyskinesia

dyslalia

dysmnesia

dysmorphic

dysosmia

dysostosis

dyspeptic

dysphagia

dysphoria

dyspnea

dysrhythmia

dysstasia

dysthanasia

dysthyroidism

dystrophy

dysuria

E

echocardiogram

echogram

echopathy

ectocardia

ectogenous

ectophyte

ectopia cordis

ectopia renis

edema

edematogenic

efferent

emetic

encephalalgia

encephalic

encephalolith

encephalomalacia

encephalomyelopathy

endangiitis

endangium

endaortitis

endarteritis

endemic

endocranium

endocrinology

endocrinotherapy

endocystitis

endodontitis

endogastritis

endometriosis

endometrium

endoneurium

endoparasite

endoscope

endosteum

endostoma

endotoscope

endotoxin

enophthalmos

enterocholecystostomy

enterocystocele

enterodynia

enteromegaly

enteromycosis

enterosepsis

enterostenosis

entopic

epicardium

epicranium

epidermitis

epigastrium

epiotic

epistaxis

epizoon

ergometer

ergophobia

erogenous

erotogenic

erotophobia

erythrism

erythrocytorrhexis

erythrocytosis

erythroleukemia

erythromelalgia

erythropenia

erythrophage

erythropoiesis

erythroprosopalgia

erythrotoxin

esophagismus

esophagocele

esthesioscopy

eubiotics

eucholia

euglycemia

eupepsia

euphonia

euphoria

eurycephalic

euthanasia

excise

excision

excrescence

exencephalia

exocardia

exodontia

exogenous

exomphalos

exotoxin

expectoration

expiration

exsanguination

externalize

extrahepatic

extrauterine

extravasation

F

facial

facial hemiplegia

faciobrachial

febrifacient

fecaloid

fecaluria

fibromyalgia

fibromyoma

fibroplasia

fibrosis

fistula

fistulatome

flexile

flexor

formation

frigolabile

frigorific

frigostabile

frigotherapy

fungi

fungicide

fungistasis

fungistatic

fungitoxic

fungoid

G

galactopoiesis

galactostasis

gastric atony

gastrocele

gastroenteralgia

gastrolithiasis

gastrology

gastropexy

gastrophrenic

gastroplegia

gastrorrhagia

gastroschisis

gastroscope

genetics

genitalia

genitoplasty

geriatric

geriatrician

geriatrics

gestosis

gingivalgia

gingivoglossitis

glossolabial

glossopyrosis

glycogeusia

glycopolyuria

gnathalgia

gnathoschisis

gonadal dysgenesis

gonadopathy

gonadotropin

gravida macromastia

gynandrism

gynandroid

gynecoid

gynecopathy

gynecophonus

gynoplasty

H

helcoid

helcoma

helcosis

helminthemesis

helminthiasis

helminthicide

helminthology

hemangiectasis

hemangioma

hemangiomatosis

hemarthrosis

hematoma

hematomphalocele

hematomyelia

hematophyte

hematopoiesis

hematosalpinx

hemialgia

hemianalgesia

hemianosmia

hemiataxia

hemic calculus

hemicephalic

hemidiaphoresis

hemidysesthesia

hemifacial

hemilaryngectomy

hemiparesis

hemocytology

hemocytozoon

hemodynamics

hemophiliac

hemosiderosis

hemostasis

hemotrophic

heparin

hepatogenous

hepatolytic

hepatomalacia

hepatomegaly

hepatomelanosis

hepatorrhexis

hepatosplenitis

hermaphrodite

herpes facialis

herpes labialis

herpetic

herpetiform

heterochromia iridis

heterodromus

heterogeusia

heterokeratoplasty

heteroprosopus

heterotoxin

hidradenitis

hidrosis

histiocyte

histiocytosis

histocyte

histokinesis

histolysis

histoma

histopathology

homeo-osteoplasty

homoerotic

homogeneous

homogenize

homolateral

homophobia

hydrocolpos

hydrometra

hydronephrosis

hydropenia

hydrophilism

hydrophthalmos

hydropneumothorax

hydrorrhachis

hydrotherapy

hymenitis

hymenorrhaphy

hypacousia

hypalgesia

hyperalgesia

hyperalgia

hypercapnia

hyperchlorhydria

hyperemesis

hyperemesis gravidarum

hyperemia

hypergenitalism

hypergeusesthesia

hyperhidrosis

hyperimmune

hyperinsulinism

hyperlactation

hypermetropia

hyperphrenia

hypertension

hyperthermalgesia

hyperthyroidism

hypertonus

hypertrichosis

hypertrophy

hyperuricemia

hypnogenic

hypnoidal

hypnotic

hypnotize

hypoalgia

hypocalcemia

hypocapnia

hypodermoclysis

hypoglossal

hypoliposis

hypologia

hypometropia

hypomnesia

hypomyxia

hyponychium

hypophrenia

hypoplasia

hypoptyalism

hyposynergia

hypotensive

hypotrichosis

hypoxemia

hysterogastrorraphy

hysterolith

hysterosalpingography

I

iatrogenesis

iatrology

icterohepatitis

icteroid

idiogram

idiopathic

idiotropic

ileocolic

ileocolostomy

ileocystoplasty

ileoproctostomy

iliocecal sphincter

immunifacient

immunobiology

immunogenic

immunology

immunotherapy

immunotoxin

inception

incipient

incise

incisor

indentation

indigestible

infracostal

inframammary

infusion

ingestant

ingestion

inguinal

inguinal reflex

inguinolabial

inguinoscrotal

inosemia

inositis

inosuria

insemination

insomnia

inspiration

insulin

insulinemia

interatrial

interauricular

internal

internalize

intra-atrial

intracranial

intraduodenal

intrapulmonary

intrauterine

introflexion

intubation

intumesce

intumescent

ipsilateral

iralgia

iridadenosis

iridocyclectomy

iridotasis

ischemia

ischesis

ischidrosis

isochromatic

isocoria

isocytosis

isocytotoxin

isodactylism

isomorphism

isotonia

J

jaundice

jejunojejunostomy

jejunostomy

K

keratectomy

keratocele

keratorrhexis

kinesiatrics

kinesioneurosis

kleptomania

kleptomaniac

kleptophobia

koniometer

L

labile

labioglossopharyngeal

labiomycosis

lacrimation

lacrimotome

lacrimotomy

lactation

lactogen

lalopathology

lalopathy

lalorrhea

laparocholecystotomy

laparoenterostomy

laparohepatotomy

laparohystero-oophorec-
tomy

laparoileotomy

laparomyitis

laparorrhaphy

laparotomy

laparotyphlotomy

laryngismus

laryngocentesis

lateroabdominal

lateroflexion

leiomyofibroma

leiomyoma

leiotrichous

leptocephalia

leptochromatic

leptomeninges

leptophonia

leukocidin

leukocoria

leukocyte

leukocytoid

leukopenia

leukopoiesis

leukopoietic

leukorrhagia

leukorrhea

leukotoxin

lienomalacia

lienopancreatic

lingula

lipemia

lipocele

lipochondroma

lipocyte

lithiasis

lithometer

lithonephritis

logagnosia

M

macrocardius
macrocheilia
macrocheiria
macrodactylia
macrolabia
macropsia
macrostoma
macrotia
malacosteon
mammogram
mammography
maniacal
mastadenitis
mastatrophia
mastochondroma
mastomenia
mazoplasia
meatometer
meatoplasty
meatoscopy
megalocystis
megalonychosis
megalophthalmus
melalgia
melaniferous
melanin
melanoglossia
melanoleukoderma
melanoma
melanomatosis
melanonychia
melanophore
melanuria
menarche
meningitis
meningoarteritis
meningococcemia

meningomyelocele
meningorrhagia
meningorrhea
meningovascular
menostaxis
mesenteriopexy
mesentery
mesocardia
mesocephalic
mesoderm
mesodiastolic
mesodont
mesogastrium
mesojejunum
metabiosis
metachromasia
metakinesis
metamyelocyte
metrectasia
metrectopia
metreurynter
microbe
microbicide
microcephalia
microdontism
microgenitalism
micrognathia
microlithiasis
micromazia
microphakia
micropsia
microstomia
monobrachius
monochromatic
monocular
monocyte
monophagia
monophasia

monorchid
monorchidism
multigravida
myasthenia
myatonia
mycethemia
mycetogenetic
mycobacterium
mycosis
myectomy
myelatelia
myelauxe
myelodysplasia
myelofibrosis
myeloid
myeloma
myelopoiesis
myeloradiculodysplasia
myodynamometer
myodynia
myoendocarditis
myofibril
myoischemia
myolipoma
myonephropexy
myoneural
myopathy
myope
myopia
myosclerosis
myotasis
myotatic
myotenontoplasty
myxadenitis labialis
myxangitis
myxochondroma
myxoid
myxoma

N

narcohypnia
narcolepsy
narcosis
narcotize
nasal
nasogastric
nasolacrimal
nasology
naso-oral
nasopharyngography
nasoseptitis
necrocytotoxin
necrogenous
necrophagous
necrosis
nematoid
nematology
neonate
neonatology
neostomy
nephralgia
nephrectomy
nephremphraxis
nephrocystanastomosis
nephrocystitis
nephrohypertrophy
nephrolithiasis
nephrolithotomy
nephropyosis
nephrosclerosis
nephrotoxin
nephrotropic
neuralgia
neurasthenia
neuritis
neurocrine

neurohistology

neuromyelitis

neurosclerosis

neurotoxin

neurotropic virus

nomogram

nomography

nonose

nonseptate

nontoxic

nosology

nosomycosis

nosophobia

nosophyte

nyctalgia

nyctamblyopia

nyctophilia

nycturia

O

occipital

occiput

occlude

oculomycosis

oculonasal

odontatrophy

odontoclasis

odontodynia

odontogenic

odontonecrosis

odontorrhagia

odynacusis

odynometer

oligodactylia

oligodontia

oligohydramnios

oligomenorrhea

oligopnea

oligospermia

oliguria

omphaloncus

omphalorrhagia

omphalorrhexis

oncology

oncolysis

onychatrophia

onychauxis

onychomycosis

onychophagy

onychorrhexis

oophorocystosis

ophthalmatrophy

ophthalmia neonatorum

ophthalmomycosis

ophthalmoplegia

optometrist

optometry

orad

orcheoplasty

orchidoncus

orchidoptosis

oreximania

orexogen

orifice

orolingual

oropharynx

orthobiosis

orthodiagraph

orthopsychiatry

orthoptic

orthosis

osmesis

osmesthesia

osmidrosis

osmodysphoria

osmonosology

ossific

ossification

ossify

ostalgia

ostempyesis

osteoarthropathy

osteochondrodystrophy

osteochondroma

osteoclast

osteogen

osteologist

osteomalacia

osteometry

osteophlebitis

osteophyte

osteoporosis

osteosclerosis

osteosynovitis

osteosynthesis

osteothrombosis

otitis

otolaryngologist

otomycosis

otoncus

otorhinolaryngology

otorhinology

ototoxic

ovariocyesis

ovariotomy

ovicide

oviduct

oxyacusis

oxycephaly

oxyesthesia

oxygeusia

oxyopia

oxypathia

oxytocin

P

pachycephalic

pachycheilia

pachyderma

pachyglossia

pachyonychia

pachyostosis

pachypleuritis

pachyrhinic

palilalia

palindromia

palingraphia

palinopsia

panasthenia

pancarditis

pancreatic

pancreatolith

pancreatoncus

pancytopenia

pandemic

panhysterocolpectomy

panophobia

panoptosis

paracanthoma

paracentesis

paracolitis

parahepatic

paranoia

paranoid

paraparesis

paraphemia

paraphrenitis

paraplegia

parasite

parasynovitis

paratyphlitis

paravesical

parenteral	periesophagitis	phoniatrics	polyneuritis
paresis	perinephrium	phonopathy	polyneuropathy
paronychomycosis	periodontal	photodysphoria	polyonychia
parorexia	periomphalic	photogenic	polyorchidism
parosmia	perionychium	photolysis	polyotia
parosphresia	perioral	photophilic	polyp
parotic	periosteitis	photopia	polyphagia
pathogenic	periosteoma	photosynthesis	polyphrasia
pathology	periosteum	phototropism	polyradiculitis
pectoral	periphrenitis	phrenicotomy	polysinusitis
pectoralgia	peripleuritis	phrenohepatic	polythelia
pectorophony	peripylephlebitis	physical	polyuria
pedatrophy	perisalpingoovaritis	physiognosis	porencephalitis
pediatrician	perispondylic	phytogenous	posteroexternal
pediculicide	peristaltic	phytotoxin	posterointernal
pediculophobia	perivaginitis	plegaphonia	posterolateral
pediculosis	perivisceritis	pleurocele	posterosuperior
pediculosis capitis	pertussis	pleuroclysis	postfebrile
pediculus	pertussoid	pneumatosis	posticteric
pedomorphism	phacoanaphylaxis	pneumocentesis	postnasal
pedorthist	phacohymenitis	pneumocephalus	postpartum
pelvicephalography	phacolysis	pneumogalactocele	postpuberty
pelvicephalometry	phacosclerosis	pneumohypoderma	prediastolic
pelvitherm	phacoscope	pneumolith	prenarcosis
penile	phage	pneumonolysis	prenatal
penischisis	phagocytolysis	pneumonorrhaphy	prepubescent
penitis	phagocytosis	podagra	presbyacusia
pepsin	phalliform	podalgia	presbyatrics
peptogenic	phalloncus	podencephalus	presbyopia
periangiitis	pharmacophobia	podocyte	presphygmic
periangiocholitis	pharmacotherapy	polioencephalitis	proctoclysis
periarteritis	pharyngismus	poliomyelitis	proctopexia
periarthritis	pharyngocele	poliovirus	proctopexy
peribronchiolitis	phlebectopia	polyadenomatosis	proencephalus
pericardiorrhaphy	phlebolith	polyarthritis	prognathous
pericarditis	phlebolithiasis	polyblennia	prolapse
pericardium	phlebomyomatosis	polycoria	prolapsus
pericholecystitis	phonasthenia	polymyositis	prophylactic

prosopodiplegia

prosoponeuralgia

prosopoplegia

prosopospasm

prosopotocia

prostatodynia

prostatomegaly

prostatorrhea

protanopia

protobiology

protoduodenum

protogaster

protoleukocyte

protopathic

protospasm

protozoa

protozoology

pseudoanemia

pseudocyesis

pseudocyst

pseudoedema

pseudohematuria

pseudoicterus

pseudopsia

pseudosmia

psychochromesthesia

psychometry

psychopharmacology

psychosis

psychosomatic

ptosis

ptyalolithiasis

pubalgia

pubarche

puberty

pubescence

pulmometry

pulmonologist

purulent

purulent conjunctivitis

purulent synovitis

pyelectasia

pyelocystostomosis

pyelogram

pyemia

pyemic

pylethrombosis

pyloroduodenitis

pylorostenosis

pyocephalus

pyohemothorax

pyoid

pyonephrosis

pyosalpinx

pyosemia

pyretolysis

pyrexia

pyrogen

pyrogenic

Q

quadriceps

quadriplegia

R

rachitis

rachitome

radiculomeningomyelitis

radix

rectocele

rectocystotomy

rectorrhaphy

rectostenosis

reflex

reflexogenic

regurgitant

relapse

renogastric

renogram

resectable

resectoscope

respiration

retinochoroid

retinodialysis

retinopathy

retroauricular

retrocecal

retrocervical

retroesophageal

retrolingual

retromorphosis

retrouterine

retroviruses

rhabdomyolysis

rhabdovirus

rhachialgia

rhinolithiasis

rhinomycosis

rhinopharyngeal

rhinoplasty

rhinorrhagia

rhinorrhea

rhinoscope

S

salpingocyesis

salpingosalpingostomy

sanguiferous

sanguine

sanguineous

sanguinopurulent

sanguirenal

saprobes

saprogenic

saprophyte

sarcoadenoma

sarcocarcinoma

sarcocele

sarcolysis

scatology

scatoscopy

schistocytosis

schistoprosopia

schistothorax

schizoblepharia

schizonychia

schizophrenia

scleradenitis

sclerencephalia

scleriasis

scleronychia

sclero-oophoritis

sclerotic

sclerotrichia

scrota

scrotitis

scrotocele

scrotoplasty

sectile

section

seminal

seminiferous

sepsis

septotome

septulum

sialadenocus

sialagogue

sialoschesis

sialosyrinx

siderofibrosis

siderogenous

sideropenia

sigmoiditis

sigmoidopexy

sincipital

sinistral

sinistraural

sinistrocerebral

sinistrocular

sinogram

sinusoid

sitophobia

sitotoxin

sitotoxism

somatic

somatocrinin

somatology

somnifacient

somniferous

somnolent

somnolentia

sone

sonic

sonogram

sonometer

spasm

spasmolytic

spermatopoietic

spermatoschesis

spermatozoicide

sphincterismus

sphygmogram

sphygmometer

spirogram

spirometry

splanchemphraxis

splanchnoptosis

splenectasia

splenemphraxis

splenicterus

splenocele

splenomegaly

spondylarthritis

spondylolysis

spondylopyosis

stabile

staphylococcemia

staphylococcus

staphylolysin

staphyloncus

stasis

stearodermia

steatolysis

steatoma

steatopathy

steatorrhea

stenocephaly

stenosis

stenostomia

stereognosis

stereology

stereometry

stereo-ophthalmoscope

stereo-orthopter

stereopsis

stereotropism

sternocostal

sternopericardial

sternoschisis

sternothyroid

sternotracheal

stethomyitis

stethoparalysis

stethoscope

stethospasm

stigmatism

stomatitis

stomatomalacia

streptococci

streptococcolysin

streptodermatitis

subaural

subfebrile

sublingual

subpulmonary

sudor

sudoresis

sudorific

superficial

supervirulent

suppurative choroiditis

supradiaphragmatic

symbiosis

symbiotic

symphysodactyly

sympodia

synalgic

synarthrosis

synchilia

syndactylism

syndactylous

syndesmopexy

synergy

synorchidism

synovectomy

synovia

synovioma

synthetic

syringocarcinoma

syringoencephalomyelia

syringoma

systole

systolic

T

tachyarrhythmia

tachycardia

tachylalia

tachyphasia

tachyphrasia

tachypnea

telangiitis

telangioma

telangiosis

tenalgia

tenodesis

tenodynia

tenontography

tenontomyotomy

tenorrhaphy

tenostosis

tensiometer

tension

thanatobiological

thanatology

thanatophobia

thelarche

theleplasty

theloncus

therapeutics

therapy

thermanesthesia

thermometry

thermostabile

thoracic

thoracoceloschisis

thoracomyodynia

thoracopathy

thrombectomy

thromboclasis

thromboendocarditis

thrombogenic

thyroaplasia

thyroplasty

thyrotome

thyrotoxicosis

thyrotropin

thyrotropism

tocophobia

topagnosis

toponarcosis

toponeurosis

topophobic

toxemia

toxic

toxicoderma

toxicodermatitis

toxicology

toxicosis

toxin

toxolysin

toxonosis

toxophylaxin

trachelismus

trachelocele

trachelodynia

trachelopexy

tracheloschisis

tracheocele

tracheomalacia

tracheotome

trachyphonia

transection

transthoracic

transtracheal

trichobacteria

trichogen

trichomycosis

trichophagia

tricuspid

trigastric

trophedema

trophic

trophocyte

tubectomy

tuboplasty

tuborrhea

tumefacient

tumefaction

tumescence

tussive

typhloempyema

U

ultramicrobe

ultrasonogram

urelcosis

ureterolithiasis

ureteroureterostomy

urethrismus

urethrostenosis

urethrotome

uricocholia

uroureter

uroxanthin

uterine

uterorectal

uterotubal

V

vaccine

vaccinotherapeutics

vaginismus

vaginodynia

vaginogenic

vaginovesical

vagitis

vagotropism

vagus

varices

variciform

varicoblepharon

varicophlebitis

varicula

vascular

vascularize

vasculitis

vasectomy

vasitis

vasoparesis

vasorrhaphy

vasovagal

venectasia

venosclerosis

venostasis

ventricle

ventricular

ventroscopy

ventrose

ventrotomy

vesicocele

vesicoclysis

vesicula seminalis

viremia

virucidal

virucide

virusemia

visceromegaly

viscerosomatic

viscerotonia

viscerotropic

viscus

X

xanthemia

xanthocyanopia

xanthocyte

xanthoderma

xanthoma

xanthophose

xanthopsia

xanthosis

xerocheilia

xeroderma

xeroma

xerostomia

xerotocia

Z

zoophilism

zoophyte

zoopsia

zymogen

zymolysis

BIBLIOGRAPHY FOR EDITION III

Definitions in this manual have been taken from the following sources:

Latin Words: Lewis, C. T., and Short, C. (eds.): *Harper's Latin Dictionary.* New York: The American Book Company, 1907.

Greek Words: Liddell, H. G., and Scott, R.: *A Greek-English Lexicon.* London (UK): Oxford University Press, 1953.

Medical Terms: Venes, D. (ed.): *Taber's Cyclopedic Medical Dictionary*, ed. 19. Philadelphia, F. A. Davis, 2001.

Aminoff, M. J., Greenberg, D. A., and Simon, R. P: *Clinical Neurology.* Stamford, CT: Appleton & Lange, 1996.

Ayers, D. M.: *English Words from Latin and Greek Elements.* Tucson: The University of Arizona Press, 1965.

Bulfinch, T.: *Bulfinch's Greek and Roman Mythology: The Age of Fable.* Mineola, NY: Dover, 2000. *www.Bulfinch.org*

Burriss, E. E., and Casson, L.: *Latin and Greek in Current Use.* Englewood Cliffs, NJ: Prentice-Hall, 1949.

Carmichael, A. G., and Razan, R. M. (eds.): *Medicine: A Treasury of Art and Literature.* New York: Harkavy Publishing Service, 1991.

Couch, M: *Greek and Roman Mythology.* New York: Metrobooks, 1997.

Dunmore, C. W., and Fleischer, R. M.: *Medical Terminology: Lessons in Etymology*, ed. 2. Philadelphia: F. A. Davis, 1985.

ecosystemworld.com. www.ecosystemworld.com

Encyclopedia Mythica. www.pantheon.org

Federative Committee on Anatomical Terminology: *Terminologia Anatomica.* Stuttgart, Germany: Georg Thieme Verlag, 1998.

Feldman, M.: *Sleisenger and Fordtran's Gastrointestinal and Liver Disease*, ed. 7. Philadelphia: W. B. Saunders, 2002.

Goldman, L., and Bennett, J.C. (eds.): *Cecil Textbook of Medicine*, ed. 21. Philadelphia: W. B. Saunders, 2000.

Grendell, J. H., McQuaid, K.R., and Friedman, S. L: *Current Diagnosis and Treatment in Gastroenterology.* Stamford, CT: Appleton & Lange, 1996.

Lewis, C. T. , and Short, C. (eds.): *Harper's Latin Dictionary.* New York: The American Book Company, 1907.

Liddell, H. G., and Robert, S.: *A Greek-English Lexicon.* London, England: Oxford University Press, 1953.

McCrum, R., Cran, W., and MacNeil, R.: *The Story of English.* New York: Viking, 1986.

Medlineplus Medical Encyclopedia. www.nlm.nih.gov/medlineplus/encyclopedia.html

Mythman's Homework Center. www.thanasis.com

Nybakken, O. E.: *Greek and Latin in Scientific Terminology.* Ames, IA: The Iowa State University Press, 1959.

Ryan, K. J., Berkowitz, R. S., and Barbieri, R. L. (eds.): *Kistner's Gynecology and Women's Health*, ed. 7. St. Louis: C. V. Mosby, 2000.

Shaw, I. (ed.): *The Oxford History of Ancient Egypt.* New York: Oxford University Press, 2000.

Tanagho, E. A., and McAninch, J. W.: *Smith's General Urology*, ed. 14. Norwalk, CT: Appleton & Lange, 1995.

Vaughan, D., Asbury, T., and Riordan-Eva, P.: *General Ophthalmology.* Stamford, CT: Appleton & Lange, 1995.

Venes, D. (ed.): *Taber's Cyclopedic Medical Dictionary*, ed. 19. Philadelphia, F. A. Davis, 2001.

Walsh, P. C. (editor-in-chief): *Campbell's Urology*, ed. 8. Philadelphia: W. B. Saunders, 2002.

Wilson, R. H.: *Williams Textbook of Endocrinology*, ed. 9. Philadelphia: W. B. Saunders, 1998.

www.ecosystemworld.com/taxa003.htm

Yanoff, M., and Duker, J.W. (eds.): *Ophthalmology.* London, England: C. V. Mosby, 1999.

BIBLIOGRAPHY FOR EDITION II

Bauer, J: *Differential Diagnosis of Internal Disease.* Grune & Stratton, New York, 1967.

Benson, RC: *Handbook of Obstetrics and Gynecology.* Lange Medical Publications, Los Altos, California, 1980.

Boggs, DR and Winkelstein, A: *White Cell Manual.* FA Davis, Philadelphia, 1975.

Geschickter, CF: *The Lung in Health and Disease.* JB Lippincott, Philadelphia, 1973.

Harker, LA: *Hemostasis Manual.* FA Davis, Philadelphia, 1974.

Harvey, AM and Cluff, LE et al: *The Principles and Practice of Medicine,* ed 17. Appleton-Century-Crofts, New York, 1968.

Hillman, RS and Finch, CA: *Red Cell Manual.* FA Davis, Philadelphia, 1974.

Holvey, DN (ed): *The Merck Manual of Diagnosis and Therapy,* ed 12. Sharp & Dohme Research Laboratories, Rahway, New Jersey, 1972.

Houston, JC, Joiner, CL, and Trounce, JR: *A Short Textbook of Medicine.* The English Universities Press Ltd., London, 1972.

Journal of the American Medical Association. Chicago, 1974, 1975, 1976.

Keefer, CS and Wilkins, RW: *Medicine, Essentials of Clinical Practice.* Little, Brown & Co, Boston, 1970.

Lewis, AE: *The Principles of Hematology.* Appleton-Century-Crofts, New York, 1970.

Nomenclature and Criteria for Diagnosis of Diseases of the Heart and Great Vessels ed 7. The Criteria Committee of the New York Heart Association. Little, Brown & Co, Boston, 1973.

Vaughan, D, Asbury, T, and Cook, R: *General Ophthalmology.* Lange Medical Publications, Los Altos, California, 1971.